1995
YEAR BOOK OF
PAIN

Statement of Purpose

The YEAR BOOK Service

The YEAR BOOK series was devised in 1901 by practicing health professionals who observed that the literature of medicine and related disciplines had become so voluminous that no one individual could read and place in perspective every potential advance in a major specialty. In the final decade of the 20th century, this recognition is more acutely true than it was in 1901.

More than merely a series of books, YEAR BOOK volumes are the tangible results of a unique service designed to accomplish the following:

- to *survey* a wide range of journals of proven value
- to *select* from those journals papers representing significant advances and statements of important clinical principles
- to provide *abstracts* of those articles that are readable, convenient summaries of their key points
- to provide *commentary* about those articles to place them in perspective

These publications grow out of a unique process that calls on the talents of outstanding authorities in clinical and fundamental disciplines, trained literature specialists, and professional writers, all supported by the resources of Mosby, the world's preeminent publisher for the health professions.

The Literature Base

Mosby subscribes to nearly 1,000 journals published worldwide, covering the full range of the health professions. On an annual basis, the publisher examines usage patterns and polls its expert authorities to add new journals to the literature base and to delete journals that are no longer useful as potential YEAR BOOK sources.

The Literature Survey

The publisher's team of literature specialists, all of whom are trained and experienced health professionals, examines every original, peer-reviewed article in each journal issue. More than 250,000 articles per year are scanned systematically, including title, text, illustrations, tables, and references. Each scan is compared, article by article, to the search strategies that the publisher has developed in consultation with the 270 outside experts who form the pool of YEAR BOOK editors. A given article may be reviewed by any number of editors, from one to a dozen or more, regardless of the discipline for which the paper was originally published. In turn, each editor who receives the article reviews it to determine whether or not the article should be included in the YEAR BOOK. This decision is based on the article's inherent quality, its probable usefulness to readers of that YEAR BOOK, and the editor's goal to represent a balanced picture of a given field in each volume of the YEAR BOOK. In addition, the editor indicates when to include figures and tables from the article to help the YEAR BOOK reader better understand the information.

Of the quarter million articles scanned each year, only 5% are selected for detailed analysis within the YEAR BOOK series, thereby assuring readers of the high value of every selection.

The Abstract

The publisher's abstracting staff is headed by a physician-writer and includes individuals with training in the life sciences, medicine, and other areas, plus extensive experience in writing for the health professions and related industries. Each selected article is assigned to a specific writer on this abstracting staff. The abstracter, guided in many cases by notations supplied by the expert editor, writes a structured, condensed summary designed so that the reader can rapidly acquire the essential information contained in the article.

The Commentary

The YEAR BOOK editorial boards, sometimes assisted by guest commentators, write comments that place each article in perspective for the reader. This provides the reader with the equivalent of a personal consultation with a leading international authority—an opportunity to better understand the value of the article and to benefit from the authority's thought processes in assessing the article.

Additional Editorial Features

The editorial boards of each YEAR BOOK organize the abstracts and comments to provide a logical and satisfying sequence of information. To enhance the organization, editors also provide introductions to sections or individual chapters, comments linking a number of abstracts, citations to additional literature, and other features.

The published YEAR BOOK contains enhanced bibliographic citations for each selected article, including extended listings of multiple authors and identification of author affiliations. Each YEAR BOOK contains a Table of Contents specific to that year's volume. From year to year, the Table of Contents for a given YEAR BOOK will vary depending on developments within the field.

Every YEAR BOOK contains a list of the journals from which papers have been selected. This list represents a subset of the nearly 1,000 journals surveyed by the publisher and occasionally reflects a particularly pertinent article from a journal that is not surveyed on a routine basis.

Finally, each volume contains a comprehensive subject index and an index to authors of each selected paper.

The 1995 Year Book Series

Year Book of Allergy, Asthma, and Clinical Immunology: Drs. Rosenwasser, Borish, Gelfand, Leung, Nelson, and Szefler

Year Book of Anesthesiology and Pain Management: Drs. Tinker, Abram, Chestnut, Roizen, Rothenberg, and Wood

Year Book of Cardiology®: Drs. Schlant, Collins, Engle, Gersh, Kaplan, and Waldo

Year Book of Chiropractic®: Dr. Lawrence

Year Book of Critical Care Medicine®: Drs. Parrillo, Balk, Calvin, Franklin, and Shapiro

Year Book of Dentistry®: Drs. Meskin, Berry, Currier, Kennedy, Leinfelder, Roser, and Zakariasen

Year Book of Dermatologic Surgery®: Drs. Swanson, Glogau, and Salasche

Year Book of Dermatology®: Drs. Sober and Fitzpatrick

Year Book of Diagnostic Radiology®: Drs. Federle, Clark, Gross, Latchaw, Madewell, Maynard, and Young

Year Book of Digestive Diseases®: Drs. Greenberger and Moody

Year Book of Drug Therapy®: Drs. Lasagna and Weintraub

Year Book of Emergency Medicine®: Drs. Wagner, Dronen, Davidson, King, Niemann, and Roberts

Year Book of Endocrinology®: Drs. Bagdade, Braverman, Horton, Kannan, Landsberg, Molitch, Morley, Nathan, Odell, Poehlman, Rogol, and Ryan,

Year Book of Family Practice®: Drs. Berg, Bowman, Davidson, Dexter, Dietrich, and Scherger

Year Book of Geriatrics and Gerontology®: Drs. Beck, Burton, Goldstein, Reuben, Small, and Whitehouse

Year Book of Hand Surgery®: Drs. Amadio and Hentz

Year Book of Hematology®: Drs. Spivak, Bell, Ness, Quesenberry, Wiernik, and Blume

Year Book of Infectious Diseases®: Drs. Keusch, Barza, Bennish, Gelfand, Klempner, Snydman, and Skolnik

Year Book of Infertility and Reproductive Endocrinology: Drs. Mishell, Lobo, and Sokol

Year Book of Medicine®: Drs. Bone, Cline, Epstein, Greenberger, Malawista, Mandell, O'Rourke, and Utiger

Year Book of Neonatal and Perinatal Medicine®: Drs. Fanaroff and Klaus

Year Book of Nephrology®: Drs. Coe, Favus, Henderson, Kashgarian, Luke, and Curtis

Year Book of Neurology and Neurosurgery®: Drs. Bradley and Wilkins

Year Book of Neuroradiology: Drs. Osborn, Eskridge, Grossman, Hudgens, and Ross

Year Book of Nuclear Medicine®: Drs. Gottschalk, Blaufox, McAfee, Wacker, and Zubal

Year Book of Obstetrics and Gynecology®: Drs. Mishell, Kirschbaum, and Morrow

Year Book of Occupational and Environmental Medicine®: Drs. Emmett, Frank, Gochfeld, and Hessl

Year Book of Oncology®: Drs. Simone, Bosl, Glatstein, Ozols, and Steele

Year Book of Ophthalmology®: Drs. Cohen, Adams, Augsburger, Benson, Eagle, Flanagan, Grossman, Laibson, Nelson, Rapuano, Reinecke, Sergott, Tasman, Tipperman, and Wilson

Year Book of Orthopedics®: Drs. Sledge, Cofield, Dobyns, Griffin, Poss, Springfield, Swiontkowski, Weisel, and Wilson

Year Book of Otolaryngology–Head and Neck Surgery®: Drs. Paparella and Holt

Year Book of Pain: Drs. Gebhart, Haddox, Jacox, Janjan, Marcus, Rudy, and Shapiro

Year Book of Pathology and Laboratory Medicine: Drs. Mills, Bruns, Gaffey, and Stoler

Year Book of Pediatrics®: Dr. Stockman

Year Book of Plastic, Reconstructive, and Aesthetic Surgery: Drs. Miller, Cohen, McKinney, Robson, Ruberg, and Whitaker

Year Book of Podiatric Medicine and Surgery®: Dr. Kominsky

Year Book of Psychiatry and Applied Mental Health®: Drs. Talbott, Breier, Frances, Meltzer, Schowalter, Tasman, and Yudofsky

Year Book of Pulmonary Disease®: Drs. Bone and Petty

Year Book of Rheumatology®: Drs. Sergent, LeRoy, Meenan, Panush, and Reichlin

Year Book of Sports Medicine®: Drs. Shephard, Drinkwater, Eichner, Torg, Col. Anderson, and Mr. George

Year Book of Surgery®: Drs. Copeland, Bland, Deitch, Eberlein, Howard, Luce, Seeger, Souba, and Sugarbaker

Year Book of Thoracic and Cardiovascular Surgery: Drs. Ginsberg, Lofland, and Wechsler

Year Book of Transplantation®: Drs. Sollinger, Eckhoff, Hullett, Knechtle, Longo, Mentzer, and Pirsch

Year Book of Ultrasound®: Drs. Merritt, Babcock, Carroll, Fagin, Finberg, and Fleischer

Year Book of Urology®: Drs. DeKernion and Howards

Year Book of Vascular Surgery®: Dr. Porter

Editors

G. F. Gebhart, Ph.D.

Department of Pharmacology, University of Iowa College of Medicine, Iowa City, Iowa

J. David Haddox, D.D.S., M.D.

Center for Pain Medicine, The Emory Clinic, Inc.; Assistant Professor, Division of Pain Medicine, Department of Anesthesiology, Emory University, Atlanta, Georgia

Ada K. Jacox, Ph.D., R.N.

Associate Dean for Research, Wayne State University College of Nursing, Detroit, Michigan

Nora A. Janjan, M.D., F.A.C.P.

Associate Professor, Radiotherapy, Division of Radiotherapy, The University of Texas, MD Anderson Cancer Center, Houston, Texas

Dawn A. Marcus, M.D.

Pain Evaluation and Treatment Institute, University of Pittsburgh Medical Center, Pittsburgh, Pennsylvania

Thomas E. Rudy, Ph.D.

Associate Professor, Departments of Anesthesiology and Psychiatry, and Associate Director, Pain Evaluation and Treatment Institute, University of Pittsburgh Medical Center, Pittsburgh, Pennsylvania

Barbara S. Shapiro, M.D.

Clinical Assistant Professor of Pediatrics, The Children's Hospital of Philadelphia, Pennsylvania; University of Pennsylvania School of Medicine, Philadelphia, Pennsylvania

Guest Editors

Eric Lang, M.D.

Pain Fellow, Center for Pain Medicine, The Emory Clinic, Atlanta, Georgia

David Van Alstine, M.D.

Pain Fellow, Center for Pain Medicine, The Emory Clinic, Atlanta, Georgia

1995

The Year Book of PAIN

Editors

G. F. Gebhart, Ph.D.

J. David Haddox, D.D.S., M.D.

Ada Jacox, R.N., Ph.D.

Nora A. Janjan, M.D.

Dawn A. Marcus, M.D.

Thomas E. Rudy, Ph.D.

Barbara S. Shapiro, M.D.

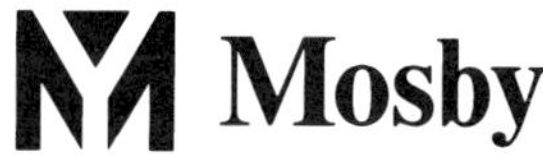

St. Louis Baltimore Boston Carlsbad Chicago Naples New York Philadelphia Portland
London Madrid Mexico City Singapore Sydney Tokyo Toronto Wiesbaden

Vice President and Publisher, Continuity Publishing: Kenneth H. Killion
Director, Editorial Development: Gretchen C. Murphy
Developmental Editor: Bernadette Buchholz
Acquisitions Editor: Jennifer Roche
Illustrations and Permissions Coordinator: Lois M. Ruebensam
Manager, Continuity–EDP: Maria Nevinger
Project Manager, Editing: Tamara L. Smith
Assistant Project Supervisor, Production: Laura Higgins
Freelance Staff Supervisor: Barbara M. Kelly
Manager, Literature Services: Edith M. Podrazik, R.N.
Senior Information Specialist: Terri Santo, R.N.
Senior Medical Writer: David A. Cramer, M.D.
Vice President, Professional Sales and Marketing: George M. Parker
Marketing Manager: Eileen M. Lynch
Marketing Specialist: Lynn D. Stevenson

1995 EDITION

Printed in the United States of America
Composition by Reed Technology and Information Services, Inc.
Printing/binding by Maple-Vail

Mosby–Year Book, Inc.
11830 Westline Industrial Drive
St. Louis, MO 63146

Editorial Office:
Mosby–Year Book, Inc.
200 North LaSalle Street
Chicago, IL 60601

International Standard Serial Number: 1070-5376
International Standard Book Number: 0-8151-3402-9

Table of Contents

Mosby Document Express

Copies of the full text of the original source documents of articles abstracted or referenced in this publication are available by calling Mosby Document Express, toll-free, at **1 (800) 55-MOSBY.**

With Mosby Document Express, you have convenient, 24-hour-a-day access to literally every article on which this publication is based. In fact, through Mosby Document Express, virtually any medical or scientific article can be located and delivered by FAX, overnight delivery service, international airmail, electronic transmission of bitmapped images (via Internet), or regular mail. The average cost of a complete, delivered copy of an article, including up to $4 in copyright clearance charges and first-class mail delivery, is $12.

For inquiries and pricing information, please call the toll-free number shown above. To expedite your order for material appearing in this publication, please be prepared with the code shown next to the bibliographic citation for each abstract.

Journals Represented

Mosby subscribes to and surveys nearly 1,000 U.S. and foreign medical and allied health journals. From these journals, the Editors select the articles to be abstracted. Journals represented in this YEAR BOOK are listed below.

AACN: Clinical Issues in Critical Care Nursing
APS Bulletin - American Pain Society
APS Journal
Acta Anaesthesiologica Scandinavica
Acta Neurochirurgica
Acta Obstetricia et Gynecologica Scandinavica
Acta Paediatrica
American Family Physician
American Journal of Critical Care
American Journal of Nursing
American Journal of Obstetrics and Gynecology
American Journal on Mental Retardation
Anaesthesia
Anaesthesia and Intensive Care
Anesthesia and Analgesia
Anesthesiology
Annals of Emergency Medicine
Annals of Rheumatic Diseases
Annals of the Royal College of Surgeons of England
Archives of Disease in Childhood
Archives of Pediatrics and Adolescent Medicine
Archives of Physical Medicine and Rehabilitation
Arthroscopy: The Journal of Arthroscopic and Related Surgery
Brain
Brain Research
British Journal of Anaesthesia
British Journal of Cancer
British Journal of Obstetrics and Gynaecology
British Journal of Ophthalmology
British Journal of Urology
Canadian Journal of Anaesthesia
Canadian Medical Association Journal
Cancer
Cancer Nursing
Cephalalgia
Clinical Journal of Pain
Clinical Orthopaedics and Related Research
Clinical Pediatrics
Critical Care Medicine
Critical Care Nurse
Dimensions of Critical Care Nursing
European Journal of Cancer
European Journal of Neuroscience
European Journal of Pharmacology
Headache
Injury
International Journal of Radiation, Oncology, Biology, and Physics
JOGNN: Journal of Obstetric, Gynecologic, and Neonatal Nursing
Journal of Acquired Immune Deficiency Syndromes
Journal of Bone and Joint Surgery (American Volume)

Journal of Clinical Anesthesia
Journal of Clinical Pharmacology
Journal of Computer Assisted Tomography
Journal of Consulting and Clinical Psychology
Journal of Dermatologic Surgery and Oncology
Journal of Developmental and Behavioral Pediatrics
Journal of Emergency Medicine
Journal of Human Hypertension
Journal of Manipulative and Physiological Therapeutics
Journal of Musculoskeletal Pain
Journal of Neurology
Journal of Neurology, Neurosurgery and Psychiatry
Journal of Neurophysiology
Journal of Neuroscience
Journal of Neuroscience Nursing
Journal of Neurosurgery
Journal of Nuclear Medicine
Journal of Occupational Rehabilitation
Journal of Oral and Maxillofacial Surgery
Journal of Orofacial Pain
Journal of Pain and Symptom Management
Journal of Pediatric Oncology Nursing
Journal of Pediatric Orthopedics
Journal of Pediatric Surgery
Journal of Pediatrics
Journal of Pharmacology and Experimental Therapeutics
Journal of Physiology
Journal of Post Anesthesia Nursing
Journal of Psychosocial Oncology
Journal of Rheumatology
Journal of Spinal Disorders
Journal of Thoracic and Cardiovascular Surgery
Journal of Trauma
Journal of Vascular Nursing
Journal of the American Academy of Child Adolescent Psychiatry
Journal of the American College of Surgeons
Journal of the American Geriatrics Society
Journal of the American Medical Association
Journal of the Neurological Sciences
Journal of the Royal Society of Medicine
Lancet
Life Sciences
Nature
Neurology
Neuropharmacology
Neuroscience
New England Journal of Medicine
Nursing Research
Oncology Nursing Forum
Orthopedics
Pain
Paraplegia
Pediatric Nursing
Pediatrics
Physical Therapy

Postgraduate Medical Journal
Proceedings of the National Academy of Sciences
Psychosomatic Medicine
RadioGraphics
Regional Anesthesia
Research in Nursing and Health
Scandinavian Journal of Rehabilitation Medicine
Scandinavian Journal of Urology and Nephrology
Scandinavian Journal of Work, Environment and Health
Schizophrenia Bulletin
Science
Somatosensory and Motor Research
Southern Medical Journal
Spine
Support Care Cancer
Surgical Neurology

Standard Abbreviations

The following terms are abbreviated in this edition: acquired immunodeficiency syndrome (AIDS), cardiopulmonary resuscitation (CPR), central nervous system (CNS), cerebrospinal fluid (CSF), computed tomography (CT), deoxyribonucleic acid (DNA), electrocardiography (ECG), health mainenance organization (HMO), human immunodeficiency virus (HIV), intensive care unit (ICU), intramuscular (IM), intravenous (IV), magnetic resonance (MR) imaging (MRI), and ribonucleic acid (RNA).

Note

The Year Book of Pain is a literature survey service providing abstracts of articles published in the professional literature. Every effort is made to ensure the accuracy of the information presented in these pages. Neither the editors nor the publisher of the Year Book of Pain can be responsible for errors in the original materials. The editors' comments are their own opinions. Mention of specific products within this publication does not constitute endorsement.

1 Neurology

Introduction

Pain is an often neglected area of study in neurology, both in medical school and in residency training. The subjective nature of complaints of pain and the inability to quantify pain variables with objective testing have contributed to disinterest in this area. For many years, patients with pain have been told that their complaints are imaginary or psychologically based because of the absence of abnormalities on medical testing. Current research has given credence to the complaints of many of these patients. Although psychological factors clearly influence pain perception, a variety of neurophysiologic changes have been demonstrated as being important for symptoms in those experiencing pain. Research has helped to quantify the pathophysiologic abnormalities and treatment outcomes for a variety of painful conditions. This increased acceptance of pain as an area that is worthy of scientific research should lead to greater clinician interest in pain and improved availability of treatment options.

An important advance in pain research has been the development of animal models of pain, which permit examination of specific lesions and their associated pain symptoms. Clinical patients with complaints of pain often have factors that contribute to their pain from a variety of changes in nerves, muscles, joints, and deconditioning. Determination of the predominant factor among these usually is difficult if not impossible. Animal models enable researchers to evaluate changes from a single known lesion. This type of information is crucial to understanding the mechanisms of pain, because pathologic data from experimental pain models cannot be obtained from human studies.

The use of experimental models and basic science research in pain has revealed a variety of physiologic changes, including neurochemical abnormalities and structural alterations such as neuronal reorganization. The research presented in this chapter supports pain models that suggest that peripheral injury to the nerve and/or muscle rapidly results in alterations of the neuronal synaptic patterns in the dorsal horn and reorganization of neural connections to peripheral muscles as well. These changes may persist despite ultimate correction of the peripheral abnormalities. This model may help to explain both the persistent nature of some chronic pain syndromes and the spread of pain into areas not involved in the original injury.

Data from the studies reviewed in this chapter help to confirm pathology in patients who have been told they cannot be experiencing pain because their radiographic, electrophysiologic, and blood tests are normal. A knowledge of underlying pathology has helped pain disorders gain acceptance as neurologic phenomena. However, it is also important to remember that pain pathology is not exclusively neurologic, because other systems, including orthopedic and psychological systems, contribute to complaints of pain as well.

Acceptance of pain disorders as being representative of physical as well as psychological pathology has increased the types of treatments that are being tested for painful conditions. Treatment options that have recently been evaluated for a variety of head, cervical, lumbar, and neuropathic pain disorders include surgery, nerve blocks, medications, and relaxation skills.

An understanding of pain disorders as conditions that have reproducible pathology with effective treatments available has made clinicians more knowledgeable and less frustrated when managing patients who have chronic pain disorders. As research continues to expand our understanding of pain and the development of a wide range of treatment options, the awareness and education of clinicians should also increase to enable patients who have painful conditions to benefit from this expanded knowledge.

Dawn A. Marcus, M.D.

Experimental Pain Models

PATHOGENESIS

Partial Sciatic Nerve Ligation Results in an Enlargement of the Receptive Field and Enhancement of the Response of Dorsal Horn Neurons to Noxious Stimulation by an Adenosine Agonist

Behbehani MM, Dollberg-Stolik O (Univ of Cincinnati, Ohio)

Pain 58:421–428, 1994 131-95-1–1

Purpose.—Peripheral nerve injury can lead to abnormal sensory processing and distorted pain perception, which is sometimes exacerbated by activation of the sympathetic nervous system. An understanding of the mechanisms of these types of sympathetic maintained pain, or reflex sympathetic dystrophy, has been hampered by the lack of a good animal model of peripheral nerve injury. Tight ligation of one third to one half of the rat sciatic nerve results in a hyperalgesia that diminishes after chemical sympathectomy; studying the physiologic changes produced by partial sciatic nerve ligation (PSNL) may improve knowledge of the mechanisms of sympathetically maintained pain. The effects of PSNL on receptive field size, baseline firing rate, and response of the spinal dorsal horn neurons to mechanical stimulation were assessed. The effects of the adenosine agonist 5′-N-ethylcarboxamide-adenosine (NECA) and the adenosine antagonist caffeine on the same variables were also evaluated.

Methods and Results.—Adult male Sprague-Dawley rats were subjected to PSNL on the right side. The animals' responses to mechanical stimulation with Von Frey filaments and a blunt probe were tested while they were unanesthetized. For rats that underwent PSNL, the mean force required to produce a paw withdrawal response was significantly less than that for animals that had not had PSNL. While the animals were under chloral hydrate anesthesia, extracellular recordings were obtained from nociceptive-specific dorsal horn neurons in laminal I-V neurons, located either ipsilateral or contralateral to the ligation site. There were no significant differences in the baseline firing rates of neurons recorded in the rats having PSNL compared with those that did not. On both sides, the mean receptive field size of neurons was significantly greater in the rats that had PSNL. Bilateral receptive fields were noted in 24% of all neurons studied in the rats that had PSNL compared with just 3% in the control group. In both groups, application of NECA and caffeine next to the recording electrode had no effect on neuron baseline firing rates and receptive field size. However, the duration of the neuronal response to noxious stimulation in the operated animals was significantly lengthened by NECA. Caffeine blocked this effect.

Conclusion.—Sprague-Dawley rats that were subjected to PSNL had hyperalgesia develop in association with an increased receptive field size. In these animals, the adenosine agonist NECA potentiated the response of nociceptive-specific neurons to noxious stimulation. As a result, PSNL appears to alter the functional characteristics of distal horn neurons, most likely through activation of silent synapses and changes in purinergic transmission in the spinal cord.

Altered Tachykinin Expression by Dorsal Root Ganglion Neurons in a Rat Model of Neuropathic Pain

Marchand JE, Wurm WH, Kato T, Kream RM (Tufts Univ, Boston)

Pain 58:219–231, 1994 131-95-1–2

Purpose.—A rat model of chronic sciatic nerve constriction injury (CCI) is used to simulate chronic pain in humans. The CCI-induced symptoms of hyperalgesia and allodynia that develop over time have been correlated with progressive morphologic changes in axons of primary sensory neurons of the dorsal root ganglia. The correlation between morphologic and biochemical changes that occur in dorsal root ganglia neurons after unilateral sciatic nerve CCI were examined.

Methods.—A CCI of the sciatic nerve was created in 15 rats. Nociceptive thresholds were measured at 2, 5, and 10 days after CCI. Time-dependent injury-induced changes in the expression of preprotachykinin (PPT) messenger RNA (mRNA) encoding substance P and other peptides in affected dorsal root ganglia neurons were quantified using in situ hybridization and histochemical methods in conjunction with computer-assisted image processing.

Results.—Early after CCI, increases in PPT mRNA levels that were associated with normal-shaped small and intermediate-size B cells were observed. Late after CCI, PPT mRNA levels in small and intermediate-size B cells were markedly decreased, and degenerative morphologic changes were noted in the cells. In addition, induction of PPT gene expression by large A cells, which was highly correlated with CCI-induced degenerative morphologic changes in B cells, was identified.

Conclusion.—The induction of PPT mRNA expression by small and intermediate-size B cells and large A cells in dorsal root ganglia neurons may be a very useful parameter for evaluating potential drugs in the treatment of neuropathic pain.

Primary Sensory Neurons Exhibit Altered Gene Expression in a Rat Model of Neuropathic Pain

Nahin RL, Ren K, De Leôn M, Ruda M (Natl Inst of Dental Research, Bethesda, Md)

Pain 58:95–108, 1994 131-95-1–3

Purpose.—The chronic constriction injury (CCI) rat model of partial sciatic nerve injury elicits behavioral changes, including hyperalgesia, over time. Previous studies have reported alterations in gene expression after complete nerve transection or crush injury. Whether the development of hyperalgesia after CCI is associated with similar alterations in gene expression was investigated.

Methods.—Dorsal root ganglia were removed at 1, 3, 7, 14, 28, and 42 days after sciatic nerve ligation. Total RNA was extracted from the dorsal root ganglia and analyzed for alterations in messenger RNA (mRNA) levels encoding growth-associated protein-43 (GAP-43), calcitonin gene-related peptide (CGRP), galanin, neuropeptide Y, substance P, and vasoactive intestinal polypeptide.

Results.—Expression of GAP-43 increased threefold over time, peaking between 7 and 14 days of post-CCI, whereas CGRP mRNA and substance P mRNA decreased to half their normally abundant baseline levels of expression within the same 7- to 14-day period. The most dramatic change was seen 3 days after CCI, when galanin, neuropeptide Y, and vasoactive intestinal polypeptide mRNAs rose dramatically from nondetectable levels.

Conclusion.—The CCI-induced hyperalgesia that develops over time causes time-dependent alterations in neuropeptide synthesis within the primary sensory neurons.

▶ Guilbaud and associates (1) produced experimental mononeuropathy in rats, using a model similar to those described in Abstracts 131-95-1–1 through 131-95-1–3. They demonstrated the simultaneous occurrence of the peak of 2 events. Two weeks after ligature placement around the sciatic nerve, the peak time of degeneration of myelinated fibers with the beginning of regeneration occurs, along with the peak of pain-related behaviors. The authors noted that although the loss of myelinated fibers may be postulated to cause suppression of spinal nociceptive inhibitory controls, pain-related behaviors disappear before recovery of myelinated fibers, which may help explain a lack of correlation between complaints of pain and lesions of large myelinated fibers in human neurologic patients. Guilbaud and associates postulated that the presence of *both* degeneration and regeneration of small-diameter fibers is necessary for the production of pain behaviors.—D.A. Marcus, M.D.

References

1. Guilbaud G, Gautron M, Jazat F, et al: Time course of degeneration and regeneration of myelinated nerve fibers following chronic loose ligatures of the rat sciatic nerve: Can nerve lesions be linked to the abnormal pain-related behaviors? *Pain* 53:147–158, 1993.

Functional Reorganization in the Rat Dorsal Horn During an Experimental Myositis

Hoheisel U, Koch K, Mense S (Institut für Anatomie und Zellbiologie, Heidelberg, Germany)

Pain 59:111–118, 1994 131-95-1–4

Introduction.—Previous studies have found that inducing an experimental arthritis in animals results in marked alterations in the discharge properties of sensory neurons at the spinal and supraspinal levels. Because of the effectiveness of muscle input in changing spinal cord reflexes and the responsiveness of dorsal horn and brain-stem neurons, a peripheral myositis would be expected to induce marked alterations at the spinal level. The effects of an induced myositis on the discharge behavior of dorsal horn neurons in rats were assessed.

Methods and Results.—An acute inflammation of the gastrocnemius-soleus (GS) muscle was induced by injection of carrageenan solution in anesthetized rats. Two to 8 hours after induction of myositis, the activity of single dorsal horn neurons was recorded using a mapping procedure. The neuron population responding to GS A-fiber input increased significantly in size. This increase was most apparent in the lateral segments L6–L3, which received little input from the GS muscle in control rats. A myositis-induced lowering of the excitability threshold was observed, as were increased latency, jitter, and input convergence. As a result, new oligosynaptic or polysynaptic connections appeared to become functional in the presence of myositis. Myositis did not significantly alter the neuronal effects induced by C fibers in the GS nerves; however, C fiber-induced activations from the peroneal and sural nerves increased in the lateral dorsal horn.

Conclusion.—Experiments in rats suggest that acute myositis quickly leads to striking changes in the functional connectivity of the dorsal horn. Excitability increased mainly in the lateral dorsal horn, with many neurons in this area acquiring new input from the inflamed muscle. This functional reorganization may play a role in the spread or referral of muscle pain.

▶ This study reports that rapid reorganization of the neurons in the dorsal horn occurs within several hours of myositis. This reorganization of the dorsal horn may help to explain the development of referred pain. A number of studies have implicated changes in the dorsal horn in the development of pain syndromes (1). Animal models have also demonstrated the development of new receptive fields in the dorsal horn in response to noxious stimulation of skeletal muscle using bradykinin injections (2). In addition, other studies have also noted the uncommon development of neuropathic abnormalities in patients who have a primary diagnosis of polymyositis (3, 4). These studies are important in increasing our understanding of the development of chronic pain conditions as well as the ability of muscle pain to spread to additional areas that were not originally involved.—D.A. Marcus, M.D.

References

1. Zochodne DW, Murray M, Nag S, et al: A segmental chronic pain syndrome in rats associated with intrathecal infusion of NMDA: Evidence for selective action in the dorsal horn. *Can J Neurol Sci* 21:24–28, 1994.
2. Hoheisel U, Mense S, Simons DG, et al: Appearance of new receptive fields in rat dorsal horn neurones following noxious stimulation of skeletal muscle: A model for referral of muscle pain. *Neurosci Lett* 153:9–12, 1993.
3. Cohn MG, Schwartz MS, Li EK, et al: Asymmetrical weakness in polymyositis associated with neuropathic involvement. *Clin Rheumatol* 10:437–439, 1991.
4. Guo YP: Polymyositis associated with peripheral nerve lesion: Clinico-pathological investigation of 8 cases. *Chung-Hua Shen Ching Ching Shen Ko Tsa Chih* 23:351–353, 1990.

TREATMENT

The Effects of Intrathecal Morphine and Clonidine on the Prevention and Reversal of Spinal Cord Hyperexcitability Following Sciatic Nerve Section in the Rat

Luo L, Puke MJC, Wiesenfeld-Hallin Z (Karolinska Inst, Stockholm; Huddinge Hosp, Sweden; Karolinska Hosp, Stockholm)

Pain 58:245–252, 1994 131-95-1–5

Introduction.—Chronic neuropathic pain, which may result from trauma or surgical procedures, is difficult to treat once it has been estab-

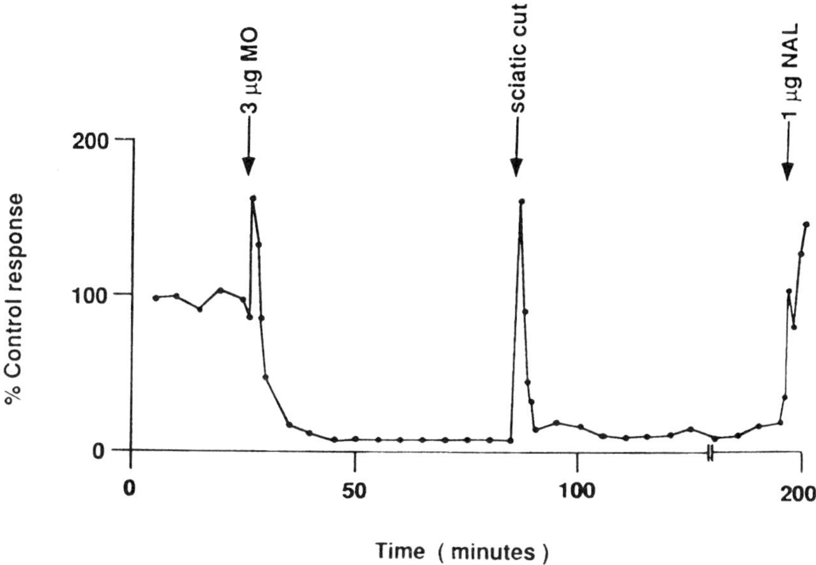

Fig 1–1.—The effects of 3 μg of morphine administered 60 minutes before sciatic nerve section. The initial effect was a brief facilitation. After sciatic nerve section, the reflex was briefly facilitated about 70% above pre-drug baseline after pretreatment. (Courtesy of Luo L, Puke MJC, Wiesenfeld-Hallin Z: *Pain* 58:245–252, 1994.)

lished. One useful behavioral model of neuropathic pain after peripheral nerve injury is autotomy in rats, in which there is self-mutilation of the limb with deafferentation. In previous experiments, it was found that intrathecal morphine, when given before sciatic nerve section, reduced the level of autotomy. Clonidine was ineffective, and neither drug was effective when given 15 minutes after nerve section. Acute physiologic experiments were performed to assess the effects of intrathecal morphine and clonidine on the development of flexor reflex hyperexcitability after sciatic nerve section.

Methods.—The flexor reflex from the hamstring muscles of decerebrate, spinalized, unanesthetized rats was recorded. Animals were pretreated with an intrathecal injection of morphine, 3 or 30 μg, or clonidine, 50 μg. The effect of sciatic nerve section on the flexor reflex without drugs was compared with that of axotomy performed 1 hour after morphine or clonidine pretreatment. The drugs' ability to reverse reflex hyperexcitability was assessed as well.

Results.—Pretreatment with both morphine doses profoundly depressed the baseline reflex (Fig 1–1). With the higher dose, reflex hyperexcitability was almost entirely abolished after nerve section. Pretreatment with clonidine was less effective than morphine, both in depressing the baseline reflex and in blocking reflex hyperexcitability. When given 15 minutes after nerve section, both drugs reversed spinal hyperexcitability.

Conclusion.—Morphine effectively blocks axotomy-induced hyperexcitability in rats, which may play a role in its ability to prevent autotomy. Clonidine is less effective in preventing spinal hyperexcitability. Neuropathic pain can develop after even a brief period of spinal cord hyperexcitability after nerve injury. These findings may have important clinical implications for the prevention of postoperative and chronic neuropathic pain.

▶ In an earlier study, two of these authors, Puke and Wiesenfeld-Hallin, demonstrated prevention of autotomy in rats when they were pretreated with morphine (1). Alpha-2-adrenoceptor agonists and saline were ineffective in pretreatment prevention of autotomy. Administering the drugs 15 minutes after nerve section was also ineffective.

Interestingly, the α2-adrenoceptor agonists clonidine and dexmedetomidine, but not morphine or saline, significantly reduced autotomy behavior when they were administered 24 hours after autotomy started. As a result, the researchers postulated that morphine should be an effective agent to prevent the development of neuropathic pain, and that α2-adrenoceptor agonists should be useful as treatment agents in those who were already experiencing neuropathic pain.

Selection of the specific opioid used for neuropathic pain may also be important. Lee and associates tested the effectiveness of opioids in reducing heat and cold allodynia and heat hyperalgesia in a rodent model of mononeuropathy (2). Morphine and selective opioids failed to alleviate thermal allodynia at antinociceptive doses. Heat hyperalgesia was reduced by morphine and the mu agonist DAMGO; this effect was lost with administration of naloxone. These results may help to explain the variable responsiveness of symptoms associated with neuropathic pain to different opioids.—D.A. Marcus, M.D.

References

1. Puke MJ, Wiesenfeld-Hallin Z: The differential effects of morphine and the alpha 2-adrenoceptor agonists clonidine and dexmedetomidine on the prevention and treatment of experimental neuropathic pain. *Anesth Analg* 77:104–109, 1993.
2. Lee SH, Kayser V, Desneules J, et al: Differential action of morphine and various opioid agonists on thermal allodynia and hyperalgesia in mononeuropathic rats. *Pain* 57:233–240, 1994.

Decreased Activity of Spontaneous and Noxiously Evoked Dorsal Horn Cells During Transcutaneous Electrical Nerve Stimulation (TENS)

Garrison DW, Foreman RD (Univ of Oklahoma, Oklahoma City)

Pain 58:309–315, 1994 131-95-1–6

Background.—Transcutaneous electrical nerve stimulation (TENS) is clinically successful in managing pain in patients with various conditions. However, the neural mechanisms that modulate pain are not well understood. Previous studies have shown changes in dorsal horn cell activity during mechanical stimulation of somatic and visceral receptive fields, electric stimulation of somatic and visceral peripheral nerves, and chemical stimulation of visceral organs. However, no data are available on the effects of conventional TENS on the discharge patterns of spontaneously firing and noxiously evoked dorsal horn cells. This information might be useful in understanding which measures are most effective in modifying the activity of dorsal horn cells and in reducing pain perception. The effects of TENS application on the activity of dorsal horn neurons in the somatic fields of cats were examined.

Methods.—A commercial unit was used to apply TENS to the somatic receptive fields in cats that were anesthetized with α-chloralose. The investigators used carbon-filament microelectrodes to make extracellular recordings from spontaneously discharging and noxiously evoked dorsal horn neurons. Action potentials were recorded from 83 spontaneously discharging cells and for 36 cells evoked with either a manual pinch or a manual clamp.

Results.—Application of TENS decreased spontaneous cell activity in 65% of the cells, increased activity in 5%, and did not affect activity in 30%. In the noxiously evoked cells, activity decreased during TENS application. Cell activity was more often decreased when high-frequency low-intensity stimulation variables were used compared with low-frequency high-intensity variables.

Conclusion.—Application of TENS appears to modify the spontaneous and noxiously evoked activity of dorsal cell neurons. The finding that the activity of dorsal cell neurons—which can potentially transmit noxious information to supraspinal levels—decreases during TENS application to somatic receptive fields is consistent with the "gate control theory of pain." Therefore, less noxious information would be involved in the pain perception process. The mechanism of the effects of TENS on dorsal horn cell activity is unknown.

► Clinical application of TENS remains controversial. A controlled study by Marchand et al. demonstrated that TENS provides short-term analgesia for up to 1 week after treatment (1). A short-term effect was also demonstrated in patients undergoing hand surgery (2). While under general anesthesia, patients who received sham TENS required 32% more anesthetic than those who received TENS treatment. However, the long-term benefit of TENS has not been demonstrated (1, 3).—D.A. Marcus, M.D.

References

1. Marchand S, Charest J, Li J, et al: Is TENS purely a placebo effect? A controlled study on chronic low back pain. *Pain* 54:99–106, 1993.

2. Bourke DL: TENS vs. placebo. *Pain* 56:122–123, 1994.
3. Herman E, Williams R, Stratford P, et al: A randomized controlled trial of transcutaneous electrical nerve stimulation (CODETRON) to determine its benefit in a rehabilitation program for acute occupational low back pain. *Spine* 19:561–568, 1994.

PAIN BEHAVIORS

Behavioural Pain-Related Disorders and Contribution of the Saphenous Nerve in Crush and Chronic Constriction Injury of the Rat Sciatic Nerve

Attal N, Filliatreau G, Perrot S, Jazat F, Giamberardino LD, Guilbaud G (INSERM, Paris, France; Service Hospitalier F Joliot, Orsay, France)
Pain 59:301–312, 1994 131-95-1–7

Introduction.—Animal models are needed to study the pathophysiologic mechanisms of pain caused by peripheral nerve injuries. Loose persistent constriction injury of the sciatic nerve in rats is accepted as a suitable model of this type, especially because behavioral studies have shown measurable behavioral disorders that seem to relate well to neuropathic pain. The morphological aspects of degeneration and regeneration after crush injury of the sciatic nerve have been well described; however, there have been few studies of the "painful" behaviors produced by this alternative model. The pain-related behaviors associated with these 2 rat models of peripheral sciatic nerve injury—transient nerve crush and chronic constriction injury (CCI)—were evaluated, as were the effects of simultaneous saphenous nerve injury.

Methods.—Adult male Sprague-Dawley rats underwent either transient crush injury or CCI of the right proximal sciatic nerve. The animals also received various lesions of the saphenous nerve to determine the role of saphenous innervation in behavioral disorders induced by sciatic nerve injuries. Various behavioral tests were performed, including assessment of responses to mechanical and thermal phasic stimulation and observation of "spontaneous" pain-related behavior.

Results.—Animals that were subjected to CCI demonstrated marked and prolonged phasic and spontaneous pain-related disorders for up to 7 weeks after injury. By contrast, rats that were subjected to crush injury showed moderate and transient hyperalgesia and allodynia to mechanical and thermal stimulation on the injured side. The behavioral findings peaked on the third day and resolved by the end of the first week. In both models, section plus ligation of the ipsilateral saphenous nerve prevented nociceptive behaviors and induced persistent mechanical and thermal analgesia or hypoesthesia of the injured paw. These effects lasted 3–4 weeks. Section without ligation of the saphenous nerve yielded similar results in rats with sciatic nerve crush injury. However, this saphenous lesion did not significantly alter nociceptive behaviors in rats with CCI.

Conclusion.—When the rat sciatic nerve is injured by crush or CCI, the injury induces nociceptive behaviors on the lesioned side. These effects are transient after crush injury, but they are persistent after CCI. Section plus ligation of the ipsilateral saphenous nerve prevents the nociceptive behaviors completely. Therefore, the adjacent saphenous nerve plays an important role in the mechanisms of pain disorders produced by sciatic nerve lesions. Pain-related behaviors are also noted in the contralateral paw, suggesting that unilateral nerve lesions induce remote modifications beyond the site of the injured nerve.

Differential Behavioral Outcomes in the Sciatic Cryoneurolysis Model of Neuropathic Pain in Rats

Willenbring S, DeLeo JA, Coombs DW (Dartmouth Med School, Lebanon, NH)

Pain 58:135–140, 1994 131-95-1-8

Purpose.—The study of neuropathic pain syndromes has been advanced by the recent development of a variety of partial or temporary nerve injury models. Peripheral nerve injury was produced by freezing the common sciatic nerve in rats using a technique called sciatic cryoneurolysis (SCN). Behavioral changes after SCN were further investigated.

Methods.—Allodynia was defined as a nocifensive response to a stimulus that was previously not noxious; hyperalgesia was defined as a reduced threshold to a previously noxious stimulus. Unilateral SCN was performed in 27 rats. Several days later, the animals were exposed to noxious thermal stimuli or tactile stimuli that were not noxious. Post-SCN mechanical allodynia and thermal hyperalgesia were compared with baseline behaviors.

Results.—After SCN, the animals displayed significant bilateral allodynia that persisted for at least 10 weeks. The finding of bilateral allodynia after SCN suggests the involvement of a central component in the development of neuropathic pain phenomena. The prolonged nature of the allodynia suggests that such hypersensitive states are caused by the sensitization of central nociceptive neurons, central disinhibition, or a combination of both. Sciatic cryoneurolysis did not cause thermal hypersensitivity. That there was no evidence of thermal hyperalgesia represents an important difference between this and other recently described neuropathic pain models.

Conclusion.—The behavioral sequelae observed in the SCN model are similar to those seen in neuropathic pain syndromes in human beings, and they differ from those seen in other neuropathic pain models.

▶ The behavioral consequences of pain have been demonstrated experimentally in a primate model as well as in the rodent (1). In primates, cold and mechanical allodynia with heat hyperalgesia were observed and noted to be similar to responses seen in humans with neuropathic pain.

Observation of pain behaviors is essential to determine pain severity in nonhuman models. In humans, these behaviors may also provide a useful tool for patient assessment and evaluation of treatment efficacy. Pain behaviors have been evaluated in a wide variety of chronically painful conditions, including diverse conditions such as sickle cell disease (2) and fibromyalgia (3). Observed pain behaviors may include changes in positioning, abnormal movements, grimacing, vocalization, and rubbing. The data obtained from these relatively objective observations have been demonstrated to be reliable and valid (4).—D.A. Marcus, M.D.

References

1. Carlton SM, Lekan HA, Kim SH, et al: Behavioral manifestations of an experimental model for peripheral neuropathy produced by spinal nerve ligation in the primate. *Pain* 56:155–166, 1994.
2. Gil KM, Phillips G, Edens J, et al: Observation of pain behaviors during episodes of sickle cell disease pain. *Clin J Pain* 10:128–132, 1994.
3. Baumstark KE, Buckelew SP, Sher KJ, et al: Pain behavior predictors among fibromyalgia patients. *Pain* 55:339–346, 1993.
4. McDaniel LK, Anderson KO, Bradley LA, et al: Development of an observation method for assessing pain behavior in rheumatoid arthritis patients. *Pain* 24:165–184, 1986.

IMMUNITY

Chronic Pain and Immunity: Mononeuropathy Alters Immune Responses in Rats

Herzberg U, Murtaugh M, Beitz AJ (Univ of Minnesota, St Paul)
Pain 59:219–225, 1994 131-95-1–9

Background.—Neurotransmitters that modulate pain and analgesia also affect immune cells, suggesting that chronic pain may affect the immune system. Although several studies have described changes in substance P and opioid peptide in chronic pain, few controlled studies have looked at the in vivo effects of chronic pain on immunity and inflammation. Possible changes in measures of immune competence were examined in a rat model of chronic pain.

Methods.—Female Sprague-Dawley rats were subjected either to sciatic nerve ligation to induce a unilateral peripheral mononeuropathy or to a sham operation. Hyperalgesia was assessed twice during the experiments using paw withdrawal latency time (PWL). Both groups were sensitized to keyhole limpet hemocyanin (KLH) 3 days after their operation, with a secondary sensitization 1 week later. Two weeks after the initial sensitization, KLH was injected into the hind footpad and vehicle into the contralateral footpad to evaluate delayed-type hypersensitivity (DTH). Testing for DTH was performed in the hind footpad ipsilateral to the ligated nerve in 1 group of animals with sciatic ligation and in the contralateral footpad in another group. The thickness of both paws was measured 24 hours later, and the animals were bled to assess the presence of anti-KLH immunoglobulins. A group of control rats was also studied; these animals underwent no surgery or hyperalgesia testing to exclude the possibility of immune alterations resulting from those procedures.

Results.—Animals undergoing sciatic nerve ligation had hyperalgesia in the operated leg on PWL testing compared with the contralateral leg. The sham-operated rats showed no differences in PWL times. The DTH response to KLH was enhanced in rats with induced mononeuropathy but not in the sham-operated or control groups. The DTH response was enhanced in both the ipsilateral and contralateral leg in the sciatic nerve-injured animals. In both cases, bupivacaine blocked this increased response. The hyperalgesic animals had lower γ-immunoglobulin levels against KLH than did the control animals, but the levels were similar to those in the sham-operated animals.

Conclusion.—These animal experiments show that chronic nociception causes identifiable changes in immune function. Generalized changes in both cell-mediated and humoral immunity responses were demonstrated. Further research is needed to evaluate the specific cell types in the immune system and the possible changes in systemic and local cytokine production.

▶ A link between nociceptive and immunologic systems has also been supported in studies in beige-J mice (1). The beige-J mutation is associated with a variety of immunologic disorders. This immune-impaired beige-J mouse model was also shown to have a selective nonresponsiveness to the analgesic effects of the mu opioid receptor. These data provide further evidence for the coexistence of immune system and nociceptive abnormalities.—D.A. Marcus, M.D.

Reference

1. Raffa RB, Mathiasen JR, Kimball ES, et al: The combined immunological and antinociceptive defects of beige-J mice: The possible existence of a "mu-repressin." *Life Sci* 52:1–8, 1993.

Head Pain

DIAGNOSIS

Assessment of International Headache Society Diagnostic Criteria: A Reliability Study

Leone M, Filippini G, D'Amico D, Farinotti M, Bussone G (Istituto Neurologico Carlo Besta, Milan, Italy)

Cephalalgia 14:280–284, 1994 131-95-1–10

Objective.—In 1988, the International Headache Society (IHS) issued new criteria for the diagnosis of migraine, tension-type headache, and other headache disorders. The diagnosis of headache is made solely on the basis of reported symptoms; therefore, the clinical diagnoses made by these criteria must be reproducible. Interobserver variability in the application of the IHS criteria was assessed.

Methods.—Two neurologists from a headache center independently reviewed the clinical records of 100 consecutive outpatients with headache. All data on the headache and associated phenomena were transferred to a form designed to reflect the IHS criteria. Interobserver agreement was assessed using kappa statistics.

Results.—In applying the diagnostic criteria of primary headaches, the observers showed "perfect" to "substantial" concordance for the first IHS digit. Kappa values were 1 for cluster headache and paroxysmal hemicrania, .88 for migraine, and .75 for tension-type headache. For the second digit, concordance was "almost perfect" to "substantial," with kappa values of .94 for cluster headache, .90 for migraine with aura, .81 for episodic tension-type headache, .78 for migraine without aura, .71 for chronic tension-type headache, and .66 for a cluster headache-like disorder that did not meet the diagnostic criteria. Concordance with only "moderate" for the migrainous disorder and tension-type headache that did not meet the criteria, with kappa values of .48 and .43, respectively.

Conclusion.—The IHS diagnostic criteria appear to be reproducible when applied by experienced neurologists who use them routinely. Although concordance is low for some pain characteristics and associated phenomena, overall diagnostic concordance is good. This means that items with the greatest level of agreement contribute disproportionately to overall agreement.

▶ The currently accepted standard for diagnosing headaches is the IHS criteria (1). Diagnosing headaches using these criteria relies on subjective symptomatic descriptions; therefore, it has a number of shortcomings. Although the IHS system has been demonstrated to be reliable when applied (2), studies have also documented inconsistent use of these criteria in both questionnaire and clinical examination formats (3, 4). Increased education about this diagnostic system is therefore essential to ensure that reliable diagnoses are being assigned to patients.—D.A. Marcus, M.D.

References

1. Headache Classification Committee of the International Headache Society: Classification and diagnostic criteria for headache disorders, cranial neuralgias and facial pain. *Cephalalgia* 8:1S–96S, 1988.
2. Granella F, D'Alessandro R, Manzoni GC, et al: International headache society classification: Interobserver reliability in the diagnosis of primary headaches. *Cephalalgia* 14:16–20, 1994.
3. Marcus DA, Nash JM, Turk DC: Diagnosing recurring headaches: IHS criteria and beyond. *Headache* 34:329–336, 1994.
4. Olesen J (ed): *Headache Classification and Epidemiology*, vol 4. New York, Raven Press, 1994.

Pathogenesis

Primary Headaches

►↓ The neurovascular, or trigeminovascular, model of recurring headaches proposed by Moskowitz describes alterations in neurochemicals, such as serotonin and norepinephrine (1). These neurochemical changes are postulated to cause the changes in blood flow, muscular contraction, and nociception that typically occur with recurring headaches. Central neurochemical alterations are believed to be the driving force behind a variety of recurring headaches, including migraine and tension-type and cluster headaches. The interrelationship of these types of recurring headaches remains controversial. Traditionally, these 3 types of recurring headaches are believed to represent different pathologic conditions; however, the much debated continuum severity model of recurring headache holds that migraine and tension-type headaches share pathophysiologic mechanisms and represent 2 extremes of a headache spectrum (2, 3).—D.A. Marcus, M.D.

References

1. Moskowitz MA, Macfarlane R: Neurovascular and molecular mechanisms in migraine headaches. *Cerebrovasc Brain Metab Rev* 5:159–177, 1993.
2. Blau JN: Diagnosing migraine: Are the criteria valid or invalid? *Cephalalgia* 13:S21–S24, 1993.
3. Marcus DA: Migraine and tension-type headaches: The questionable validity of current classification systems. *Clin J Pain* 8:28–36, 1992.

Platelet ^{3}H-Imipramine Binding and Sulphotransferase Activity in Primary Headache

Marazziti D, Bonuccelli U, Nuti A, Toni C, Pedri S, Palego L, Pavese N, Lucetti C, Muratorio A, Cassano GB (Inst of Psychiatry, Pisa, Italy; Inst of Neurology, Pisa, Italy)

Cephalalgia 14:210–214, 1994 131-95-1–11

Background.—Serotonin (5-hydroxytryptamine, 5HT) plays an indefinite role in migraine and tension-type headache (TH). The similarities of kinetic properties between platelet 5HT uptake and that of the presynaptic serotonergic neuron allows the use of platelets to study the pharmacology of the serotonergic system. In migraine, platelets show decreased 5HT uptake and ^{3}H-imipramine binding (^{3}H-IMI). The enzyme sulphotransferase that is (ST) present in platelets appears to be similar to that in the brain. Sulphotransferase occurs in 2 forms: thermolabile (TL) and thermostable (TS). The binding of ^{3}H-IMI and the activity of ST in the platelets of patients with migraine without an aura (MWoA) and patients with TH were investigated.

Methods.—Patients consecutively admitted to the headache unit of a day hospital were given a diagnosis according to the International Headache Society criteria. The 14 MWoA patients (13 women with a mean age of 32 years) had a mean period of headaches of 15 years. The 10 patients with TH (7 women with a mean age of 28 years) had a mean period of headaches of 9 years. The 20 healthy controls (12 women with a mean age of 29 years) had negative personal and family histories for chronic headaches. Platelet membrane preparation and ^{3}H-IMI binding were done according to a World Health Organization (WHO) protocol. The ST activity was measured according to a modification of the Foldes and Meek method.

Results.—The means of ^{3}H-IMI binding were as follows: The B_{max}. (fmol/mg protein) was 321 in the MWoA patients and 351 in the patients with TH (no significant difference). The mean level in the controls was 902, which was significantly higher than that in the 2 patient groups). The mean TL ST level in the controls was also significantly higher than those in the 2 patient groups (table). The TS ST levels did not show any significant intergroup difference.

Conclusion.—The decreased number of ^{3}H-imipramine binding sites confirmed the involvement of 5HT in primary headaches and suggested a presynaptic 5HT dysfunction. The decreased ST activity may cause changes in the levels of sulphated biogenic amines, which can affect some aspects of primary headaches. The similar abnormalities in the platelet markers in the patients with MWoA and TH suggest a continuum between these 2 types of primary headache.

3H-Imipramine Binding Parameters (B_{max} and Kd) and Sulphotransferase Activity (TL and TS Forms) in Patients and Controls

	^{3}H-Imipramine binding		Sulphotransferase	
	B_{max}	Kd	TL	TS
Patients with MWoA	321* ± 144	1.43 ± 0.66	6.3† ± 3.8	4.0 ± 2.5
Patients with TH	351* ± 151	1.451 ± 0.681	4.4† ± 3.0	2.0 ± 1.9
Controls	902 ± 201	1.23 ± 0.45	10.7 ± 7.6	3.9 ± 4.17

* Significant vs. controls: F = 3, $P < .02$.
† Significant vs. controls: F = 4, $P < .01$.
Abbreviations: B_{max}, fmol/mg protein; *Kd*, nM; *MWoA*, migraine without aura; *ST*, pmol/min/mg protein; *TH*, tension headache; *TL*, thermolabile form of sulphotransferase; *TS*, thermostable form of sulphotransferase.
(Courtesy of Marazziti D, Bonuccelli U, Nuti A, et al: *Cephalalgia* 14:210–214, 1994.)

Plasma Serotonin Increase During Episodes of Tension-Type Headache

Jensen R, Hindberg I (Gentofte Hosp, Hellerup, Denmark; Frederiksberg Hosp, Denmark)

Cephalalgia 14:219–222, 1994 131-95-1–12

Purpose.—Serotonin (5HT) is thought to play a role in the pathogenesis of migraine. Although the clinical features of tension-type headaches (TH) differ from those in migraine, it has been proposed that 5HT could also play a role in the pathogenesis of TH.

Patients.—Levels of 5HT were measured in platelet-poor plasma obtained from 13 women (age, 28–62 years) during and between TH episodes, and from 29 healthy controls (age, 31–60 years). Blood samples were drawn at the same time of the day to avoid diurnal variation. The intensity of the headache was recorded on a 100-mm visual analogue scale.

Results.—The median plasma 5HT concentration in patients with TH who were free of headache did not differ from that in healthy controls (Fig 1–2), but plasma 5HT concentrations were significantly increased during a headache episode (Fig 1–3).

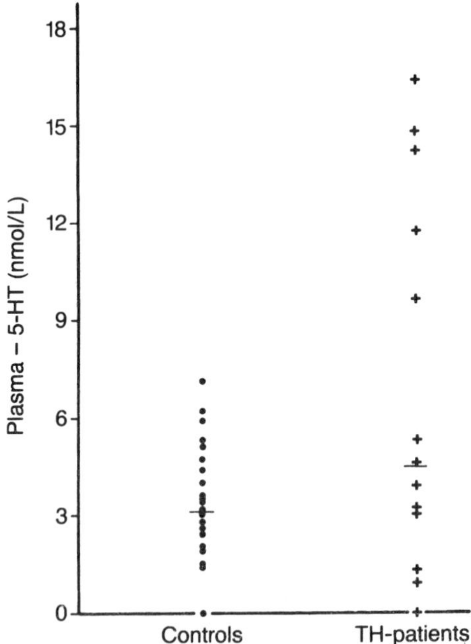

Fig 1–2.—Plasma 5HT concentrations in healthy controls and patients with TH who were free of headache. The median values are indicated with a *horizontal bar*. (Courtesy of Jensen R, Hindberg I: *Cephalalgia* 14:219–222, 1994).

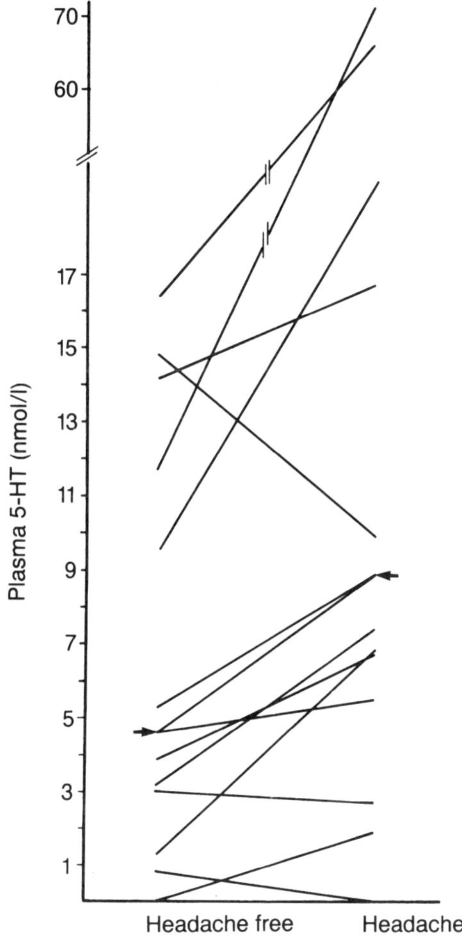

Fig 1–3.—Individual plasma 5HT concentrations in patients with TH who were free of headache and during a headache episode. The *arrows* indicate median values. (Courtesy of Jensen R, Hindberg I: *Cephalalgia* 14:219–222, 1994).

Conclusion.—Although 5HT may be involved in the pathogenesis of TH, its mechanism of 5HT involvement differs from that in migraine.

▶ Changes in neurochemicals have been well documented for migraine headaches. More recently, changes in both 5HT (1) and norepinephrine (2) have also been investigated in patients with TH (or what used to be called muscle contraction). The findings of those TH are quite similar to those found in individuals with migraine. Therefore, TH probably also represents more of a biochemical than a muscular condition.—D.A. Marcus, M.D.

References

1. Rolf LH, Wiele G, Brune GG: 5-Hydroxytryptamine in platelets of patients with muscle contraction headache. *Headache* 21:10–11, 1981.
2. Gallai V, Gaiti A, Sarchielle P, et al: Evidence for an altered dopamine-hydroxylase activity in migraine and tension-type headache. *Acta Neurol Scand* 86:403–406, 1992.

Lignocaine and Headache: An Electrophysiological Study in the Cat With Supporting Clinical Observations in Man

Kaube H, Hoskin KL, Goadsby PJ (The Prince Henry Hosp, Sydney, Australia)
J Neurol 241:415–420, 1994 131-95-1–13

Introduction.—Intravenous administration of lidocaine has been suggested as a useful option to control chronic daily headache (CDH), which is a particularly difficult type of headache to manage because of its uncertain pathophysiology. These patients often demonstrate excessive use of compound analgesics, such as those with codeine phosphate, and they often have psychological problems or stressors that aggravate their difficulties. Lidocaine is a local anesthetic, the action of which derives from blockade of fast Na+ channels.

Methods.—Nineteen patients who, for 6 or more months, had CDH with continuous pain that included at least weekly exacerbations and whose symptoms fulfilled the International Headache Society diagnostic criteria for migraine without aura received an initial bolus of lidocaine, 1 mg/kg, followed by an infusion of 2 mg/min for the next 2 days. In 5 cats, the effect of lidocaine was examined through craniovascular nociception, where electrical stimulation of the superior sagittal sinus (SSS) was used. Single-unit activity and sensory evoked potentials were recorded in the spinal trigeminal nucleus in the upper cervical spinal cord of the anesthetized cats.

Results.—Lidocaine rendered 26% of the patients pain free, with another 42% having at least a 50% improvement in pain. Prophylaxis with a tricyclic antidepressant or monoamine oxidase inhibitor after completion of the lidocaine infusion was used with continued benefit. In the cats, lidocaine substantially reduced (by more than 25%) the probability of cell firing and the size of the trigeminal evoked potential.

Conclusion.—The data suggest that CDH is likely to be a disorder of central craniovascular nociceptive control and that lidocaine interrupts a part of the pathway involved, but it is unlikely to act at the central generator of the disorder. Lidocaine ameliorated CDH. In the cat model of craniovascular pain evoked by electrical stimulation of the SSS, IV lidocaine blocked central trigeminal neurons in a dose-dependent manner.

Human In Vivo Evidence for Trigeminovascular Activation in Cluster Headache: Neuropeptide Changes and Effects of Acute Attacks Therapies

Goadsby PJ, Edvinsson L (The Prince Henry Hosp, Sydney, Australia; Univ Hosp of Lund, Sweden)

Brain 117:427–434, 1994 131-95-1–14

Introduction.—The symptoms and extreme pain associated with cluster headaches have been well characterized, but the pathogenesis and pathophysiology are poorly understood. The signs and symptoms suggest involvement of the ipsilateral trigeminal nociceptive pathways, regional parasympathetic nerves, and the ipsilateral cervical sympathetic nerves. The hypothesized mediational role of the trigeminovascular pathways was investigated by measuring peptide markers during an acute attack and after resolution.

Methods.—Blood samples were taken from the external jugular vein of 13 patients with verified episodic cluster headache immediately and 15 minutes after treatment with oxygen inhalation, sumatriptan, or meperidine. The plasma levels of neuropeptide Y, substance P, calcitonin gene-related peptide (CGRP), and vasoactive intestinal polypeptide (VIP) were compared with levels in age- and sex-matched controls.

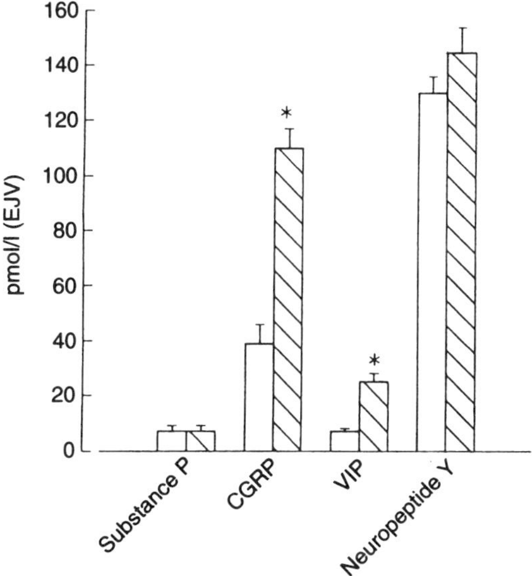

Fig 1–4.—Combined data for all patients, comparing control neuropeptide levels with those found in the external jugular vein (EJV) during an acute spontaneous attack of cluster headache. Substance P, calcitonin gene-related peptide (CGRP), vasoactive intestinal peptide (VIP), and neuropeptide Y levels are expressed in pmol/L on the ordinate. *Open bar* represents control; *crossed-hatched bar,* headache phase. Significant increases in both CGRP and VIP are seen during headache. (Courtesy of Goadsby PJ, Edvinsson L: *Brain* 117:427-434, 1994.)

Results.—All the treatment modalities resulted in clinical improvement. The quickest resolution was obtained with sumatriptan, and the slowest came with opiates. During headaches, the CGRP and VIP levels were significantly higher in patients than in controls, whereas substance P and neuropeptide Y levels were similar (Fig 1–4). The levels of CGRP and VIP were normalized in patients 15 minutes after treatment with sumatriptan or oxygen, but not with pethidine.

Discussion.—These data indicate that the trigeminovascular system is activated during acute attacks of cluster headache and that this activation is terminated with resolution. The elevated VIP levels suggest a parasympathetic activation. Elevation of both CGRP and VIP suggests that both afferent and efferent brain-stem reflexes may be activated, thereby affecting both the trigeminal nerve and the seventh nerve's cranial outflow. Sumatriptan and oxygen administration successfully terminate both an attack and trigeminovascular activity. Opiate administration brings relief of pain but not of the other autonomic features, and it does not quickly terminate trigeminovascular activation.

▶ Increased understanding of the role of the trigeminal system in headache is important to better understand pathogenesis and allow the development of treatments that more specifically act at the site of pathology. Recently, several medical (1) and surgical (2, 3) treatments that are designed to influence the trigeminal system have been successfully tested in cluster headache patients.—D.A. Marcus, M.D.

References

1. Nicolodi M: Nostril capsaicin application as a model of trigeminal primary sensory neuronal activation. *Cephalalgia* 14:134–138, 1994.
2. Morgenlander JC, Wilkins RH: Surgical treatment of cluster headache. *J Neurosurg* 72:886–871, 1990.
3. Rowed DW: Chronic cluster headache managed by nervus intermedius section. *Headache* 30:401–406, 1990.

Secondary Headaches

Cervical Musculoskeletal Dysfunction in Post-Concussional Headache

Treleaven J, Jull G, Atkinson L (Univ of Queensland, Australia; Princess Alexandra Hosp, Brisbane, Queensland, Australia)

Cephalalgia 14:273–279, 1994 131-95-1–15

Background.—Patients with minor head injury or concussion commonly experience a chronic, persistent headache, but the mechanisms of these postconcussional headaches (PCH) are poorly understood. It is possible that they are related to simultaneous injury of structures of the

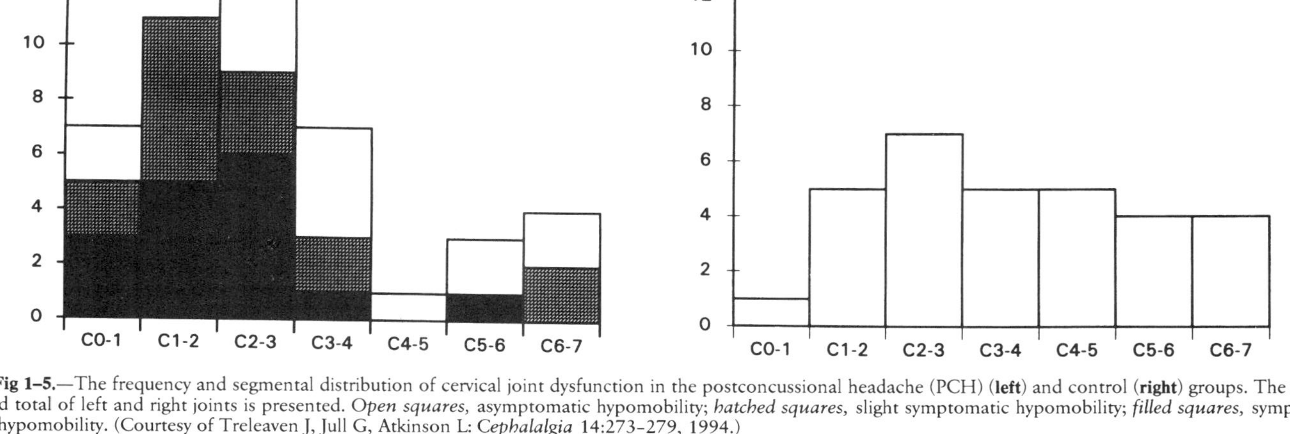

Fig 1–5.—The frequency and segmental distribution of cervical joint dysfunction in the postconcussional headache (PCH) (**left**) and control (**right**) groups. The combined total of left and right joints is presented. *Open squares*, asymptomatic hypomobility; *hatched squares*, slight symptomatic hypomobility; *filled squares*, symptomatic hypomobility. (Courtesy of Treleaven J, Jull G, Atkinson L: *Cephalalgia* 14:273–279, 1994.)

cervical spine. Postural, cervical muscle, and cervical joint function were assessed in patients with PCH vs. controls.

Methods.—The PCH group consisted of 12 patients with a history of cerebral concussion or mild head injury and PCH for at least 6 weeks afterward, with at least 1 headache per week. Those with a premorbid history of headache or a previous neck injury or condition were excluded. An age- and sex-matched group of healthy controls was studied as well. Both groups underwent a physical examination that included measurements of natural head posture, active range of cervical movement, manual assessment of cervical segmental motion, assessment of muscle lengths, and a measure of the endurance capacity of the neck flexors.

Findings.—Patients in the PCH group demonstrated signs of cervical articular and muscular dysfunction compared with the control group. Those in the PCH group had a painful dysfunction of the upper cervical segmental joint (Fig 1–5), reduced endurance of the neck flexor muscles, and a greater incidence of moderately tight neck musculature. There were no group differences in active range of cervical motion or postural attitude. The patients with PCH received no treatment of the cervical spine, excluding any causative relationship.

Conclusion.—The common problem of PCH may include a cervicogenic component. The main abnormal finding in these patients is a symptomatic cervical segmental joint dysfunction, particularly in the upper 3 cervical joints. The findings support the performance of a precise physical examination of the cervical spine in patients with persistent headache after concussion.

The Effect of Manipulation (Toggle Recoil Technique) for Headaches With Upper Cervical Joint Dysfunction: A Pilot Study

Whittingham W, Ellis WB, Molyneux TP (RMIT, Melbourne, Australia)
J Manipulative Physiol Ther 17:369–375, 1994 131-95-1–16

Background.—Clinical results show that the cervical spine can be a source of headaches, but the relative prevalence of these headaches is not known. Manipulation of the neck may help relieve headaches originating in the cervical spine. The effectiveness of a manipulative technique (toggle recoil) in the treatment of chronic headaches of cervical origin was investigated. For purposes of this trial, all headaches in patients with upper cervical joint dysfunction were categorized as cervical headaches.

Methods.—Twenty-six of 30 respondents to a newspaper advertisement for patients with chronic headaches were accepted for the study. The 16 females (mean age, 42 years) and 10 males (mean age, 52 years) all had experienced headaches for more than 3 months. All the patients had upper cervical joint dysfunction in the C1–2 complex, which was

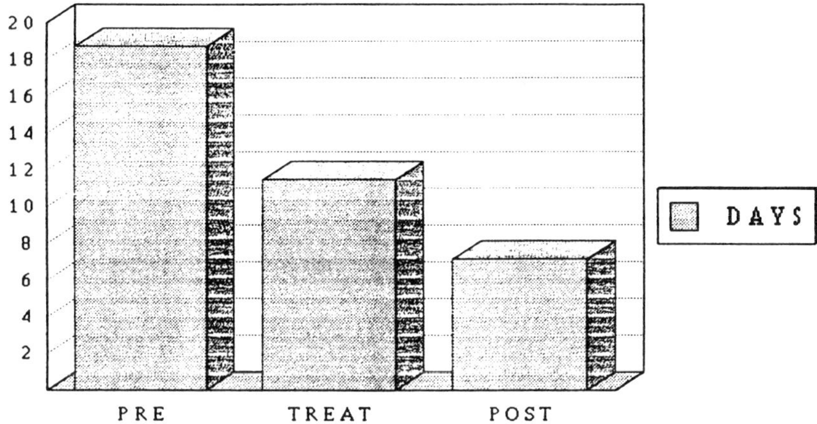

Fig 1–6.—Frequency of headache (summed total of days of headache) for pretreatment group, treatment group, and post-treatment group. (Courtesy of Whittingham W, Ellis WB, Molyneux TP: *J Manipulative Physiol Ther* 17:369–375, 1994.)

shown by motion palpation and cervical spine radiography. Aberrant motion and/or obvious rotational displacement in the upper cervical spine was used to make both the motion palpation and radiographic diagnosis. After completing a baseline history, questionnaire, physical examination, and cervical spine radiography, each patient received 4 upper cervical toggle recoil adjustments during a 2-week period. Questionnaires were completed at the end of the treatment period and again 2 weeks after treatment stopped. Patients served as their own historical controls.

Results.—All but 2 of the patients had statistically significant improvements in headache frequency, duration, and severity. The overall duration of headaches decreased by 77% (from 110 hours to 25 hours). The perceived pain improved by 60%. At the time of the 2-week post-treatment follow-up, the frequency of headaches had been decreased by half in 14 of the patients (Fig 1–6).

Conclusion.—The clinical efficacy of manipulation for chronic headaches of cervical origin was not proven by this pilot study, because it was not adequately controlled. However, the significant improvement of these patients as a group suggests that a randomized, controlled clinical trial is warranted.

▶ The important role of musculoskeletal abnormalities in a variety of chronic headaches has been explored (1, 2). Electromyographic recordings demonstrate increased muscular activity in individuals with either migraine or tension-type headache (3). The identification of these musculoskeletal changes may suggest treatments designed to affect these specific abnormalities. As discussed in this study by Whittingham and associates, controlled studies are needed before recommendations can be offered.—D.A. Marcus, M.D.

References

1. Kidd RF, Nelson R: Musculoskeletal dysfunction of the neck in migraine and tension headache. *Headache* 33:566–569, 1993.
2. Wilson PR: Cervicogenic headache. *APS J* 1:259–264, 1992.
3. Lichstein KL, Fischer SM, Eakin TL, et al: Psychophysiological parameters of migraine and muscle-contraction headaches. *Headache* 31:27–34, 1991.

Third Occipital Nerve Headache: A Prevalence Study

Lord SM, Barnsley L, Wallis BJ, Bogduk N (Univ of Newcastle, Australia)

J Neurol Neurosurg Psychiatry 57:1187–1190, 1994 131-95-1–17

Objective.—Third occipital nerve headache is said to be present in patients with chronic headache whose pain is relieved by selective blockade of the third occipital nerve. The pain is believed to be caused by post-traumatic arthropathy of the C2–3 zygapophyseal joint. Although the nerve block technique used to diagnose this type of headache is target specific and valid, only small numbers of patients have been assessed in poorly controlled studies. The prevalence of third occipital nerve headache was determined in patients who had chronic neck pain after whiplash.

Methods.—One hundred consecutive patients with more than 3 months of neck pain after whiplash injury were studied. Headache associated with neck pain was a complaint in 71 of these patients and was the main complaint of 40. The 71 patients with headache underwent double-blind, controlled diagnostic blocks of the third occipital nerve. Two blocks were performed on separate occasions, 1 using lidocaine and 1 bupivacaine in random order. Only when both blocks completely relieved the patient's upper neck pain and headache and when the relief lasted longer with bupivacaine was third occipital nerve headache diagnosed.

Results.—Third occipital nerve headache was present in 27% of the overall sample of patients with whiplash and in 53% of those with headache as their dominant complaint. Among patients in whom headache was a secondary complaint, the prevalence was only 19%. No history or physical examination finding could lead to a definitive diagnosis before the nerve blocks were performed. However, patients with a positive diagnosis of third occipital nerve headache were more likely to have tenderness over the C2–3 zygapophyseal joint.

Conclusion.—Among patients with chronic neck pain and headache after whiplash injury, third occipital nerve headache is a common condition. It is particularly frequent for patients in whom headache is the dominant complaint. The diagnosis can only be made by third occipital nerve block. No valid treatment for this condition is yet available, but a controlled trial of percutaneous radiofrequency neurotomy of the third occipital nerve is being conducted.

▶ After whiplash injury, prolonged head and neck pain, respectively, have been reported, in 42% and 66% of individuals (1). Uomoto and Esselman identified a variety of chronic pain complaints, including head, neck, shoulder girdle, and back, after even minor head injury (2). Persistent headache 6 months after whiplash is more likely to occur in patients with pretraumatic headaches, associated neck pain, and depression (3).—D.A. Marcus, M.D.

References

1. Norris SH, Watt I: The prognosis of neck injuries resulting from rear-end vehicle collisions. *J Bone Joint Surg (Br)* 65:608–611, 1983.
2. Uomoto JM, Esselman PC: Traumatic brain injury and chronic pain: Differential types and rates by head injury severity. *Arch Phys Med Rehabil* 74:61–64, 1993.
3. Radanov BP, Sturzenegger M, DiStefano G, et al: Factors influencing recovery from headache after common whiplash. *BMJ* 307:652–655, 1993.

Prospective Study of Sentinel Headache in Aneurysmal Subarachnoid Haemorrhage

Linn FHH, Wijdicks EFM, van der Graaf Y, Weerdesteyn-van Vliet FAC, Bartelds AIM, van Gijn J (Univ Dept of Neurology, Utrecht, The Netherlands; Univ Dept of Epidemiology, Utrecht, The Netherlands; Netherlands Inst of Primary Health Care, Utrecht, The Netherlands)

Lancet 344:590–593,1994 131-95-1–18

Background.—It is generally believed that minor hemorrhages (warning leaks) associated with an acute severe headache precede aneurysmal subarachnoid hemorrhage (SAH). Furthermore, many neurologists and neurosurgeons believe that early recognition and surgical repair of aneurysms can lead to improved disease outcome. In this propsective study, the association and precedence of acute severe headache with SAH were examined to evaluate such headaches as indicators and early warning of aneurysm.

Methods.—One hundred forty-eight patients with an acute severe headache starting within 1 minue and lasting at least 1 hour were followed up for 1 year.

Results.—Four patients died before further investigation and were considered to have probably had SAH. Thirty-three of 110 patients who were investigated further had SAH. Other significant neurologic abnormalities were diagnosed in 18, whereas no cause for the headache was found in 59. In 103 of the 148 patients, headache was the only symptom, including 12 patients with SAH and 4 with another CNS disease. Previous headache was reported in only 2 of the 37 patients with confirmed or probable SAH. No patient with acute, severe headache who did not have a diagnosis of SAH or other serious neurologic disorder subsequently had SAH develop during the 1 year follow-up. Acute, severe headache was indicative of severe neurologic disorder in 37% of the affected patients and of SAH in 25% of the patients with headache as the only symptom. Good outcome at 1 year was reported in 56% of initially surviving patients with SAH, a value similar to those published in hospital-based reports.

Conclusion.—Acute, severe headache is a common symptom of SAH; however, the occurrence of warning leaks as premonitory to serious SAH is not supported by this study. Instead, most first hemorrhages are serious. In this study group, vigilance and early recognition of SAH did not significantly improve the outcome of affected patients.

▶ Headache as a possible warning of a cerebral aneurysm and impending SAH is a serious concern for clinicians. Broderick and colleagues reported morbidity and mortality data for 80 first-ever SAH patients (1). The 30-day mortality after bleed was 45%, with approximately 60% of these patients dying within 2 days of the bleed from the initial hemorrhage. Delayed arterial vasospasm contributed to mortality in only about 5% of cases. Several other recent and interesting studies have also examined factors important in determining outcome after SAH (2–4).—D.A. Marcus, M.D.

References

1. Broderick JP, Brott TG, Duldner JE, et al: Initial and recurrent bleeding are the major causes of death following subarachnoid hemorrhage. *Stroke* 25:1342–1347, 1994.
2. O'Sullivan MG, Dorward N, Whittle IR, et al: Management and long-term outcome following subarachnoid hemorrhage and intracranial aneurysm surgery in elderly patients: An audit of 199 consecutive cases. *Br J Neurosurg* 8:23–30, 1994.
3. Rosenorn J, Eskesen V: Patients with ruptured intracranial saccular aneurysms: Clinical features and outcome according to the size. *Br J Neurosurg* 8:73–78, 1994.
4. Sano K: Grading and timing of surgery for aneurysmal subarachnoid haemorrhage. *Neurological Res* 16:23–26, 1994.

MEDICATIONS

Headache Treatments

Combined Oral Lysine Acetylsalicylate and Metoclopramide in the Acute Treatment of Migraine: A Multicentre Double-Blind Placebo-Controlled Study

Chabriat H, Joire JE, Danchot J, Grippon P, Bousser MG (Hôpital Saint Antoine, Paris; Synthélabo France, Meudon La Forêt, France)

Cephalalgia 14:297–300, 1994 131-95-1–19

Introduction.—The combination of aspirin and metoclopramide is widely used in the clinical management of migraine. However, only 1 placebo-controlled study has found this combination to be effective. The efficacy and safety of oral combined lysine acetylsalicylate (LAS)—a highly soluble aspirin salt—and metoclopramide (MCP) for the treatment of migraine attacks were assessed in a multicenter, double-blind, placebo-controlled study.

Methods.—The study included 266 adult patients with migraine, as diagnosed by the International Headache Society criteria, at 46 French centers. All patients had 2–6 attacks of migraine per month, with or without aura. Under the parallel group study design, the patients were to treat 2 migraine attacks with either LAS-MCP or placebo. The LAS-MCP treatment consisted of 1,620 mg of LAS, which is equivalent to 900 mg of aspirin, and 10 mg of metoclopramide. Headache relief was defined as a reduction in severity from grade 3 or 2 to grade 1 or 0.

Results.—The LAS-MCP combination was twice as effective as placebo in relieving headache for both attacks, 56% compared with 28%. It was also superior to placebo in terms of the secondary outcome measures of complete headache relief, 18% and 7%; nausea; 28% and 44%; vomiting, 3% and 11%; and use of rescue medication, 47% and 68%, respectively. Global efficacy with LAS-MCP was judged to be good or excellent 32% of the time compared with 14% with placebo. In both groups, tolerability was rated as good in 94% of attacks. Headache recurrence rates did not significantly differ.

Conclusion.—The combination of LAS-MCP is an effective and well-tolerated short-term treatment for migraine attacks. The benefits in terms of nausea and vomiting are probably related to MCP. Because of the good efficacy and tolerance ratio and the cost-effectiveness of LAS-MCP, it should be considered as one of the first types of therapy for migraine attacks.

Chronic Tension-Type Headache: Amitriptyline Reduces Clinical Headache-Duration and Experimental Pain Sensitivity But Does Not Alter Pericranial Muscle Activity Readings

Göbel H, Hamouz V, Hansen C, Heininger K, Hirsch S, Lindner V, Heuss D, Soyka D (Christian-Albrechts-Univ, Kiel, Germany)

Pain 59:241–249, 1994 131-95-1–20

Background.—Substantial controversy exists concerning the etiology of the chronic tension-type headache (CTTH). Excessive muscle contraction, abnormal serotonin activity, increased pericranial pain sensitivity, shortened late suppression periods during exteroceptive suppression of the temporal muscle, and decreased contingent negative variation (CNV) amplitude have all been described in patients with CTTH. Although amitriptyline has been used to treat CTTH, the results of clinical trials have yielded conflicting results regarding its efficacy. Furthermore, the mechanism of action of amitriptyline in relieving CTTH is not known. The efficacy of amitriptyline in relieving symptoms of CTTH and abolishing associated muscular and CNS abnormalities was evaluated.

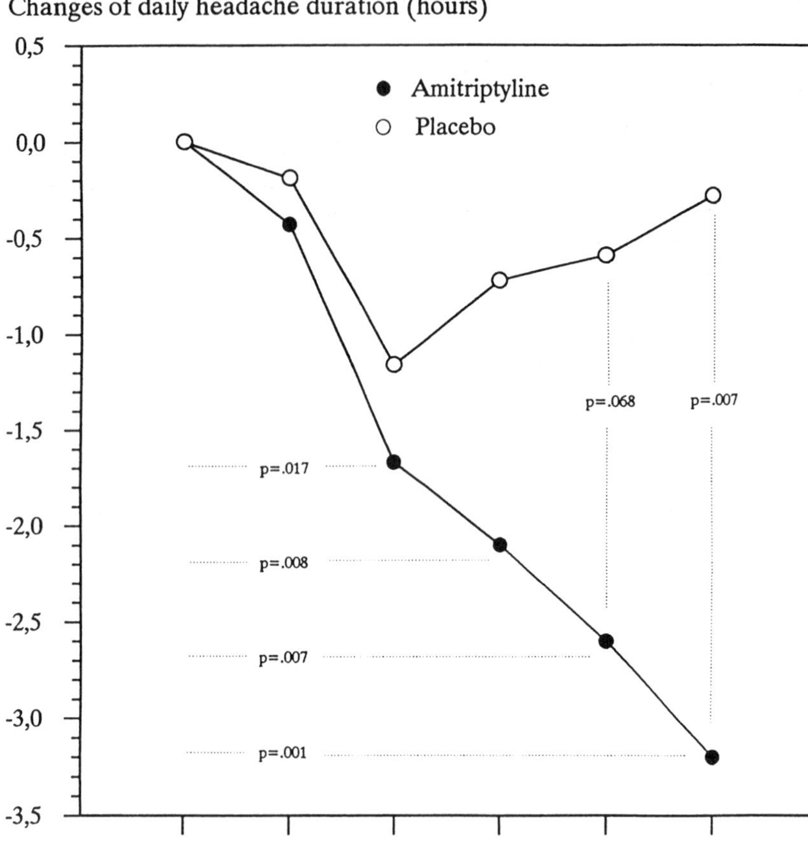

Fig 1–7.—Reduction in the average daily duration of headache in the amitriptyline and the placebo groups during weeks 2–6 in comparison with the first week. Significance in the *t* test. (Courtesy of Göbel H, Hamouz V, Hansen C, et al: *Pain* 59:241–249, 1994.)

Methods.—Fifty-three patients with a history of CTTH were treated with either amitriptyline-HCL or a placebo for 6 weeks. The amitriptyline dose was increased from 25 mg during week 1 to 50 mg in week 2 and to 75 mg in weeks 3–6. A headache diary was kept by each patient during the 6-week treatment, and electromyographic activity and exteroceptive suppression of the temporal muscles, CNV, and sensitivity to induced headache were assessed at the beginning and end of the treatment period.

Results.—Mean daily headache duration decreased significantly by week 3 in the amitriptyline group and continued to decline until week 6. There was no significant effect in the placebo group (Fig 1–7). The average reduction in headache duration during weeks 4–6 was 1.6 hours for the placebo group and 7.82 hours for the amitriptyline group. Among the neurophysiologic parameters measured, only sensitivity to suprathreshold pain differed between the groups, declining in the amitriptyline group during the course of treatment. The drug was well tolerated, with dryness of the mouth and mild drowsiness being the only significant side effects.

Conclusions.—Amitriptyline, which is well tolerated, can decrease the duration of CTTH but will not abolish it. Although the mechanism of action of amitriptyline in ameliorating the duration of CTTH cannot be determined from the results of this experiment, the decreased pain sensitivity in the amitriptyline group suggests the possibility that the drug has a direct analgesic effect.

A Differential Response to Treatment With Divalproex Sodium in Patients With Intractable Headache

Rothrock JF, Kelly NM, Brody ML, Golbeck A (Univ of Calif, San Diego; San Diego Headache Ctr, Calif; San Diego State Univ, Calif)

Cephalalgia 14:241–244, 1994 131-95-1–21

Introduction.—Although the mechanisms that generate migraine and other primary headache syndromes are still unknown, it seems that serotoninergic cells of the midbrain dorsal raphe nuclei play a role in establishing a headache "threshold." In theory, divalproex sodium, a 1:1 mixture of valproic acid and valproate sodium, can raise the headache threshold.

Methods.—Seventy-five patients with intractable headache syndromes were divided into 3 groups: 18 frequent migraine (FM), 43 transformed migraine (TM), and 14 tension-type headache (TT); 58 (77%) were women. All patients were treated with divalproex sodium, 500 mg twice daily.

Results.—Thirty-six patients (49%) reported a 50% or greater reduction in headache frequency. The 3 groups had significantly different treatment response rates, with 11 of 18 (61%) patients with FM reporting the highest rate of improvement; 22 of 43 (51%) patients with TM, an intermediate rate; and 3 of 14 (21%) patients with TT, the lowest response rate. Thirty-four (45%) of the 75 patients who began treatment reported side effects, and 5 reported multiple side effects. The most common side effects were gastrointestinal and chiefly involved nausea, which at times was profound and accompanied by vomiting.

Conclusion.—Prophylactic therapy with divalproex may be effective in selected patients with intractable headache syndromes. A response to treatment may be predicted by identifying clinically distinct headache subtypes. Because of the significant 20% dropout rate among the patients and the absence of any control group, confirmation of the efficacy of divalproex must be obtained through a prospective, placebo-controlled trial.

▶ Traditionally, certain medications have been used to treat migraine headache, and a different set of medication options were used to treat TT headache. The controversy over the classification of migraine and TT headaches as 2 distinct syndromes vs. 2 extremes of a severity spectrum or continuum model has led researchers to test "migraine" medications in patients who were given a diagnosis of TT headache. The efficacy of sumatriptan (1), ergotamine (2), antidepressants (3), and β-blockers (4) has been demonstrated for patients with TT, in addition to those with migraine. Therefore, clinicians may wish to broaden their armamentarium of treatment options for the patient with TT headache. Although there is a shared usefulness of many "migraine" medications in TT headache, it is important to remember that divalproex sodium, in the study by Rothrock and associates (Abstract 131-95-1–21), is more effective in patients who have migrainous characteristics to their headache descriptions.—D.A. Marcus, M.D.

References

1. Brennum J, Kjeldsen M, Olesen J: The 5-HT1-like agonist sumatriptan has a significant effect in chronic tension-type headache. *Cephalalgia* 12:375–379, 1992.
2. Horton BT, Ryan R, Reynolds JL: Clinical observations on the use of E. C. 110, a new agent for the treatment of headache. *Mayo Clin Proc* 23:105–108, 1948.
3. Lance JW, Curran DA: Treatment of chronic tension headache. *Lancet* 1:1236–1239, 1964.
4. Mathew NT: Prophylaxis of migraine and mixed headache: A randomized controlled study. *Headache* 21:105–109, 1981.

Medication-Induced Headaches

Octreotide Dependency and Headache: A Case Report

May A, Lederbogen S, Diener HC (Univ of Essen, Germany)
Cephalalgia 14:303–304, 1994 131-95-1–22

Objective.—The analgesics used to treat migraine or tension-type headaches can sometimes lead to chronic headache. More than half the patients with acromegaly have headache as a prominent symptom. Use of the long-acting somatostatin analogue octreotide to treat acromegaly has been reported to provide dramatic relief of chronic severe headache. A patient with acromegaly who experienced octreotide-induced headache (the first such case) was reported.

Case Report.—Woman, 33, started octreotide treatment for acromegaly after having undergone surgery and radiotherapy. She began experiencing a daily frontal, dull, pressing headache that increased with physical activity. The headache resolved quickly after subcutaneous administration of octreotide. The pain responded to octreotide but not to treatment with antirheumatic or antimigraine drugs. However, the headaches continued to occur every 4 to 6 hours, even at octreotide doses of 700 and 800 μg/day. Cholelithiasis developed as a complication of octreotide treatment, and the patient's growth hormone level normalized. However, she could not stop hormonal treatment of her severe recurrent headaches. There seemed to be no structural cause for the headaches; the MRI appearance of the pituitary adenoma was unchanged. The patient was admitted for cessation of octreotide treatment. Her worsening headaches were treated with oral naproxen and metamizol and IV acetylsalicylic acid. The headaches improved within 2–3 days. The medications were tapered and stopped over the next few weeks, and the patient was pain free at discharge.

Discussion.—Increasing octreotide dosage may lead to an upregulation of substance P receptors. This would explain the analgesic effect of octreotide as well as the occurrence of headache upon its withdrawal.

Ergotamine-Induced Headache Can Be Sustained by Sumatriptan Daily Intake

Catarci T, Fiacco F, Argentino C, Sette G, Cerbo R (La Sapienza Univ, Rome)

Cephalalgia 14:374–375, 1994 131-95-1–23

Objective.—Sumatriptan is an effective drug for the treatment of migraine attacks and drug-induced headache. It has also been recommended for a rebound headache induced by ergotamine. A patient with migraine who overused ergotamine, replaced it with sumatriptan, and continued to have a constant headache with superimposed migraine-like episodes was described.

Case Report.—Woman, 42, with a long history of migraine, was seen after 10 months of daily sumatriptan intake. She had been taking ergotamine, about 10 mg per week, for several years. After the first year, however, she began having headaches almost daily. They were of mild intensity but became episodically severe, and they were relieved only by ergotamine plus caffeine. Severe headache with nausea and vomiting prevented the patient from stopping ergotamine.

The patient replaced ergotamine with sumatriptan when it first became available. This drug relieved her episodic severe headaches but not the constant mild pain. In addition, the severe headaches were now occurring every 24 hours and were resolving only in response to sumatriptan, of which the patient was taking 7 or 8 tablets per week. The patient was asked to stop taking sumatriptan and was given a prescription for daily and as-needed nonsteroidal anti-inflammatory drugs. She had 3 migraine attacks per week in the subsequent 4 weeks. Various preventive treatments were started over the next 2 years all of which were ineffective. Eventually, she again began taking sumatriptan on a daily basis. She started a trial of acupuncture and soon reported dramatic improvement. She was having only 1 migraine attack per week, which promptly resolved with ingestion of 1 sumatriptan tablet.

Discussion.—Daily sumatriptan intake is well tolerated by patients with migraine. However, misuse of the drug may sustain the constant daily headache initiated by ergotamine. It is recommended that sumatriptan intake be limited to 1 or 2 doses per week in such patients.

▶ A variety of medications have been implicated in the development of headaches or the worsening of pre-existing headaches, including cardiac medications, estrogen supplementation/replacement, gonadotropin, and pain medications. Although the use of daily pain medications may be beneficial for certain types of chronically painful conditions, long-term daily or near daily use of ergotamine, sumatriptan, narcotic, or analgesic preparations in patients with headache is often associated with a worsening of headaches or the development of a chronic daily headache.

This headache pattern is called analgesic overuse or a drug rebound headache. In addition, the concomitant use of daily pain medications *prevents* effective headache treatment with headache-preventive medications, such as antidepressants and β-blockers (1). Overuse of prescription or over-the-counter pain medications should be considered in all patients with chronic daily headache and in patients for whom a variety of headache-preventive treatments have failed.—D.A. Marcus, M.D.

Reference

1. Mathew NT, Kurman R, Perez F: Drug induces refractory headache-clinical features and management. *Headache* 30:634–638, 1990.

Psychological Factors

Migraine and Major Depression: A Longitudinal Study

Breslau N, Davis GC, Schultz LR, Peterson EL (Henry Ford Health Sciences Ctr, Detroit; Case Western Reserve Univ, Cleveland, Ohio)
Headache 34:387–393, 1994 131-95-1–24

Objective.—Recent epidemiologic studies suggest a possible association between migraine and major depression, prompting a study of this association in a random sample of 1,007 HMO patients 21–30 years of age. All but 3% were available to be reinterviewed 3.5 years later.

Methods.—Psychiatric disorder was identified using the National Institute of Mental Health-Diagnostic Interview Schedule as revised to cover the *Diagnostic and Statistical Manual of Mental Disorders, Third Edition, Revised,* disorders. Migraine was diagnosed on the basis of International Headache Society criteria, which include at least 5 episodes of headache lasting longer than 4 hours; the occurrence of nausea and vomiting or photophobia/phonophobia; and at least 2 of the following symptoms: unilateral pain, pulsation, interference with daily activities, and worsening on routine physical activity.

Findings.—At age 30 years, the cumulative incidence of migraine was 23.8% in women and 9.4% in men. The cumulative rates of major depression at age 30 were 24% for women and 13% for men. The cumulative incidence of major depression at age 33 years was 53% in individuals with migraine and 15.9% in those without migraine, for a relative risk of 3.8. The relative risk for major depression associated with previous migraine was significantly increased in both men and women. The relative risk of migraine associated with previous major depression was 4.5 in men and 2.9 in women.

Conclusion.—An explanation for the bidirectional influences of major depression and migraine on each other would require that each disorder lead to the other by a distinct mechanism. Although this is not inconceivable, no such complex explanation is readily available. Another possibility is that comorbid migraine cases are distinct from cases of isolated migraine.

Headache and Depression: Confounding Effects of Transdiagnostic Symptoms

Holm JE, Penzien DB, Holroyd KA, Brown TA (Univ of North Dakota, Grand Forks; Univ of Mississippi, Jackson; Ohio Univ, Athens; et al)

Headache 34:418–423, 1994 131-95-1–25

Objective.—It has long been recognized that there is a link between chronic headache and depression. However, previous studies of this relationship have failed to address the potential impact of transdiagnostic symptoms, i.e., those indicating both depression and headache—on correlations between measures of the 2 problems. The relationship between self-reported depressive symptoms and headache activity was studied.

Methods.—The research subjects were 229 patients with recurrent headaches—either vascular or tension—who sought treatment at 2 university-based clinics. At their first visit, each patient completed the Beck Depression Inventory (BDI), a 21-item assessment of the extent of depressive symptoms. Measures of headache activity were derived from daily patient monitoring data.

Results.—Factor analysis identified 2 distinct factors. The first appeared to reflect the cognitive and affective component of depression, whereas the second appeared to tap the somatic manifestation. However, instead of being independent, these 2 factors were strongly related. On correlational analysis, there were consistent relationships between the somatic symptom factor and measures of headache activity. However, the cognitive/affective factor appeared to be unrelated to headache activity. Patients who had clinically significant reductions in headache activity after treatment also had significant reductions in BDI scores, mostly on items in factor 2.

Conclusion.—Use of the BDI to assess depressive symptoms in patients with recurrent headaches can be improved by recognition of the 2 factors identified. Items that comprise the somatic factor may be indicators of both headache and depression and therefore may not be appropriate indicators of depression in recurrent headache samples. The 2 factors should be studied further for their differential effectiveness as indicators of depression in patients with recurrent headache.

▶ Co-existing depression alters patients' perceptions of their pain complaints (1). In addition, Jacob and colleagues identified depression as being an important prognostic indicator for the outcome of relaxation treatment in headache patients (2). A poor prognosis was recorded after relaxation therapy in patients with headache who had pretreatment BDI scores of 8 or higher, representing at least mild depressive symptoms. Identification and management of coexisting depression may help improve the response to headache treatments.—D.A. Marcus, M.D.

References

1. Krause SJ, Wiener RL, Tait RC: Depression and pain behavior in patients with chronic pain. *Clin J Pain* 10:122–127, 1994.
2. Jacob RG, Turner SM, Szekely BC, et al: Predicting outcome of relaxation therapy in headaches: The role of "depression." *Behav Ther* 14:457–465, 1983.

Factors Influencing Treatment-Seeking Behavior in Problem Headache Sufferers

Rokicki LA, Holroyd KA (Univ of Mississippi, Jackson)
Headache 34:429–434, 1994 131-95-1–26

Introduction.—Most studies of recurrent headache disorders include only those patients who seek and receive treatment. The external validity of the findings of these studies may be threatened if treatment-seeking patients are not representative of the larger population of individuals with recurrent headaches. Factors related to treatment-seeking behavior among young patients with recurrent headaches were studied.

Methods.—Two groups of young adult patients with recurrent tension-type or migraine headaches were studied: 81 patients who had sought treatment for their problem and 109 who had not. Headache variables were compared between these 2 groups. In addition, a group of 129 research subjects without headache were studied. The 3 groups were compared on various factors associated with treatment-seeking behavior in other populations, including psychological symptoms/neuroticism, coping strategies, and cognitive variables.

Results.—On comparison of headache variables, those who sought treatment had more frequent headaches and had problem headaches for a longer time than those who did not seek treatment. However, those in the 2 headache groups were no different in their psychological symptoms, coping strategies, or beliefs about their headache problems. Patients in the 2 headache groups, regardless of their treatment-seeking behavior, had more depression and physical symptoms than did research subjects without headaches.

Conclusion.—Among young patients with recurrent headache, the most important determinant of treatment-seeking behavior appears to be the severity of the headache. Treatment-seeking behavior does not appear to relate to psychological symptoms, beliefs about headaches, or coping strategies.

▶ This study addresses the important issue of extrapolating data from a research sample to the general population. A research study group, such as a group of healthy medical students, may present a very different population from that found in a particular clinical practice. These dissimilar groups may show important differences in psychological profiles, associated behaviors, levels of motivation, educational background, and other factors that can strongly influence treatment outcome.

Therefore, when assigning medication or nonmedication (such as biofeedback and relaxation) treatments to an individual patient with headache, these psychosocial variables should be considered in addition to the patient's headache diagnosis to maximize the response to the prescribed treatment.—D.A. Marcus, M.D.

Cervical Pain

Evaluation

Cervical Spine Nerve Root Compression: An Analysis of Neuroforaminal Pressures With Varying Head and Arm Positions

Farmer JC, Wisneski RJ (Univ of Pennsylvania, Philadelphia; Princeton Orthopaedic Associates, NJ)

Spine 19:1850–1855, 1994 131-95-1–27

Background.—Cervical disk herniation with nerve root involvement is a relatively common syndrome that is diagnosed in part by clinical signs and patient responses to a variety of dynamic tests. Although the head, neck, and arm positions used in the tests are assumed to increase or decrease nerve compression or traction these assumptions have not been adequately tested. Pressure changes within intervertebral foramina of C5–7 were described with positional changes of the neck, shoulder, and arm.

Methods.—An anterior approach to the cervical spine was made in 8 fresh cadavers that had no histories of spinal or shoulder surgeries or spinal disease. A balloon catheter with an attached pressure transducer was placed in the neural foramina. Pressures within the foramina were determined with the neck variously flexed or extended, with the arm in neutral position and the shoulder abducted maximally.

Results.—Neck extension of 20 and 40 degrees resulted in significant increases in pressures of all nerve roots tested. Neck flexion resulted in significant pressure increases at C5 at both 20 and 40 degrees but insignificant changes at C6 or C7. With the neck extended at 20 or 40 degrees, pressure decreased in all nerve roots, as the arm was moved from neutral to abduction. Similar arm movement resulted in no significant pressure changes when the neck was flexed or in the neutral position.

Conclusion.—The exacerbation of clinical signs of cervical disk herniation with radicular involvement by neck extension and their amelioration by shoulder abduction were consistent with changes in pressure within intervertebral foramina. The effect of neck flexion on these pressures is less clear.

▶ This study helps explain the physical basis for the often useful shoulder abduction relief sign (1, 2). The patient with cervical radiculopathy notes pain improvement when abducting the shoulder with a flexed arm and placing the palm on the head. This seemingly unusual desirable posture can provide a strong indication that the patient's pain complaints are radicular.—D.A. Marcus, M.D.

References

1. Beatty RM, Fowler FD, Hanson J: The abducted arm as a sign of ruptured cervical disc. *Neurosurgery* 21:731–732, 1987.
2. Davidson RI, Dunn DJ, Metzmaker JN: The shoulder abduction test in the diagnosis of radicular pain in cervical extradural compression monoradiculopathies. *Spine* 6:441–446, 1981.

TREATMENT

Long-Term Results of Cervical Epidural Steroid Injection With and Without Morphine in Chronic Cervical Radicular Pain

Castagnera L, Maurette P, Pointillart V, Vital JM, Erny P, Sénégas (Hôpital Pellegrin, Bordeaux, France)

Pain 58:239–243, 1994 131-95-1–28

Introduction.—Cervical epidural steroid injection (CESI) has been used to manage patients with chronic cervical pain, spinal stenosis, documented compressive lesions, and cervical radicular pain (CRP). However, CESI techniques vary, and success rates range from 40% to 64%. Previous reports have also indicated that patients with low-back pain had better long-lasting pain relief when morphine was co-administered with steroids.

Methods.—In a prospective and randomized study, the short-, mid-, and long-term effectiveness of a single CESI that was performed with or without morphine was assessed in 24 patients with chronic CRP of noncompressive and nonmalignant origin whose indications did not require surgery. The patients had CRP for more than 12 months. With an increasing volume (10 mL maximum) of isotonic saline solution, the cervical epidural space was injected (C7–D1 with an 18-gauge needle) to exacerbate the patient's radicular pain. Fourteen patients (the steroid group) received an equivalent volume of .5% lidocaine plus triamcinolone acetonide (10 mg/mL), and 10 patients (the steroid plus morphine group) received the same combination as well as 2.5 mg of morphine sulfate.

Results.—Between the 2 groups, the anthropometric data were similar. In the steroid group, the mean volume injected in the epidural space was 6.6 mL, and in the steroid plus morphine group, the mean volume injected was 6.3 mL, which exacerbated pain in 21 of 24 patients. The long-term results of pain relief did not differ, despite observation of a better transient improvement the day after CESI in the steroid plus morphine group. In the steroid group, the success rate was 78.5%, with a pain relief of 86.8%, and in the steroid plus morphine group, the success rate was 80%, with a pain relief of 86.9%. With time, pain relief remained stable (mean follow-up, 43 months).

Conclusion.—A single CESI performed in patients with CRP produces long-lasting pain relief, which is not improved when morphine is combined with steroids.

▶ Ferrante and colleagues performed a retrospective analysis of patients who received cervical epidural steroids for neck pain and radiculopathy, and they also identified predictors of outcome (1). A most favorable outcome occurred in patients who had radiculopathy associated with neck pain.—D.A. Marcus, M.D.

Reference

1. Ferrante FM, Wilson SP, Iacobo C, et al: Clinical classification as a predictor of therapeutic outcome after cervical epidural steroid injection. *Spine* 18:730–736, 1993.

Lumbar Pain

INTRODUCTION

▶ Low back pain represents a significant health and economic problem that in 1990 cost in excess of $50 billion dollars (1). Frank recently published a comprehensive review of low back pain, describing its etiology, evaluation, and treatment options (2). Although the presence of disk disease is typically explored in patients with complaints of low back pain, Cassisi and associates recently noted greater reports of pain, disability, and psychological distress in patients who were given a diagnosis of myofascial pain compared with those who had herniated disks (3).

Therefore, our understanding and investigation of patients with complaints of low back pain require a comprehensive, multisystem evaluation. Failure to identify neurologic disease should not lead the clinician to the often incorrect assumption that the patient should be pain free, because musculoskeletal structures also contribute to the complaint of chronic low back pain.—D.A. Marcus, M.D.

References

1. Cats-Baril WL, Frymoyer JW: The economics of spinal disorders, in Frymoyer JW (ed): *The Adult Spine: Principles and Practice,* New York, Raven Press, 1991, pp 85–106.
2. Frank A: Low back pain. *BMJ* 306:901–909, 1993.
3. Cassisi JE, Sypert GW, Lagana L, et al: Pain, disability, and psychological functioning in chronic low back pain subgroups: Myofascial versus herniated disc syndrome. *Neurosurgery* 33:379–385, 1993.

PATHOGENESIS

Experimental Lumbar Radiculopathy: Immunohistochemical and Quantitative Demonstrations of Pain Induced by Lumbar Nerve Root Irritation of the Rat

Kawakami M, Weinstein JN, Spratt KF, Chatani K-I, Traub RJ, Meller ST, Gebhart GF (Wakayama Med College, Japan; Univ of Iowa Hosps and Clinic Iowa City; Kyoto Prefectural Univ of Med, Japan)
Spine 19:1780–1794, 1994 131-95-1–29

Objective.—The mechanisms of development of low back and leg pain after lumbar disk herniation and/or lumbar canal stenosis are unknown. Such an understanding requires experimental models of lumbar radiculopathy. The design and validation of a rat model of lumbar radiculopathy was reported.

Methods.—Two basic nerve trauma approaches were considered: direct compression damage and introduction of foreign materials leading to inflammation and chronic symptoms. A suture ligature around the nerve was considered analogous to nerve root entrapment. Initial studies compared 5 distinct treatments: a sham operation, nerve root clipping, a 4-0 silk ligature around the nerve roots, a 4-0 chromic gut ligature around the nerve roots, and 4-0 chromic gut suture material adjacent to the nerve roots. The 5 methods were compared for their differential effects over time, including their effects on animal function and biochemistry.

Results.—Animals that received large amounts of chromic gut ligature had differential results on the injured and noninjured sides that were consistent with lumbar radiculopathy. Thermal hyperalgesia related to neuropathic pain, initial mechanical hypoalgesia, and motor dysfunction were all significantly worse on the injured side. Two weeks postoperatively, c-*fos* counts were significantly increased on the injured side, but they returned to baseline within 12 weeks. The dorsal root ganglia showed significantly increased vasoactive intestinal polypeptide (VIP) concentrations at 2 weeks that did not resolve by 12 weeks. Vasoactive intestinal polypeptide depletion of the spinal cord was noted at 2 weeks, and it did not return to baseline until 12 weeks. The animals' behavior and functional patterns correlated with the quantitative and qualitative changes in c-*fos* and VIP.

Conclusion.—These experiments provide the first evidence linking outcome behaviors and function to the underlying neurochemical processes in lumbar radiculopathy resulting from nerve root irritation. With further refinements, the animal model described should be very useful in explaining the process of injury and repair and in facilitating effective treatment interventions. More research is needed to define the exact mechanism underlying the development of neuropathic pain.

Experimental Lumbar Radiculopathy: Behavioral and Histologic Changes in a Model of Radicular Pain After Spinal Nerve Root Irritation With Chromic Gut Ligatures in the Rat

Kawakami M, Weinstein JN, Chatani K-I, Spratt KF, Meller ST, Gebhart GF (Wakayama Med College, Japan; Univ of Iowa Hosp & Clinics, Iowa City; et al)

Spine 19:1795–1802, 1994 131-95-1–30

Purpose.—The pathophysiologic mechanisms underlying pain in lumbar radiculopathy are unknown. A rat model of this condition was developed in which the L4 to L6 nerve roots were loosely ligated with silk or chromic gut sutures. This model was associated with motor paresis and thermal hyperalgesia of the affected hind limb and evidence of spontaneous pain. It was used in a direct investigation of the pathophysiologic mechanisms associated with lumbar radiculopathy.

Methods.—The study included 3 different nerve root treatments. The first was a sham operation in which the nerve roots and dorsal root ganglion were exposed, followed by standard closing procedures. In the second, 2 loose 4-0 silk ligatures were placed around the nerve root. In the third treatment, four .3-cm pieces of 4-0 chromic gut were placed adjacent to the nerve roots and secured loosely with 2 ligatures of 4-0 chromic gut. The effects of the 3 treatments in terms of animal function were assessed over time. The histologic findings of the ipsilateral and contralateral nerve roots, dorsal root ganglia, and spinal nerves were assessed and correlated with the behavioral changes.

Results.—The behavioral changes were similar to those observed in the study in which the model was developed. Prolonged thermal hyperalgesia was observed in rats treated with chromic gut but not with silk. This effect was maximal at 2 weeks postoperatively and persisted for up to 12 weeks. However, the 2 groups showed similar histologic changes in the nerve roots, dorsal root ganglia and spinal nerves, the ipsilateral spinal nerves, dorsal root ganglia, and nerve roots, with significantly decreased numbers of large-diameter myelinated fibers. The behavioral changes did not correlate with the histologic changes.

Conclusion.—Mechanical constriction of the L4–L6 spinal nerve roots produces a loss of myelinated fibers. However, the histologic changes are insufficient to produce the behavioral effects observed in the new rat model of lumbar radiculopathy. Chemical factors from the chromic gut may play a role in the pathophysiology and development of the behavioral but not the histologic changes that occur in this model.

Pain From the Lumbar Zygapophysial Joints: A Test of Two Models

Schwarzer AC, Derby R, Aprill CN, Fortin J, Kine G, Bogduk (Univ of Newcastle, Callaghan, New South Wales, Australia; Spinecare, Daly City, Calif; Magnolia Diagnostics Inc, New Orleans, La; et al)

J Spinal Disord 7:331–336, 1994 131-95-1–31

Background.—The lumbar zygapophyseal joints can cause both back pain and referred pain to the lower extremities, but the clinical diagnosis of this pain continues to pose a frustrating problem. Some reports conclude that "facet arthrosis syndrome" is characterized by morning stiffness and pain that is aggravated by rest and extension and relieved by gentle movement and flexion. Others have found no such clinical features, and they express doubt about the existence of this syndrome. The predictive value of the clinical features and a rating system similar to that of Helbig and Lee were examined.

Methods.—The clinical criteria were tested in 176 consecutive patients with chronic low back pain. Clinical features were assessed by history and physical examination. In addition, each patient underwent a series of zygapophyseal joint injections of blocks of the medial branches of the dorsal ramus using lidocaine. Patients who responded to these blocks received confirmatory blocks with bupivacaine.

Results.—Forty-seven percent of the patients had at least a definite response to a lidocaine block at 1 of more levels. Of 71 patients who underwent confirmatory blocks with bupivacaine, 15% reported a 50% or greater improvement in their pain. The L5–S1 and L4–5 levels were the most commonly involved, and interobserver agreement was high. None of the predictive clinical features—pain that was increased by sitting, pain that was relieved by walking, pain in the thigh, back pain produced by straight leg raising, or pain on forward flexion—was associated with zygapophyseal joint pain in the study population. Scoring was likewise unreliable in distinguishing pain of zygapophyseal joint origin from pain of other origins.

Conclusion.—Previously reported clinical criteria cannot discriminate lumbar zygapophyseal joint pain from other forms of back pain. There is a need for some way of identifying the subgroup with zygapophyseal joint pain without having to perform diagnostic blocks in all patients.

▶ Chronic back pain is a common complaint, and as Abstracts 131-95-1–29 through 131-95-1–31 demonstrate, multiple structures often influence the seemingly simple complaint of back pain. Abnormalities can be identified in nerves, joints, and muscles. Therefore, complete examination of patients who complain of lumbar pain requires attention to all these areas.—D.A. Marcus, M.D.

EVALUATION

The Occurrence and Inter-Rater Reliability of Myofascial Trigger Points in the Quadratus Lumborum and Gluteus Medius: A Prospective Study in Non-Specific Low Back Pain Patients and Controls in General Practice

Njoo KH, Van der Does E (Erasmus Univ, Rotterdam, The Netherlands)

Pain 58:317–323, 1994 131-95-1–32

Background.—The myofascial pain syndrome is a regional pain complaint for which the presence of a trigger point is considered essential. Distinct criteria for the presence of trigger points in the quadratus lumborum and gluteus medius muscles were identified by investigating the occurrence and interrater reliability of trigger point symptoms.

Patients and Methods.—Symptoms and signs defined by Simons and 2 other previous sets of criteria were used. Sixty-one patients with nonspecific low back pain and 63 controls were examined in general practice by 5 observers who worked in pairs.

Results.—The 2 major criteria defined in Simons' 1990 report were localized tenderness and referred pain. Of these, only localized tenderness showed good discriminative ability and interrater reliability (Figs 1-8 and 1-9). No evidence for the clinical usefulness of "referred pain," which showed neither of these abilities, was noted. The "jump sign" and "patient recognition" criteria also had good discriminative ability and interrater reliability when localized tenderness was present. Trigger points defined by the eligible criteria permitted significant distinction between the patients with nonspecific low back pain and the controls; the same was not true of trigger points defined by Simons' 1990 criteria. Reliability in the 2 different criteria sets also significantly differed.

Conclusion.—The clinical value of trigger points was increased when localized tenderness, coupled with the jump sign or the patient's recognition of pain, were used as criteria for the presence of trigger points in the quadratus lumborum and gluteus medius muscles.

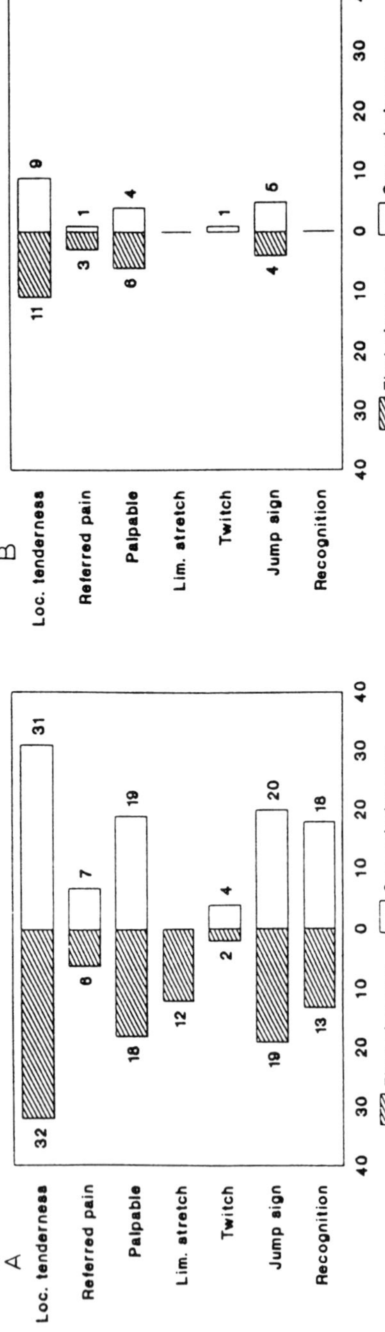

Fig 1–8.—*Musculus quadratus lumborum.* **A,** patients with low back pain. **B,** controls. (Courtesy of Njoo KH, Van der Does E: *Pain* 58:317–323, 1994.)

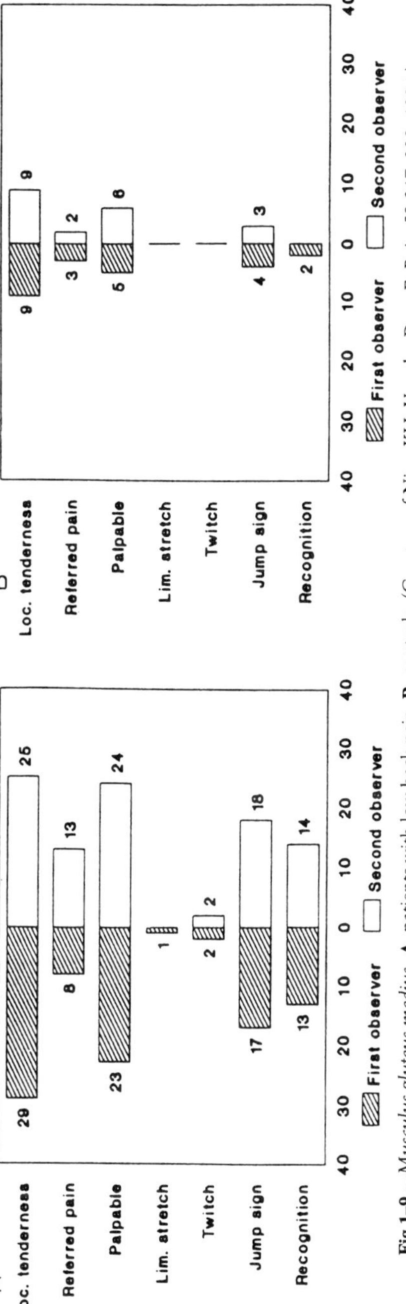

Fig 1–9.—*Musculus gluteus medius.* **A,** patients with low back pain. **B,** controls. (Courtesy of Njoo KH, Van der Does E: *Pain* 58:317–323, 1994.)

Thermal Deficit in Lumbar Radiculopathy: Correlations With Pain and Neurologic Signs and Its Value for Assessing Symptomatic Severity

Takahashi Y, Takahashi K, Moriya H (Chiba Univ, Japan)

Spine 19:2443–2450, 1994 131-95-1–33

Background.—Thermography reportedly demonstrates "hot spots" at sites of low back pain and a thermal deficit in areas of sciatica, presumably reflecting decreased cutaneous blood flow. Thermal deficits were related to the distribution of symptoms in 109 patients with low back pain and evidence of unilateral lumbar radiculopathy secondary to a herniated intervertebral disk. Sixty-eight healthy men also were examined.

Methods.—Thermograms were recorded with infrared telethermography at temperatures of 24°C to 29°C. The responses in delimited areas of the lumbar region and lower extremities were compared with ratings of pain, other symptoms, muscle tenderness, and motor weakness in the same areas.

Findings.—Rates of thermal deficit in patients with radiculopathy ranged from 10% in the lower back to 40% in the lateral region of the lower extremity. Forty patients (37%) exhibited a significant decrease in temperature over the entire surface, and 40% had 3 or more areas of thermal deficit. Only 23% of painful areas were thermally defective. Pain, muscle tenderness, sensory disorder, and motor weakness corresponded with areas of thermal deficit in 61% to 72% of instances. A thermal deficit was approximately 30% sensitive to symptoms and signs, but it was 80% specific. A temperature reduction in the affected extremity correlated at a moderate level (.57) with the Japanese Orthopedic Association score.

Implications.—Thermal deficit is an independent indicator of lumbar radiculopathy. Normal thermographic findings may indicate an asymptomatic region. Estimates of thermal deficit in the affected extremity reflect the severity of radiculopathic symptoms.

The False-Positive Rate of Uncontrolled Diagnostic Blocks of the Lumbar Zygapophysial Joints

Schwarzer AC, Aprill CN, Derby R, Fortin J, Kine G, Bogduk N (Univ of Newcastle, Callaghan, Australia; Magnolia Diagnostics, New Orleans, La; Spinecare, Daly City, Calif; et al)

Pain 58:195–200, 1994 131-95-1–34

Background.—Debate continues regarding the epidemiologic and clinical significance of zygapophyseal joint pain. This form of back pain is commonly diagnosed by blocks of the zygapophyseal joints, the reliability of which must be determined before formal studies of the prevalence of lumbar zygapophyseal joint pain can be performed. The false positive rate of single diagnostic blocks of the lumbar zygapophyseal joints was assessed.

Methods.—The study sample included 176 consecutive patients with chronic low back pain and no history of previous lumbar surgery. Diagnostic blocks using lidocaine were performed in all patients. Those who had definite or complete relief with lidocaine block then underwent confirmatory blocks using .5% bupivacaine. All blocks were performed under fluoroscopic control.

Results.—Forty-seven percent of the patients had at least a definite response to the initial lidocaine block at 1 or more levels. However, only 15% had at least a 50% response to the confirmatory bupivacaine block. When the response to confirmatory blocks was used as the criterion standard, uncontrolled diagnostic blocks had a false positive rate of 38% and a positive predictive value of only 31%.

Conclusion.—Uncontrolled diagnostic blocks of the lumbar zygapophyseal joints have an unacceptably low positive predictive value. This will always be there, because the positive predictive value of a test is lower when the prevalence is low, and the prevalence of lumbar zygapophyseal joint pain is likely to be less than 50%. As a result, uncontrolled blocks are diagnostically unreliable not only in epidemiologic studies but also in any given patient.

▶ Because abnormalities of a variety of physical structures can contribute to lumbar pain, numerous clinical and laboratory tests have been developed to assess these varying areas of possible pathology. Whenever a clinician orders, performs, or interprets a test, it is essential that he understand the test's flaws and limitations. Low reliability has been demonstrated for physical examinations (1–3). Objective laboratory tests may also provide inaccurate information.

Structural abnormalities on MRI have been demonstrated in asymptomatic adults, with herniated disks seen in 24% and spinal stenosis in 4%; bulging disks can be identified in 54% of asymptomatic adults younger than 60 years of age and 79% of those older than age 60 (4). Limitations of electrophysiologic testing, thermography, and nerve blocks have also been reviewed (5). Clinicians should remember that available testing is best used to confirm a clinical diagnosis that was determined from the history and examination and that it should not be used to replace the clinical examination.—D.A. Marcus, M.D.

References

1. Agre JC, Magness JL, Hull A, et al: Strength testing with portable dynamometer: Reliability for upper and lower extremities. *Arch Phys Med Rehabil* 68:454–458, 1987.
2. Nelson MA, Allen P, Clamp SE, et al: Reliability and reproducibility of clinical findings in low back pain. *Spine* 4:97–101, 1979.
3. Dreyfuss P, Dryer S, Griffin J, et al: Positive sacroiliac screening tests in asymptomatic adults. *Spine* 19:1138–1143, 1994.

4. Boden SD, Davis DO, Dina TS, et al: Abnormal magnetic-resonance scans of the lumbar spine in asymptomatic subjects. *J Bone Joint Surg* 72A:403–408, 1990.
5. Verdugo RJ, Ochoa JL: Use and misuse of conventional electrodiagnosis, quantitative sensory testing, thermography, and nerve blocks in the evaluation of painful neuropathic syndromes. *Muscle Nerve* 16:1056–1062, 1993.

TREATMENT

The Short-Term Effect of a Spinal Manipulation on Pain/Pressure Threshold in Patients With Chronic Mechanical Low Back Pain

Côté P, Mior SA, Vernon H (Royal Univ Hosp, Saskatoon, Sask, Canada; Canadian Mem Chiropractic College, Toronto)
J Manipulative Physiol Ther 17:364–368, 1994 131-95-1–35

Background.—There is little information in the literature on objective quantitative measurement of spinal manipulation efficacy in managing back pain. To what extent and for how many minutes manipulation increases the pain/pressure threshold of specific myofascial points was studied in patients with chronic mechanical lumbosacral back pain.

Methods.—Thirty adults (mean age, 31 years) with chronic lumbosacral back pain (mean duration of pain, 74 months) who visited a chiropractic outpatient clinic were studied. Selection criteria included chronic unilateral lumbosacral or sacroiliac back pain of mechanical origin for more than 2 months, reported pain over the lumbosacral area, pain that could be reproduced by digital palpation, and at least 2 of several other clinical criteria. Sixteen patients were randomized to the manipulation group and 14 to the mobilization group. Manipulation was done with the patient lying on his side. The mobilization procedure was an assisted knee-to-chest maneuver. A pressure algometer was used to quantify the pain over 3 selected myofascial points that were the same for each patient (L5, posterior sacroiliac ligament, and gluteus). Pressure was slowly increased at about 100 g/sec until the patient verbally reported pain. Measurements were taken 15 minutes before the allocated treatment and immediately after, and they were repeated 15 and 30 minutes later. The treating clinician and the clinician doing the measurements were blinded from each other's procedures.

Results.—Statistical analysis of the algometer measurements for the 3 myofascial points did not reveal significant differences between the 2 treatments or between treatment and the time of the measurement.

Conclusion.—Failure to detect any significant effect of the manipulative treatment of chronic lumbosacral back pain may be the result of problems with the selection of myofascial points, the insensitivity of the instrument to small changes, the differences in baseline measures, and/or the lack of effect from only one manipulative intervention.

▶ The Agency for Health Care Policy and Research of the U.S. Department of Health and Human Services published recommendations for clinical assessment and treatment of *acute* low back pain in adults in December 1994 (1). Its literature review supported the short-term use of spinal manipulation during the first month of symptoms in patients with acute low back pain without radiculopathy. Data regarding the effectiveness of spinal manipulation for chronic low back pain are insufficient to permit recommendation (2).—D.A. Marcus, M.D.

References

1. Bigos S, Bowyer O, Braen G, et al: *Acute Low Back Problems in Adults: Clinical Practice Guidelines* No. *14*. Rockville, Md: Agency for Health Care Policy and Research, Public Health Service; December 1994. US Dept of Health and Human Services, AHCPR publication 95-0642.
2. Shekelle PG, Adams AH, Chassin MR, et al: Spinal manipulation for low-back pain. *Ann Intern Med* 117:590–598, 1992.

Effects of Methylprednisolone on Nucleus Pulposus–Induced Nerve Root Injury

Olmarker K, Byröd G, Cornefjord M, Nordborg C, Rydevik B (Univ of Gothenburg, Sweden; Sahlgren Hosp, Gothenburg, Sweden)

Spine 19:1803–1808, 1994 131-95-1-36

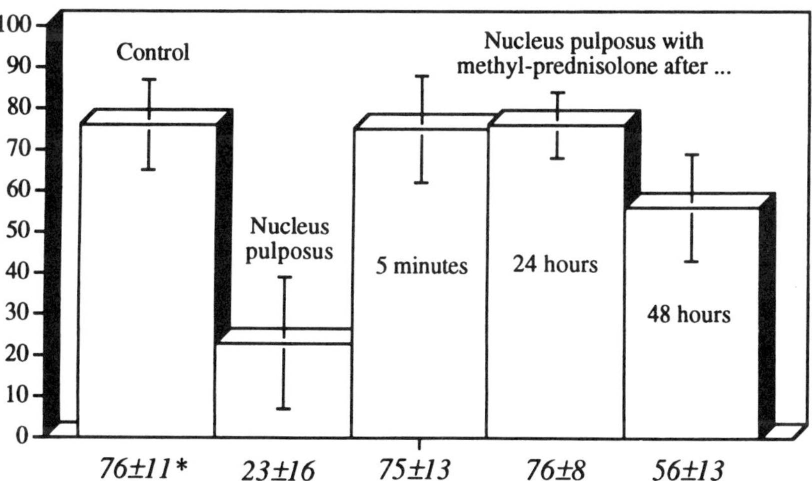

Fig 1–10.—Nerve conduction velocity in the different subseries, 7 days after application of nucleus pulposus. Results from control-application (retroperitoneal fat) from a previous study are presented for comparison. (Courtesy of Olmarker K, Byröd G, Cornefjord M, et al: *Spine* 19:1803–1808, 1994.)

Introduction.—Intravenous injection of methylprednisolone was studied to evaluate how its effects reduce the nerve root injury after epidural application of autologous nucleus pulposus. According to results of previous studies, if it is applied epidurally, autologous nucleus pulposus may induce significant change in nerve root morphology and function.

Methods.—An experimental model on the pig cauda equina in 20 animals was conducted. Nucleus pulposus was harvested from a lumbar disk. The pH of the nucleus pulposus was lowered to 3.5, and it was placed onto the sacrococcygeal cauda equina. A single IV injection of methylprednisolone, 30 mg/kg, was given to 15 pigs at 5 minutes, 24 hours, or 48 hours after the application. The nerve conduction velocity was determined, and biopsy specimens of the cauda equina were examined by light microscopy. Five pigs formed the control group.

Results.—In the control group, nerve conduction velocity was reduced; however, it was normal in the pigs treated 5 minutes and 24 hours after nucleus pulposus application (Fig 1–10). Nerve conduction velocity was reduced only slightly in pigs that were treated after 48 hours. Significant changes occurred in all series at the light microscopic level. When nucleus pulposus at pH 3.5 had been applied without steroid treatment, the conduction velocity was significantly lower than that observed in a previous study for retroperitoneal fat control.

Conclusion.—The nucleus pulposus-induced effects on nerve function can be reduced dramatically by high-dose methylprednisolone administration within 5 minutes to 24 hours in an experimental pig model after epidural application of autologous nucleus pulposus. The effect of methylprednisolone was less pronounced when steroids were injected after 48 hours. For the nerve function, the light microscopic changes were probably not significant. A morphological explanation on a subcellular level should probably be sought.

Percutaneous Nucleotomy in the Treatment of Lumbar Disc Herniation: Results After a Mean Follow-Up of 2 Years

Kotilainen E, Valtonen S (Turku Univ Central Hosp, Finland)

Acta Neurochir (Wien) 128:47–52, 1994 131-95-1–37

Background.—The technique of percutaneous nucleotomy was developed to avoid the major tissue trauma of conventional disk operations. The clinical outcome of the first patients who underwent surgery using this technique for a single-level lumbar disk herniation was described.

Methods.—A total of 53 consecutive patients underwent percutaneous nucleotomy between 1989 and 1992. The 45 patients (85%) who responded to a follow-up questionnaire in 1993 were studied. Preoperatively, all patients (28 women, 17 men; mean age, 46 years) were evaluated for possible segmental instability of the lumbar spine using the symptom of "apprehension" as a clinical criterion (positive in 24%), and

TABLE 1.—Postoperative Recovery of Low Back Pain and Sciatica at the 2-Week Follow-Up

Recovery	Number (%) of patients	
	Low back pain	Sciatica
Completely recovered	14 (31)	25 (56)
Markedly diminished	23 (52)	14 (31)
Unchanged	6 (13)	6 (13)
Worse	2 (4)	0
Total	45 (100)	45 (100)

(Courtesy of Kotilainen E, Valtonen S: *Acta Neurochir (Wien)* 128:47–52, 1994.)

TABLE 2.—Postoperative Recovery of Low Back Pain and Sciatica at the Mean Follow-Up After 2 Years

Recovery	Number (%) of patients	
	Low back pain	Sciatica
Completely recovered	9 (20)	13 (28)
Markedly diminished	25 (56)	25 (56)
Unchanged	9 (20)	4 (9)
Worse	2 (4)	3 (7)
Total	45 (100)	45 (100)

(Courtesy of Kotilainen E, Valtonen S: *Acta Neurochir (Wien)* 128:47–52, 1994.)

TABLE 3.—Postoperative Working Capacity of Patients at the Mean Follow-Up After 2 Years

Working capacity	Number of Patients	Frequency (%)
In work	35	78
On sick leave	1	2
Retired because of the back	7	16
Retired because of another disease	2	4
Total	45	100

(Courtesy of Kotilainen E, Valtonen S: *Acta Neurochir (Wien)* 128:47–52, 1994.)

the diagnosis of lumbar disk herniation was confirmed by either CT scan or MRI. The patients had a history of back pain for an average of 7 years and sciatic pain for 5 months. The selection criteria included disk herniation that was radiologically graded as a protrusion or small prolapse at the levels of L3–4 (4%), L4–5 (94%), or L5–S1 (2%). The patients were examined 2 weeks after surgery and were sent a follow-up questionnaire an average of 2 years postoperatively.

Results.—Intraoperative diskography showed a protrusion in 51% and a prolapse in 49% of patients. The sciatica had markedly improved or totally disappeared in 87% of patients at 2 weeks (Table 1) and in 84% of patients at 2 years (Table 2). At 2 years after surgery, 78% of patients were working (Table 3). Forty-five percent of the patients with preoperative instability were postoperatively retired or were taking sick leave because of back problems compared with 15% of patients without preoperative instability. The postoperative diskitis that developed in 4% of patients responded well to antibiotics.

Conclusion.—The outcome of most patients who underwent percutaneous nucleotomy for single-level lumbar disk herniation was successful. However, preoperative lumbar spine instability was significantly associated with an unsatisfactory outcome. Also, patients who underwent surgery for a prolapse usually had a better outcome than those who were operated on for a protrusion. In the future, an optimal treatment will be better defined for different subgroups of patients.

▶ Conventional surgery has been shown to be effective for the majority of patients with herniated disks or nerve root canal stenosis (1, 2). The prognostic factors associated with a favorable outcome after lumbar surgery include lack of neurologic deficits, preoperative use of autotraction, and sedentary work requirements (3). Jonsson and Stromqvist reported outcome results for 93 patients who were prospectively followed after repeated conventional lumbar surgery (4). Repeat surgeries to treat recurrent disk herniation or bony compression showed good results, whereas surgeries for scarring did poorly.—D.A. Marcus, M.D.

References

1. An HS, Vaccaro A, Simeone FA, et al: Herniated lumbar disc in patients over the age of fifty. *J Spinal Disord* 3:143–146, 1990.
2. Postacchini F, Cinotti G, Perugia D: Microdiscectomy in treatment of herniated lumbar disc. *Ital J Ortho Traumatol* 18:5–16, 1992.
3. Barrios C, Ahmed M, Arrotegui JI, et al: Clinical factors predicting outcome after surgery for herniated lumbar disc: An epidemiological multivariate analysis. *J Spinal Disord* 3:205–209, 1990.
4. Jonsson B, Stromqvist B: Repeat decompression of lumbar nerve roots: A prospective two-year evaluation. *J Bone Joint Surg (Br)* 75:894–897, 1993.

Caudal Epidural Blocks for Elderly Patients With Lumbar Canal Stenosis

Ciocon JO, Galindo-Ciocon D, Amaranath L, Galindo D (Cleveland Clinic Florida, Fort Lauderdale; Veterans Affairs Med Ctr, Miami, Fla; Univ of Miami, Fla)

J Am Geriatr Soc 42:593–596, 1994 131-95-1–38

Background.—Population-based studies have shown that one fourth to one half of elderly individuals have significant pain. Musculoskeletal conditions are the main source of the pain. The effectiveness of caudal epidural blocks (CEB) in alleviating pain and the duration of pain relief with CEB in elderly persons with degenerative lumbar canal stenosis (LCS) were investigated.

Methods.—Thirty patients, with a mean age of 76 years, were enrolled in a descriptive, prospective study. All had leg discomfort with or without back pain and LCS documented by MRI. None had had CEB or surgery for their leg discomfort, nor did they have pain relief from analgesics alone. Treatment consisted of 3 doses per week of .5% lidocaine (Xylocaine) with 80 mg of methylprednisolone (Depo-Medrol) into the caudal epidural space through the sacral hiatus.

Findings.—On admission, LCS was moderate in 66.7% of the patients, mild in 23.3%, and severe in 10%. A mean of 2.4 lumbar vertebrae were involved. The degree of LCS was directly correlated with the pain level before CEB. After CEB, the mean pain level changed from 3.43 to 1.5. Pain relief was significant for up to 10 months. The duration of pain relief ranged from 4 to 10 months.

Conclusion.—Caudal epidural block can significantly relieve pain in elderly patients with degenerative LCS. This treatment alternative appears to be particularly important for patients who respond poorly to drug treatment and those who cannot or will not have surgery.

▶ It is unfortunate that this study did not use outcome assessment variables other than pain scores. Ideally, post-treatment assessments would also investigate functional improvements such as increased ability (speed, distance) to ambulate, increased activities of daily living, and improved sleep.

The use of epidural steroids in chronic pain is an area of hot debate, with a recent focus article and commentaries being published in the *APS Journal* (1–3). Hopwood and Abram investigated prognostic factors for success using lumbar epidural steroids and reported a poor outcome to be associated with nonradicular pain, constant and long duration pain, a reduction in recreational and work activities, sleep disturbance, smoking, lower levels of education, and psychological distress (4).—D.A. Marcus, M.D.

References

1. Risk versus benefit of epidural steroids: Let's remain objective. *APS J* 3:28–30, 1994.
2. Hammonds WD: Epidural steroid injections: An unproven therapy for pain. *APS J* 3:31–32, 1994.
3. Rowlingson JC: Epidural steroids: Do they have a place in pain management? *APS J* 3:20–27, 1994.
4. Hopwood MB, Abram SE: Factors associated with failure of lumbar epidural steroids. *Reg Anesth* 18:238–243, 1993.

Hyaluronidase in the Management of Pain Due to Post-Laminectomy Scar Tissue

Borg PAJ, Krijnen HJ (Academic Hosp Groningen, The Netherlands)
Pain 58:273–276, 1994 131-95-1–39

Background.—Otherwise successful laminectomy with decompression of the involved lumbar nerve root is sometimes complicated by recurrent radicular pain caused by scar tissue that traps the involved nerve root. Surgery is usually followed by recurrent scar tissue and root compression; conservative therapies bring sufficient relief in some but not all patients. The use of locally applied hyaluronidase to dissolve scar tissue in a patient with cicatrical radiculopathy was studied.

Case Report.—Man, 31, was treated for a rebound radicular syndrome resulting from postlaminectomy scarring in the intervertebral foramen and epidural space. Various drug treatments—including baclofen, clorazepate, diazepam, carbamazepine, clonazepam, and amitriptyline—were ineffective. The patient, whose *visual analogue scale* (VAS) socres remained at 7, refused further oral medication. He gave informed consent to try local hyaluronidase treatment. Hyaluronidase, 150 units in 3 mL of normal saline, was injected through a 20-gauge spinal needle into the L4–5 intervertebral foramen on the affected side. Correct needle placement was confirmed with the use of an image intensifier. There was no response to the initial injection, so another treatment was given one month later. For the next 2 weeks, the patient's pain decreased to a VAS score of 3. A total of 9 injections were given, with hyaluronidase doses of up to 600 units and correspondingly longer durations of reduced pain. The addition of radiopaque dye showed unhindered spread into the epidural space, as had been suggested by the decreasing resistance to injection. One week after the last injection, the VAS score was 2, and straight leg-raising was unlimited on both sides.

Conclusion.—Local hyaluronidase injection may be a useful treatment for the management of pain associated with postlaminectomy scar tissue. Further trials of this treatment, using higher doses to establish a dose-effect relationship, are planned. If hyaluronidase proves to be safe and effective, it may represent a valuable early therapeutic option with a favorable cost-benefit ratio.

▶ Postoperative scarring is associated with morbidity for a variety of surgeries. Interestingly, powdered surgical gloves promote excessive scarring (1), and the use of powder-free gloves might prove helpful in minimizing the development of painful scar tissue. The use of the scar lysis enzyme hyaluronidase has also been applied to pain related to endodontic treatment (2). The concomitant use of hyaluronidase with nonsteroidal anti-inflammatory drugs (NSAIDs) was associated with a greater number of pain-free patients after treatment when compared with the use of NSAIDs alone.—D.A. Marcus, M.D.

References

1. Ellis H: Pathological changes produced by surgical dusting powders. *Ann R Coll Surg Engl* 76:5–8, 1994.
2. Negm MM: Effect of intracranial use of nonsteroidal anti-inflammatory agents on posttreatment endodontic pain. *Oral Surg, Oral Med, Oral Pathol* 77:507–513, 1994.

Risk Factors of Chronicity in Lumbar Disc Patients: A Prospective Investigation of Biologic, Psychologic, and Social Predictors of Therapy Outcome

Hasenbring M, Marienfeld G, Kuhlendahl D, Soyka D (Univ Hosp of Kiel, Germany)

Spine 19:2759–2765, 1994 131-95-1–40

Objective.—It would be very helpful to find a way of predicting which patients with lumbar disk prolapse or protrusion will have chronic pain develop. One hundred eleven consecutive patients with acute radicular pain were studied to learn whether various psychological factors have predictive value.

Patients.—All participants had a radiographic diagnosis of prolapsed or protruded lumbar disk. The average patient age was 42 years, but patients ranged in age from 17 to 72 years. About 60% of patients were males. Nearly half the affected disks were at the L5–S1 level. Two thirds of the patients underwent surgery.

Methods.—The Beck Depression Inventory (BDI) was administered as well as Kiel tests of daily hassles and pain coping strategies. The Health locus of control was also administered. The social parameters measured included social status, occupational setting, and time away from work. Patients were assessed at the time of discharge and 6 months later.

Findings.—Psychological variables, notably the degree of depressive mood and specific strategies for coping with pain, accounted for 38% of the variance in pain intensity at the time of discharge. Social support, daily hassles, and social status also contributed to the early outcome. The degree of disk displacement was a key factor both at discharge and 6 months later. Scoliosis was a factor in the 6-month outcome. Strategies for coping with pain were important factors, as was social status. Whether patients had applied for early retirement at the 6-month follow-up was best predicted by depression and work-related stress.

Conclusion.—An assessment of psychological and social status at the time patients are treated for acute lumbar back pain can help predict whether chronic symptoms and disability will ensue.

▶ Attempts to identify risk factors associated with low back pain have not produced conclusive recommendations (1). Interestingly, cigarette smoking has been consistently associated with low back pain (1–4), and it has been postulated to affect pain because of changes in neurochemicals associated with nicotine, altered blood flow, and associated behavioral changes.

Predictors of chronicity include sciatic symptoms, pain duration and recurrence, and age (1). Poor treatment outcome in patients with chronic pain is associated with abnormalities in spinal flexibility, trunk strength, and psychological variables, such as coping skills, fear of pain, and job satisfaction (1).—D.A. Marcus, M.D.

References

1. Skovron ML: Epidemiology of low back pain. *Baillieres Clin Rheumatol* 6:559–573, 1992.
2. Jackson RP, McManus AC: Radiologic analysis of sagittal plane alignment and balance in standing volunteers and patients with low back pain matched for age, sex, and size: A prospective controlled clinical study. *Spine* 19:1611–1618, 1994.
3. Jamison RN, Stetson BA, Parris WC: The relationship between cigarette smoking and chronic low back pain. *Addict Behav* 16:103–110, 1991.
4. O'Connor FG, Marlowe SS: Low back pain in military basic trainees: A pilot study. *Spine* 18:1351–1354, 1993.

Effects of Work-Oriented Fitness Courses in Lumberjacks With Low Back Pain

Leino P, Kivekäs J, Hänninen K (LEL Employment Pension Fund, Helsinki)
J Occup Rehabil 4:67–76, 1994 131-95-1–41

Background.—The work of a lumberjack is physically demanding, and disability resulting from musculoskeletal disease and back pain is common among workers of this profession. Rehabilitation programs for patients with musculoskeletal disorders are gaining popularity in Finland; however, there is little information regarding the efficacy of such intervention. The effects of work-oriented fitness courses on the performance and musculoskeletal health of lumberjacks with a history of back pain were explored.

Methods.—Eighty-seven Finnish lumberjacks who had experienced short-term disability resulting from lower back pain within the past year were recruited to take 1-week fitness courses emphasizing leisure time exercise and ergonomic work performance. A similar cohort of 61 lumberjacks that did not attend the course served as controls. A questionnaire regarding work ability, health, working conditions, and lifestyle was sent to all lumberjacks who were employed by 2 timber companies before the study took place, and a follow-up questionnaire was sent to members of the study groups 1 year after the courses ended. The frequency and causes of sickness allowances were assessed in members of each group both before and 1 year after the courses ended.

Results.—At follow-up, increases in fitness, ability to work, and perceived health and decreases in symptoms of distress such as heartburn, abdominal pain, insomnia, and headache were greater in those in the intervention group than in the controls. There were no differences between the groups in health, ergonomic strain, or back or musculoskeletal symptoms. There was no significant change in the number of spells or days of sickness allowance caused by lower back pain in either group, although there was a trend toward fewer spells in the intervention group.

Conclusion.—The fitness courses evaluated in this study decreased the occurrence of distress symptoms, a factor associated with development of future back pain, and increased perceived ability to work, a factor associated with the reduced risk of early retirement. This suggests that these courses may also decrease the frequency of sickness allowances resulting from low back pain; however, this effect cannot be regarded as conclusive. Larger studies are required to describe more fully the effects of work-oriented fitness courses.

▶ Lehmann and associates evaluated long-term disability in 55 patients with work-related acute back pain (1). About 16% of their patients did not return to work; 13% returned after 1 month, and 80% had returned within 7 months of injury. Married patients tended to return to work more quickly. Identification of high-risk groups for back injury with disability is an important first step in reducing this disability.

Risk factors for work-related injury with disability have been evaluated for a variety of occupations and include previous disability and heavy lifting (2). Interestingly, a history of previous back injury alone was not an important risk factor. For nurses, risk factors also included heavy work, the strength of quadriceps, Health Locus of Control, and height in 1 study (3); and evening shift and weight more than 200 pounds in another study (4).

A variety of studies have evaluated the effectiveness of back injury prevention programs used in high-risk groups with mixed results (5, 6). One study that evaluated high-risk government employees demonstrated a modest decrease in the prevalence of back pain after participation in education, exercise, and ergonomic training (7). A significant reduction in risky behaviors and an increase in satisfaction were also reported. An economic assessment of the program revealed a net benefit of more than $160,000, which represented a net return on investment of 179%. Further research into the prevention of back injuries and disability is important to help to reduce employee health care costs and improve worker satisfaction and productivity.—D.A. Marcus, M.D.

References

1. Lehmann TR, Spratt KF, Lehmann KK: Predicting long-term disability in low back injured workers presenting to a spine consultant. *Spine* 18:1103–1112, 1993.
2. Zwerling C, Ryan J, Schootman M: A case-control study of risk factors for industrial low back injury: The utility of preplacement screening in defining high-risk groups. *Spine* 18:1242–1247, 1993.
3. Klaber-Moffett JA, Hughes GI, Griffiths P: A longitudinal study of low back pain in student nurses. *Int J Nurs Stud* 30:197–212, 1993.
4. Garrett B, Singiser D, Banks SM: Back injuries among nursing personnel: The relationship of personal characteristics, risk factors, and nursing practices. *AAOHN J* 40:510–516, 1992.
5. Daltroy LH, Iversen MD, Larson MG, et al: Teaching and social support: Effects on knowledge, attitudes, and behaviors to prevent low back injuries in industry. *Health Educ Q* 20:43–62, 1993.
6. King PL: Back injury prevention programs: A critical review of the literature. *J Occup Rehabil* 3:145–158, 1993.
7. Shi L: A cost-benefit analysis of a California county's back injury prevention program. *Public Health Rep* 108:204–211, 1993.

Neuropathic Pain

PATHOGENESIS

Extra-Territorial Pain in Rats With a Peripheral Mononeuropathy: Mechano-Hyperalgesia and Mechano-Allodynia in the Territory of an Uninjured Nerve

Tal M, Bennett GJ (Hebrew Univ, Jerusalem, Israel; Natl Inst of Dental Research, Bethesda, Md)

Pain 57:375–382, 1994 131-95-1–42

Background.—Peripheral neuropathies can cause abnormal pain sensations in a distribution that is not consistent with the territories of nerves or posterior roots. Patients with this "extraterritorial" pain are often thought to have a psychoneurosis rather than an organic neurologic dysfunction. Tying ligatures around the sciatic nerve of a rat produces the chronic constriction injury (CCI), a model of painful peripheral neuropathy that produces symptoms similar to those of patients with traumatic nerve injury. The CCI model was used to study extraterritorial pain in rats.

Methods.—Four loosely constricting ligatures were tied around the sciatic nerve of rats at the mid-thigh level. Each animal had the contralateral sciatic nerve exposed without tying the ligature as a control. For behavioral testing, animals were placed on a perforated floor, which permitted mechanical stimuli to be applied to the hindpaw from below. Mechanohyperalgesia was assessed with a pinprick; mechanoallodynia was assessed by touching the skin with von Frey hairs.

Results.—Starting on postoperative day 1 and continuing for more than 17 days, exaggerated withdrawal reflexes to pinprick stimulation (mechanohyperalgesia) were present on the side of the nerve injury in the hindpaw territories of both the sciatic nerve and the uninjured saphenous nerve. Starting on postoperative day 4 and continuing for longer than 20 days, the withdrawal responses to von Frey hairs occurred at a much lower threshold (mechanoallodynia). The time course and severity of the mechanoallodynia were similar in the territories of both nerves. Mechanoallodynia in the saphenous nerve territory was obliterated by an acute saphenous transection but not by a sciatic transection. Mid-plantar sciatic territory-evoked mechano-allodynia was obliterated by an acute sciatic transection but not by a saphenous transection.

Conclusion.—Rats that have a painful experimental peripheral mononeuropathy have extraterritorial pain similar to that seen in individuals with traumatic nerve injury. A peripheral nerve injury can cause extraterritorial pain by evoking dysfunction of pain-processing neurons in the CNS.

Referred Pain of Peripheral Nerve Origin: An Alternative to the "Myofascial Pain" Construct

Quintner JL, Cohen ML (St John of God Med Centre, Perth, Western Australia; St Vincent's Hosp, Sydney, Australia; Univ of New South Wales, Sydney, Australia)

Clin J Pain 10:243–251, 1994 131-95-1–43

Introduction.—The myofascial pain syndrome (MPS) hypothesis is built around the trigger point (TrP), a location within a muscle that, on palpation, evokes local and remote pain. Myofascial pain is thought to be caused by TrPs. Activation of latent, secondary, and satellite TrPs causes spread and chronicity of pain. A system of empirical treatment for MPS is often accepted uncritically. It has been argued on clinical, epistemologic, and pathophysiologic grounds that the MPS theory is invalid and that the pertinent clinical phenomena are better explained as secondary hyperalgesia of peripheral neural origin.

Arguments.—Problems with the MPS hypothesis include the fact that the definition of the syndrome incorporates the hypothesis of causation. This error in logic has resulted in a system of diagnosis and treatment that is entirely anecdotal. The TrPs lack clinical reliability and validity. When blinded as to diagnosis, experts in the MPS field could detect active TrPs in only 18% of examinations of patients with a diagnosis of MPS. There are many predisposing, precipitating, and perpetuating factors of MPS. Biopsies, electromyographic, and thermographic studies of painful muscles have not shown significant abnormalities in TrPs. Animal models and human muscle injury studies do not support the MPS hypothesis. The TrPs are an operational hypothesis that has been elevated to the status of theory by circular reasoning. The anatomical distribution of pain referred from TrPs bears a close relationship to the course of peripheral nerves, and the MPS pain is clinically indistinguishable from nerve trunk pain—an example of somatic-referred pain. Sympathetic dysfunction is described both with the MPS and with pain of peripheral neural origin. Neurologic examination and conventional electrodiagnostic tests can be normal in pain of peripheral neural origin. Intolerance of muscles to stretch most likely is caused by a reflex spasm secondary to nociception elsewhere (e.g., the peripheral nerve).

Conclusion.—All MPS phenomena are better understood as secondary hyperalgesia of peripheral neural origin than as trigger points within muscles. This explanation for the clinical phenomena can be tested to obtain external validation.

Norepinephrine and Epinephrine Levels in Affected Versus Unaffected Limbs in Sympathetically Maintained Pain

Harden RN, Duc TA, Williams TR, Coley D, Cate JC, Gracely RH (Northwestern Univ, Chicago; Med Univ of South Carolina, Charleston; Natl Insts of Neural Research, Bethesda, Md; et al)

Clin J Pain 10:324–330, 1994 131-95-1–44

Background.—The conventional hypothesis regarding the mechanism of sympathetically maintained pain (SMP) holds that there is a long-term increase in pathologic sympathetic tone in the affected extremity. However, recent studies have suggested that SMP is associated with upregulation of peripheral sensitivity to norepinephrine that is released at the terminals of sympathetic efferents or circulating norepinephrine and epinephrine. This increased sensitivity could lead to the clinical features of SMP. To evaluate the central hypothesis of relative sympathetic hyperactivity, serum norepinephrine and epinephrine levels were measured in the affected and unaffected sides in patients with SMP.

Methods.—Study patients were 16 women and 7 men with SMP (mean age, 44 years). This diagnosis was based on the finding of a greater than 50% reduction in pain in response to a paravertebral sympathetic block. In addition, all patients met the International Association for the Study of Pain criteria for either reflex sympathetic dystrophy or causalgia. The investigators obtained venous pool samples from a site located just proximal to the affected area and from the same site on the unaffected side. They then used high-pressure liquid chromatography with electrochemical detection to measure serum norepinephrine and epinephrine levels in these samples.

Results.—Seventy percent of patients had lower plasma norepinephrine levels in the venous pools of the affected side. Overall, mean plasma norepinephrine levels were 44 pg/mL lower on the affected side. By contrast, there was no significant difference between epinephrine levels on the affected and unaffected sides.

Conclusion.—In patients with SMP, plasma norepinephrine levels were lower in the venous pool of the affected extremity than in those of the unaffected extremity. These findings are inconsistent with the conventional hypothesis of segmental sympathetic hyperactivity in the affected limb. Instead, they support a hypothesis of peripheral receptor upregulation with a pathologic response to circulating catecholamines. Larger studies using a more definitive staging system are advocated.

▶ A number of authors have presented a model of altered central processing as an explanation for the persistent symptoms of peripheral neuropathy (1–3). Peripheral nerve injury is thought to result in alterations in the excitability of the spinal cord, with structural reorganization of synaptic connections resulting in central sensitization. Abnormalities have also been identified in sympathetic postganglionic innervation in neuropathic rats (4). Mao and co-workers identified increases in calcium-mediated neuronal plasticity with increased membrane-bound protein kinase C in neuropathic rats (5). Spinal administration of the protein kinase C inhibitor GM1 ganglioside reversed both increases in protein kinase C and neuropathic pain behaviors.

Data from Abstracts 131-95-1–42 through 131-95-1–44 help to support the importance of central mechanisms in the development and maintenance of neuropathic pain. This type of a model makes it easier to explain the failure of treatments that are designed to address only changes in the periphery in patients with chronic neuropathic pain.—D.A. Marcus, M.D.

References

1. Gracely RH, Lynch SA, Bennett GJ: Painful neuropathy: Altered central processing maintained dynamically by peripheral input. *Pain* 51:175–194, 1993.
2. Woolf CJ: The pathophysiology of peripheral neuropathic pain: abnormal peripheral input and abnormal central processing. *Acta Neurochir Suppl (Wien)* 58:125–130, 1993.
3. Yaksh TL: New horizons in our understanding of the spinal physiology and pharmacology of pain processing. *Semin Oncol* 20:6S–18S, 1993.
4. Chung K, Kim HJ, Na HS, et al: Abnormalities of sympathetic innervation in the area of an injured peripheral nerve in a rat model of neuropathic pain. *Neurosci Lett* 162:85–88, 1993.
5. Mao J, Price DD, Mayer DJ, et al: Pain-related increases in spinal cord membrane-bound protein kinase C following peripheral nerve injury. *Brain Res* 588:144–149, 1992.

TREATMENT

Deafferentation Pain Exacerbated by Subarachnoid Lidocaine and Relieved by Subarachnoid Morphine

Iacono RP, Boswell MV, Neumann M (Loma Linda Univ, Calif; Case Western Reserve Univ, Cleveland, Ohio)
Reg Anesth 19:212–215, 1994 131-95-1–45

Background.—Chronic neuropathic pain syndromes are often resistant to conventional drug therapy, including systemic opioids. It has been suggested that subarachnoid administration of opioids may be effective for some forms of neuropathic pain.

Case Report.—Woman, 44, who had a 16-year history of deafferentation pain of the legs and who had been resistant to multidisciplinary pain clinic management, including spinal cord stimulation, agreed to undergo differential spinal anesthesia with lidocaine and morphine. Evoked potential monitoring was used to evaluate the intensity of the spinal anesthetic block. A subarachnoid injection of lidocaine exacerbated the leg pain, but a subarachnoid morphine injection provided rapid pain relief. Long-term control of pain has been maintained with an implanted spinal infusion device. At 18 months after pump implantation, the patient continued to have satisfactory pain relief and had returned to work.

Conclusion.—The dramatic pain relief obtained with subarachnoid opioids in a patient with chronic deafferentation pain suggests involvement of a segmental, opioid-sensitive dorsal horn mechanism.

The Resolution of Neuropathic Hyperalgesia Following Motor and Sensory Functional Recovery in Sciatic Axonotmetic Mononeuropathies

Kingery WS, Lu JD, Roffers JA, Kell DR (Veteran's Affairs Med Ctr, Palo Alto, Calif; Stanford Med School, Calif)

Pain 58:157–168, 1994 131-95-1–46

Background.—The surgical treatment of chronic nerve injury-induced pain remains controversial. Some authors have had good results with direct reanastomosis of the damaged nerve or bridging the resected nerve ends with a nerve graft, but others have been unable to duplicate these results. The temporal relationship between recovery of function and nociceptive threshold changes in 2 axonotmetic mononeuropathy rat models was examined.

Methods.—Crush injury (CI) of the sciatic nerve was induced with forceps. Chronic constrictive injury (CCI) was induced by loose ligature ligation. A sciatic CI and a sciatic CI with a 3-cm distal section were compared with a contralateral sham operation and a contralateral sciatic nerve transection. A sciatic CCI was compared with a contralateral sham operation.

Results.—Both CC and CCI injuries caused transient loss of function. Crush injury caused motor loss and sensory loss, whereas CCI caused motor loss and a saphenous-mediated adjacent neuropathic hyperalgesia (ANH). After CI, extensive recovery of motor function occurred over days 23–38, and the functional recovery was associated with the resolution of hyperalgesia. By contrast, motor function did not recover, and hyperalgesia did not resolve when nerve regeneration after a CI was prevented by nerve transection. After CCI, motor function recovery occurred primarily between days 23–59, and the functional recovery was associated with the resolution of hyperalgesia and saphenous-mediated ANH.

Conclusion.—Successful nerve regeneration after CI or CCI can initiate the resolution of neuropathic hyperalgesia. It is postulated that the resolution of hyperalgesia in rats after a CI or CCI correlates with the reversal of nerve injury-induced neuropathic pain in humans.

▶ Medical treatment of neuropathic pain has typically relied on antidepressants and anticonvulsants (1). Poor response of neuropathic pain to opioids has been reported in a number of studies (2). As in the study by Iacono and associates (Abstract 131-95-1–45), the effectiveness of opioids for relief of neuropathic pain was also reported by Desmeules and colleagues, who demonstrated good antinociceptive effects in neuropathic rats who received an IV injection of selective opioids (3). Recently, there have been a number of trials of additional medications for use in neuropathic pain, including cannabinoid (a nonpsychotropic derivative of tetrahydrocannabinol) (4), capsaicin (5), dextrorphan (6), ketamine (7), lidocaine (8), and salmon calcitonin (9). The effectiveness of neurosurgical treatments for neuropathic or nerve injury pain have also been reviewed, with mixed results (10, 11).—D.A. Marcus, M.D.

References

1. Ollat H: Pharmacological treatment of neuropathic pain. *Rev Neurol* 148:521–531, 1992.
2. Kenner DJ: Pain forum: Part 2. Neuropathic pain. *Aust Fam Physician* 23:1279–1283, 1994.
3. Desmeules JA, Kayser V, Guilbaud G: Selective opioid receptor agonists modulate mechanical allodynia in an animal model of neuropathic pain. *Pain* 53:277–285, 1993.
4. Zeltser R, Seltzer R, Eisen A, et al: Suppression of neuropathic pain behavior in rats by a non-psychotropic synthetic cannabinoid with NMDA receptor-blocking properties. *Pain* 47:95–103, 1991.
5. Meller ST, Gebhart GF, Maves TJ: Neonatal capsaicin treatment prevents the development of the thermal hyperalgesia produced in a model of neuropathic pain in the rat. *Pain* 51:317–321, 1992.
6. Tal M, Bennett GJ: Dextrorphan relieves neuropathic heat-evoked hyperalgesia in the rat. *Neurosci Lett* 151:107–110, 1993.
7. Backonja M, Arndt G, Gombat KA, et al: Response of chronic neuropathic pain syndromes to ketamine: A preliminary study. *Pain* 56:51–57, 1994.
8. Devulder JE, Ghys L, Dhondt W, et al: Neuropathic pain in a cancer patient responding to subcutaneously administered lignocaine. *Clin J Pain* 9:220–223, 1993.
9. Kovcin V, Jelic S, Babovic N, et al: A pilot study to assess the efficacy of salmon calcitonin in the relief of neuropathic pain caused by extraskeletal metastases. *Support Care Cancer* 2:71–73, 1994.
10. Burchiel KJ, Johans TJ, Ochoa J: Painful nerve injuries: Bridging the gap between basic neuroscience and neurosurgical treatment. *Acta Neurochir Suppl (Wien)* 58:131–135, 1993.

11. Gybels J, Kupers R, Nuttin B: What can the neurosurgeon offer in peripheral neuropathic pain? *Acta Neurochir Suppl* (*Wien*) 58:136–140, 1993.

Long Term Follow Up of Dorsal Root Entry Zone Lesions in Brachial Plexus Avulsion

Thomas DGT, Kitchen ND (Natl Hosp for Neurology and Neurosurgery, London)

J Neurol Neurosurg Psychiatry 57:737–738, 1994 131-95-1–47

Objective.—Dorsal root entry zone (DREZ) lesioning is indicated for pain relief in a number of injuries. Long-term results were evaluated in 44 patients who underwent the DREZ procedure for relief of pain resulting from brachial plexus avulsion injury.

Methods.—The 44 patients, aged 19–66 years, had unilateral deafferentation pain. Drug therapy, stellate ganglion blockade, surgery, and transcutaneous stimulation had not been effective in relieving pain.

Results.—After an average of 63 months of follow-up, 30 patients had good pain relief, 5 had fair pain relief, and 9 had poor pain relief. Ten patients had postoperative motor deficits.

Conclusion.—In 64% of patients who had the DREZ procedure, pain relief was good or fair. Only 1 patient had a reduction in pain relief one year after the procedure.

Cervical Dorsal Column Stimulation Relieves Pain of Brachial Plexus Avulsion

Bennett MI, Tai YMA (St James Univ Hosp, Leeds, England; Guest Hosp, Dudley, England)

J R Soc Med 87:5–6, 1994 131-95-1–48

Introduction.—Avulsion injury of the brachial plexus can lead to marked burning pain in the hand and arm that is sometimes associated with trophic changes. The causalgia-like pain, which is a result of deafferentation, is hard to treat effectively.

Patients.—Five patients who had incurred avulsion injuries of the brachial plexus 5–16 years earlier and who had continued to have debilitating limb pain underwent insertion of a cervical epidural dorsal column stimulation device. The patients had failed to respond to repeated stellate ganglion blocks, cervical epidural injections, and attempts at rehabilitation.

Technique.—Cervical epidural electrodes are inserted percutaneously under fluoroscopic control, usually in the D6–7 interspace, and are advanced cephalad to overlie the cervical spine at the C5–7 levels. The final electrode position is determined by the patient's verbal responses to stimulation using an external pulse generator. After a brief trial period, an internal pulse generator is placed in the iliac fossa using general anesthesia.

Results.—All 5 patients had substantial relief of pain. The mean reduction in pain at 13.5 months, as determined using a visual analogue scale, was significant. Most patients were able to reduce their oral analgesic intake, and their mood scores also improved.

Discussion.—Persistent relief of long-lasting pain secondary to avulsion injury of the brachial plexus may be possible with cervical dorsal column stimulation. In contrast to coagulation of the dorsal root entry zone, the stimulation procedure has been free of complications.

▶ Dreval also noted good long-term results for brachial plexus avulsion in 87% of a series of 127 patients who were undergoing ultrasonic dorsal root entry zone operations (1). Nerve transposition has also been investigated in the treatment of brachial plexus injuries. Battiston and colleagues reported good axonal regeneration and muscle reinnervation in rats with brachial plexus lesions that underwent nerve transfer from experimentally lesioned radial nerve to axillary nerve (2). Good functional restoration has also been demonstrated in humans after nerve transposition that follows brachial plexus avulsion (3).—D.A. Marcus, M.D.

References

1. Dreval ON: Ultrasonic DREZ-operations for treatment of pain due to brachial plexus avulsion. *Acta Neurochir (Wien)* 122:76–81, 1993.
2. Battiston B, Guizzi P, Vigasio A, et al: Experimental investigation of cross-nerve transfers relating to repair of brachial plexus avulsion injuries. *Microsurgery* 11:91–94, 1990.
3. Friedman AH, Nunley JA II, Goldner RD, et al: Nerve transposition for the restoration of elbow flexion following brachial plexus avulsion injuries. *J Neurosurg* 72:59–64, 1990.

2 Pediatrics

Introduction

The assessment and treatment of pain in infants, children, and adolescents continue to be subjects of concern to clinicians and investigators. This concern is reflected by the number of articles that have appeared in a variety of journals and other publications during the past year. Those of us who work with children know that they are vulnerable to undertreatment of pain and other subjective symptoms.

This vulnerability in children is a model for the problems of inadequate management of pain in all patients. Children are physically and psychologically dependent on others. They depend on adults to understand their needs and advocate for appropriate intervention. The communication styles of children differ from those of adults, and their attempts at communication may not be heard or understood. However, the same is true for other vulnerable groups, such as individuals who are cognitively impaired or severely emotionally disturbed and those whose culture or language significantly differs from that of the health care professional.

The selections in this chapter represent a sampling from the literature. Most articles pertain to acute postoperative pain and procedural pain. Several articles, however, address areas that previously have not been a primary focus. These areas include neonatal pain; pain associated with chronic illnesses, such as sickle cell disease; chronic pain unrelated to disease; and pain in individuals with developmental disabilities.

Most instances of pain in children (and adults) could be assessed and treated effectively using currently available and relatively well understood interventions. Clinical practice lags far beyond knowledge, however, and one of the most pressing needs in the management of pediatric pain is the development of interventions to narrow this gap. A few articles in this chapter address clinical practice. Hopefully, the future will bring more reports of successful (and unsuccessful) interventions, so that the knowledge gained can be used by a wide variety of concerned and dedicated clinicians.

Barbara S. Shapiro, M.D.

Assessment

Incidence of Significantly Altered Pain Experience Among Individuals With Developmental Disabilities

Biersdorff KK (Vocational and Rehabilitation Research Inst, Calgary, Alberta, Canada)

Am J Ment Retard 98:619–631, 1994 131-95-2–1

Background.—Individuals who are developmentally disabled do not always show basic pain behaviors when they need medical care, suggesting that their experience of pain may be absent or significantly altered. Pain insensitivity or indifference is rare in the general population; if it is relatively frequent among those who are developmentally disabled, it would significantly affect their health care. The prevalence of a significantly altered pain threshold among individuals who are developmentally disabled and its effect on their health and quality of life were assessed using third-party reports.

Methods.—One hundred twenty-four developmentally disabled clients of a large rehabilitation agency were included. At least 2 respondents—family members and rehabilitation staff members—were sought for each client. These respondents were asked to describe a time when the client was ill or injured in a way expected to be painful and to describe his or her behavior at that time. Supplementary information was gathered from agency files.

Results.—Fifty-two percent of clients were found to have typical pain responsiveness, 11% were found to be hyperresponsive, and 37% were found to be hyporesponsive. In the latter group, 25% had a consistently and significantly elevated pain threshold. Seven percent were categorized as stoic, and 4% as having slow reaction times. Individuals with moderate-to-severe mental disability were significantly more likely to have a significantly elevated pain threshold. Medications and communication ability had no effect on pain sensitivity. The characteristics and effect of pain insensitivity and indifference varied, but the potential consequences included prolonged contact with hazards; delayed reporting of illness; avoidable death, depending on the physician's response to the patient; self-injurious behavior; impaired response to temperature extremes; paradoxic use of pain behaviors; and nonspecific pain responses. Several respondents mentioned that the search for an emotional cause of hyperactivity often led to the discovery of a painful physical problem.

Conclusions.—A significant proportion of individuals who are developmentally disabled may be insensitive or indifferent to pain. Because they do not recognize and respond to conditions that would be painful in others, these individuals risk avoidable death and increased physical disability. Rehabilitation professionals should educate other health care professionals in this problem and provide compensatory training for individuals at risk.

▶ The assessment and treatment of pain in children with developmental disabilities have received little attention in the pain or pediatric literature. This neglected group is potentially at high risk for the undertreatment of pain and other subjective experiences. Barriers to adequate treatment include physiologic and neurologic differences that affect the ability to communicate, our lack of understanding of these potential differences, and a lack of advocacy. It is often easier to interpret pain behaviors in a neonate than in a young adult with severe mental retardation.

Patients with developmental disabilities may have a variety of altered responses to pain, including pain insensitivity, pain indifference, delayed responses to pain, and an ability to feel but not respond to pain. They may also have responses that are not easily understood by others as being secondary to pain. This article focuses on pain indifference and insensitivity, and it adds to our understanding of the potential difficulties encountered in assessment.—B.S. Shapiro, M.D.

Acute Pain

Postoperative Analgesics for Children and Adolescents: Prescription and Administration

Tesler MD, Wilkie DJ, Holzemer WL, Savedra MC (Univ of California, San Francisco; Univ of Washington, Seattle)

J Pain Symptom Manage 9:85–95, 1994 131-95-2-2

Background.—The undertreatment of children who experience postoperative pain has been well established for more than 25 years and remains a major ethical concern. The prescription and administration patterns of analgesics received by children and adolescents after complex surgeries were evaluated to determine the appropriateness of the dose based on body weight, the effect of the drug at the time pain was assessed, and the association between dose of equianalgesics and intensity of pain.

Patients and Methods.—One hundred thirty-one patients, aged 8–17 years, were included. Pain was measured with the Adolescent Pediatric Pain Tool (APPT), and analgesic treatment was assessed over 5 postoperative days. Analgesic data were converted to 10 mg of IM morphine-equivalent doses (IMMSEQ). Treatment was defined as either appropriate or inappropriate based on body weight.

Results.—Children reported moderate-to-severe levels of pain in many body locations. Analgesics were initially prescribed for all but 2 patients and were ultimately given to all but 1 patient. Intravenous morphine was the most frequently administered analgesic on days 1 and 2, followed by acetaminophen with codeine on days 3 and 4, and acetaminophen with or without codeine on day 5. Both the prescribed and administered doses were frequently less than the recommended doses based on body weight. Most children were beyond analgesic action at each APPT pain assessment. The IMMSEQ doses and pain intensity scores demonstrated weak to moderately strong associations on each of the 5 postoperative days.

Conclusions.—Although some progress has been made within the past 25 years, children with postoperative pain continue to be undertreated. Unrelieved pain is associated with both physiologic and psychological consequences and may adversely affect a child's immediate and future response to medical treatment.

▶ Although we have progressed, the undertreatment of pain in children continues, even in large institutions known for excellent pediatric care. On a positive note, all but 2 children had orders for analgesics, morphine was the most frequently prescribed parenteral analgesic, and IM analgesics were prescribed in only 12% of children. Unless there are extenuating circumstances, however, 12% of children should not have to receive IM injections. Without a closer scrutiny of the data, the significance of dose prescriptions outside the usual recommended range is difficult to ascertain. Doses must be titrated to effect. Finally, after major surgery, analgesics should be prescribed around the clock, rather than as needed (unless clinical circumstances are unusual). This is a cardinal principle for adequate pain management. Although data on prescribed schedule were not reported, most children were beyond the temporal duration of analgesia at the time of evaluation.

If education and improvement of quality were responsible for the changes seen, then more of both are needed.—B.S. Shapiro, M.D.

▶ This study indicates that significant progress has been made in acknowledging and controlling children's pain after surgery. Although the authors state that their findings "reaffirm the undertreatment of children's pain that has apparently changed only slightly in 25 years," their data suggest substantial improvement. The earliest study cited in their paper was published in 1977 and showed that postoperative analgesics were prescribed in only 4% of children (1). In contrast, the current study showed that analgesics were prescribed in all but 2 of 131 children. Additionally, appropriate drugs and routes of administration were generally prescribed. Seventy-seven percent of children had prescribed doses that fell within the recommended range, 16% of doses were below the recommended range, and 4% were above the range. Considering that these data were likely collected before the release of the Agency for Health Care Policy and Research Guidelines for the Management of Pain in Children (2), the study indicates that remarkable progress has been made in pain management. Despite this progress, there still are areas of improvement needed in the management of children's pain.—A.K. Jacox, R.N., Ph.D.

References

1. Eland JM, Anderson JE: The experience of pain in children, in Jacox AK (ed): *Pain: A Sourcebook for Nurses and Other Health Professionals.* Boston, Little Brown & Co, 1977, pp 453–473.
2. US Department of Health and Human Services: *Quick Reference Guide for*

Clinicians. *Acute Pain Management in Infants, Children, and Adolescents: Operative and Medical Procedures.* Rockville, Md, Agency for Health Care Policy and Research (AHCPR). Public Health Service 92-0020, 1992.

Preoperative and Postoperative Pain Control

Howard R (Hosp for Sick Children, London)

Arch Dis Child 69:699–703, 1993 131-95-2-3

Introduction.—Responses to analgesics vary with age, and side effects are unpredictable. The treatment of acute pain in children is, therefore, a challenge. In addition, pain in preverbal children may be difficult to evaluate.

General Principles.—Rather than using a linear visual analogue scale to quantify postoperative pain, as in adults, some type of observer assessment most often is used to gauge pain in children. Several observer-rated behavioral scales are available. The age, physical state, and capabilities of the patient all are important when planning analgesic management. The presence of pain and anxiety before surgery and the site and extent of surgery must be considered. The concept of balanced analgesia involves the use of several agents together in moderate dosage to achieve maximal analgesia with minimal side effects.

Treatment.—Paracetamol and nonsteroidal anti-inflammatory drugs may be used to control pain after minor surgery. They may also be used with a local anesthetic nerve block. In major surgery, these drugs may complement opioid analgesics. Local analgesic methods range from a simple peripheral nerve block to a more complex central block, such as continuous epidural analgesic. If a local block is not feasible, infiltrating the surgical incision with a local anesthetic may lower the subsequent need for analgesics. Epidural analgesic may be used over several days to produce profound analgesia with few systemic side effects. Hypotension is rare in children, and postoperative respiratory function is well preserved. Respiratory function must be closely monitored in children given opioid analgesics after surgery. Patient-controlled analgesia is being used increasingly in older children. In younger children, the same apparatus may be used to deliver a continuous opiate infusion in the form of nurse-controlled analgesia.

▶ This is a nice review for pediatricians and pediatric nurses. Unfortunately, the degree to which children hate and fear IM injections is not emphasized, nor is the importance of around-the-clock, rather than as-needed, administration of analgesics while the pain is severe.—B.S. Shapiro, M.D.

Lidocaine as a Diluent for Ceftriaxone in the Treatment of Gonorrhea: Does It Reduce the Pain of the Infection?

Schichor A, Bernstein B, Weinerman H, Fitzgerald J, Yordan E, Schechter N (Saint Francis Hosp, Hartford, Conn; Univ of Connecticut Health Ctr, Farmington)

Arch Pediatr Adolesc Med 148:72–75, 1994 131-95-2-4

Introduction.—Intramuscular injection of ceftriaxone sodium is the recommended treatment for uncomplicated gonococcal infection. Adolescents are the second most frequent age group to acquire this sexually transmitted disease, and the pain of the injection may deter some of these patients from actively seeking therapy. Sterile water, 5% dextrose, normal saline, and 1% lidocaine are all recommended as diluents for ceftriaxone; none is recommended over the others. The pain associated with ceftriaxone sodium injection was assessed prospectively using 2 different diluents—lidocaine hydrochloride and sterile water.

Methods.—Twenty-seven female and 12 male adolescents and young adults (mean age, 18 years) who were culture positive for gonorrhea were included. All were treated at an urban, hospital-based adolescent medical service. Most were black or hispanic. The patients were randomized to receive ceftriaxone sodium, 250 mg, diluted with either sterile water or 1% lidocaine without epinephrine. Using a visual analogue scale, the patients predicted their pain response before treatment and rated it 5 times after the injection.

Results.—The 2 groups were no different in their preinjection predictions of pain. However, the lidocaine group reported significantly less pain at the 10-minute, 20-minute, and 6-hour intervals after the injection. The diluent effect on pain was significant on repeated-measures analysis of variance models. The patients who received an injection diluted with sterile water described it as the "worst ever," whereas those who received lidocaine were more likely to report "no pain at all." Only adolescents receiving sterile water experienced such sequelae as muscle spasms or antalgic gait.

Conclusions.—Compared with sterile water, lidocaine can significantly reduce the amount of pain experienced with IM injection of ceftriaxone. Lidocaine, which poses no threat of toxicity at the dosage used and has no effect on the bioavailability of ceftriaxone, should be considered as the diluent of choice. It may also be useful for IM injection of other medications, each of which will have to be studied separately.

▶ This is a nice, simple, and clinically relevant study. The results should be distributed to every emergency department and clinic that treats adolescents. Adolescents who are seeking treatment for sexually transmitted diseases have enough problems without having the pain of the treatment added to their suffering.—B.S. Shapiro, M.D.

Mothers' Management of Adenoid-Tonsillectomy Pain in 4- to 8-Year-Olds: A Preliminary Study

Gedaly-Duff V, Ziebarth D (Oregon Health Sciences Univ, Portland; California State Univ, San Bernardino)

Pain 57:293–299, 1994 131-95-2-5

Objective.—No studies have addressed how families manage a child's postoperative pain at home. Mothers were asked how they reacted to and influenced their children's pain after adenoid-tonsillectomy.

Methods.—Seven mothers of children aged 4.5–8 years were interviewed 2–3 times about plans and expectations of home care and managing tonsillectomy pain after day surgery.

Results.—Mothers described the duration and intensity of pain as being worst in the first 12–36 hours, decreased on days 3–5, and virtually absent by days 5–7. The pattern of pain was more intense in the morning and during meals and decreased after analgesics were given. Mothers associated not drinking, facial grimace, crying, tiredness, and decreasing movement with pain. Mothers worried about drug addiction and treated pain by "trial and error."

Conclusion.—The pain management techniques used by mothers are similar to those used by health professionals. These techniques can be useful in families with children who experience pain fromchronic or life-threatening health problems.

▶ It is nice to read a qualitative study. More such studies are needed to develop hypotheses and clinical interventions.

The mothers seemed to have received no education about pain management before being sent home with their children. A little education in these situations would go a long way. Simple written material could save parents from using trial and error to assess pain and medication needs and could assuage fears of addiction. Hopefully, this study will inspire the development of simple educational efforts. The authors also point out that further qualitative studies should involve the entire family unit.—B.S. Shapiro, M.D.

Comparison of the Ventilatory Effects of Morphine and Buprenorphine in Children

Hamunen K, Olkkola KT, Maunuksela E-L (Univ of Helsinki)

Acta Anaesthesiol Scand 37:449–453, 1993 131-95-2-6

Introduction.—The use of opioid analgesics in pediatric patients is partly limited by fear of ventilatory depression. Buprenorphine provides comparable postoperative analgesia as morphine, although somewhat longer lasting, in children. The ventilatory effects of equianalgesic doses of intravenously administered buprenorphine and morphine on postoperative pain in children were compared.

Study Design.—Twenty children, aged 5–8 years, who were undergoing elective ophthalmic surgery were studied prospectively. Thirty minutes after discontinuation of anesthetic gases, the patients received a single equianalgesic IV dose of morphine hydrochloride, 100 μg/kg, or buprenorphine, 3 μg/kg, for postoperative analgesia.

Outcome.—Buprenorphine resulted in a greater decrease in ventilatory rate, a greater and longer-lasting increase in end-tidal carbon dioxide concentration, and a greater acute decrease in oxygen saturation. The mean oxygen saturation recovered longer after buprenorphine, but no child had apnea or hypoventilation requiring assistance. For both drugs, the time, magnitude, and duration of ventilatory changes varied appreciably among the children, although buprenorphine had a slower onset and longer duration of maximal ventilatory effect.

Conclusions.—Acute administration of buprenorphine depresses ventilation to a greater degree than morphine. With buprenorphine, maximal ventilatory effect occurs later and ventilatory depression may develop late. Its use should not be discouraged, however, because its long duration of action and possibility for sublingual administration offer considerable advantages in pediatric practice. For safety, all children given intravenously administered opioids should be observed until they are fully responsive and ventilatory control has stabilized.

▶ Morphine remains the drug of first choice. Respect, not fear, is indicated in its use for postoperative pain.—B.S. Shapiro, M.D.

Epidural Versus Patient-Controlled Analgesia With Morphine for Postoperative Pain After Orthopaedic Procedures in Children

Goodarzi M, Shier N-h, Ogden JA (Shriners Hosp for Crippled Children, Tampa, Fla; Univ of South Florida, Tampa)

J Pediatr Orthop 13:663–667, 1993 131-95-2-7

Objective.—Pain after orthopedic surgery is one of the most severe types of postoperative pain. The effect of intermittent epidural morphine (EM) was compared with that of patient-controlled analgesia using intravenously administered morphine. The dosage of drug needed for equal relief of pain and the incidence and severity of side effects in pediatric patients after orthopedic surgery were determined.

Study Design.—Forty pediatric patients received either EM or morphine by the patient-controlled analgesia machine (PCAM). Age, weight, height, anesthesia, and duration of operation were similar in the 2 groups. In the special care unit, trained observers evaluated the patient's level of pain for the first 30 hours after surgery using the Visual Pain Scale and a pain relief questionnaire. The drug dose was titrated until the Visual Pain Scale was less than 2.

Outcome.—The quality of pain relief did not differ significantly between the EM and PCAM groups. However, the postoperative morphine requirement for good analgesia was much less in the EM group (1.7 vs. 77.8 mg for the 30-hour postoperative period). Good to excellent pain control was achieved in 80% to 85% of patients in the EM group and in 70% to 80% of those in the PCAM group. The EM group had a higher incidence of nausea and vomiting and pruritus, whereas the PCAM group spent significantly more time asleep or drowsy. Urinary retention was common in both groups. None of the patients had severe respiratory insufficiency or an episode of apnea.

Conclusions.—Morphine provides effective analgesia of comparable quality when infused either epidurally or by PCAM. Epidural morphine requires lower morphine dosage than PCAM but has a higher incidence of nonrespiratory side effects.

▶ The epidural vs. PCA debate has been going on for a while. So far, the definitive study has not emerged, and clinicians continue to practice according to their own interpretations of the data. The criticism of this study is likely to be that an alternative epidural regimen might have been more effective and might have had fewer side effects.

This study shows a significant difference in side effects between the 2 groups, with patients who received epidural analgesia experiencing more pruritus, nausea, and vomiting. Although the authors say that urinary retention was common in both groups, 10% of patients receiving PCA had urinary retention, compared with 55% of those receiving epidural analgesia. This is a very significant difference.

The higher incidence of sedation in patients who receive PCA may not be clinically significant, as long as ventilation, recovery, and ambulation are not impeded. Likewise, the lower dose of morphine required by patients who receive epidural analgesia does not seem clinically significant, looking at the profile of side effects.

This is an important area of study. Competent pain management for children is crucial. At the same time, we must be aware of costs and of the problems attached to high-tech approaches. Patient outcome is the decisive factor.—B.S. Shapiro, M.D.

Complications of Continuous Epidural Infusions for Postoperative Analgesia in Children

Wood CE, Goresky GV, Klassen KA, Kuwahara B, Neil SG (Univ of Calgary, Alta, Canada)

Can J Anaesth 41:613–620, 1994 131-95-2–8

Background.—Treatment of postoperative pain in children has been based on the use of parenteral opioids. This approach provides improved tolerance of pain but does not eliminate it. Because of the limitations, complications, and side effects of parenteral opioids, epidural analgesia is an attractive alternative for the management of postoperative pain. The incidence of side effects and complications of epidural analgesia is not known. The management, side effects, and complications of epidural analgesia in infants and children were reviewed retrospectively.

Methods.—The management, side effects, and complications of each epidural infusion administered to 190 children (mean age, 5.6 years) during a 2-year period were recorded. Epidural infusions of bupivacaine .125% or bupivacaine .1% with epinephrine were given.

Results.—The mean duration of epidural infusions was 4.7 days. There were 203 complications recorded in 127 patients. Complications included nausea and vomiting in 23% of patients, motor blockage in 15.8%, oversedation in 6.3%, and pruritus in 5.3%. In 4 patients, there were complications possibly related to toxic effects of bupivacaine or resistance to it; serum levels of bupivacaine were 3.86, 5.5, 2.1, and 2.34 $\mu g/mL^{-1}$. In 41 patients, the infusion was discontinued early; the most common reason was technical problems with the epidural catheter. There were 3 potentially serious complications, but none had lasting consequences.

Conclusions.—Although the high incidence of complications associated with this analgesic modality necessitates close follow-up of patients and regular monitoring, most complications were minor and easily remedied. With increased experience, technical problems with epidural infusions may diminish, and consistency and reliability should improve.

▶ This is a retrospective study, whereas the previous study (Abstract 131-95-2–7) was prospective and randomized. Thus, data about side effects are subject to the vagaries of reporting in the charts. This method is particularly problematic for subjective side effects, such as pruritus and nausea.

I have a problem with calling the side effects minor and easily remedied. Children who experience severe pruritus or nausea would not call these symptoms minor, nor would their families. A urinary catheter is not a minor event to a child (or to an adult). The accidental or unplanned discontinuation of epidural analgesia may also become a major problem for the patient, particularly if it occurs in the middle of the night, when the timely provision of adequate alternative analgesia may be problematic.—B.S. Shapiro, M.D.

An Audit of Extradural Infusion Analgesia in Children Using Bupivacaine and Diamorphine

Wilson PTJ, Lloyd-Thomas AR (Hosp for Sick Children, London)

Anaesthesia 48:718–723, 1993 131-95-2–9

Objective.—The use of extradural analgesia by continuous infusion in children at the Hospitals for Sick Children, London, was investigated prospectively.

Methods.—During a 15-month period, 150 extradural infusions of diamorphine and bupivacaine were used for relief of pain after major surgery in children. The median age of the patients was 25 months, and 69% were younger than 5 years of age. Lumbar extradural block was performed on 125 patients, and a thoracic block was performed in 25. Bupivacaine .125% and diamorphine at 3, 5, and 10 mg were used. The median duration of infusion was 47 hours (range, 4–96 hours). Only 47 children received supplementary intraoperative opioid.

Outcome.—Analgesia was assessed or self-rated as "very good" by 77% of patients. The most common reasons for a "fair" or "poor" assessment were technical complications and unpleasant side effects. Technical complications resulted in premature cessation of extradural therapy in 16.7% of infusions and included leakage in 11, occlusions in 19, and catheter connector disconnections in 5. Eight patients had unsatisfactory sedation. Urinary retention developed in 11% of patients, particularly among those aged 5–10 years. Pruritus occurred in 10%, more frequently in older children. Only 1 patient, a premature infant born at 39 weeks' gestation, experienced respiratory depression that required intervention.

Summary.—Extradural analgesia by continuous infusion of a mixture of opioid and local anesthetic provides successful analgesia after surgery in children. The complexity of the technique, however, demands significant medical and nursing time, particularly to overcome technical problems. In addition, side effects may complicate the postoperative course. These findings suggest the need for comparative studies of extradural and IV infusions of opioid analgesia. The use of the former can only be justified, given its greater technical complexity and morbidity, if the quality of analgesia is markedly superior to that achieved with IV infusions.

▶ I absolutely agree with the authors' conclusions. The original article is worth reading, particularly the discussion.—B.S. Shapiro, M.D.

Comparison of Different Bolus Doses of Morphine for Patient-Controlled Analgesia in Children

Doyle E, Mottart KJ, Marshall C, Morton NS (Royal Hosp for Sick Children, Glasgow, Scotland)

Br J Anaesth 72:160–163, 1994 131-95-2-10

Objective.—In pain-controlled analgesia (PCA) treatment of acute pain in children, bolus doses of morphine usually range from 10 to 50 µg/kg. No studies have been done to compare the effectiveness of different doses. The effectiveness of bolus doses of 10 vs. 20 µg of morphine per kg was compared.

Methods.—Forty children, aged 6–14 years, who were undergoing appendicectomy were included. They were randomly selected to receive a bolus dose of either 10 (group B10) or 20 (group B20) μg of morphine per kg with a lockout interval of 5 minutes and a background infusion of 4 μg/kg/hr. Oxygen saturation, ventilatory frequency, sedation score, pain score, and nausea score were measured. The number of demands and volume of solution were recorded every hour.

Results.—Group B20 administered significantly more morphine than did group B10 and had significantly less pain during movement. There was no significant difference in resting pain scores between groups. Group B10 had significantly more oxygen saturation scores below 94% than did group B20. There were no significant differences between groups in the incidence of vomiting, time sleeping, or oversedation.

Conclusion.—These results were similar to those found in adults. Patients do not use PCA to reach a satisfactory level of analgesia. Pain scores at rest are not useful for assessing pain scores or for determining the amount of analgesia necessary for relief of pain.

▶ Pain-controlled analgesia is not a panacea, and it must not be frustrating for the patient if it is to work well. The authors' method of assessing movement-related pain as well as pain at rest seems clinically and conceptually sound.—B.S. Shapiro, M.D.

Prevention of Postoperative Nausea and Vomiting With Transdermal Hyoscine in Children Using Patient-Controlled Analgesia

Doyle E, Byers G, McNicol LR, Morton NS (Royal Hosp for Sick Children, Glasgow, Scotland)

Br J Anaesth 72:72–76, 1994 131-95-2–11

Objective.—Postoperative nausea and vomiting (PONV), although common, seems to be less of a problem in children who use pain-controlled analgesia (PCA). Hyoscine has been shown to be an effective antiemetic. The effectiveness of transdermal hyoscine in preventing PONV after surgery in children using PCA morphine was evaluated.

Methods.—Before abdominal surgery, 40 children, aged 6–14 years, received either a hyoscine patch (group H) or a placebo patch (group P). After surgery, patients received PCA morphine, 20 μg/mL/kg, with a 5-minute lockout period. Oxygen saturation, ventilatory frequency, and sedation, nausea, and pain scores were recorded.

Results.—Group H had significantly less PONV and had a significant antiemetic effect during the first 48 hours compared with group P. There was no significant difference between groups with regard to pain scores. Group H had a significantly higher sedation score and incidence of dry mouth than did group P.

Conclusion.—During the first 48 hours, transdermal hyoscine is effective as a postoperative antiemetic in children who are undergoing abdominal surgery and receiving PCA morphine.

▶ This could be a useful intervention. It would help to know the severity of dry mouth in weighing alternative antiemetic regimens, as this is a common and sometimes very bothersome symptom.—B.S. Shapiro, M.D.

Postoperative Analgesia in Children Using Continuous S.C. Morphine

McNicol R (Royal Hosp for Sick Children, Glasgow, Scotland)

Br J Anaesth 71:752–756, 1993 131-95-2-12

Objective.—Morphine, given by continuous subcutaneous infusion, has proved effective in relieving postoperative pain in adults. This approach was evaluated in 60 children (mean age, 6½ years) who underwent major abdominal, urologic, or orthopedic surgery with the use of balanced general anesthesia.

Methods.—Analgesia was established intraoperatively after induction of anesthesia, using extradural or peripheral bupivacaine to produce a regional nerve block. After surgery, morphine was infused subcutaneously at a rate of 20 μg/kg/hr for a mean of 38.8 hours. Pain, sedation, and nausea and vomiting were monitored along with oxygen saturation.

Results.—Only 6% of pain scores indicated more than mild pain. Eleven patients had severe pain at some time after surgery. None of the children were unrousable at any time. All but 3% of oxygen saturation values exceeded 94%. Thirteen patients had varying degrees of nausea or vomiting. There were no cannula-related complications.

Discussion.—Nurses have been enthusiastic regarding the use of subcutaneous infusion of morphine to control postoperative pain in children. Pulse oximetry should be used routinely if available.

▶ This method could be an alternative when the IV route is not available. Usually, children who require parenteral morphine also require parenteral fluids, so IV access is already in place. If IV access is available, no advantage of subcutaneous administration is evident.—B.S. Shapiro, M.D.

Pain Management for Children Following Selective Dorsal Rhizotomy

Geiduschek JM, Haberkern CM, McLaughlin JF, Jacobson LE, Hays RM, Roberts TS (Univ of Washington, Seattle)

Can J Anaesth 41:492–496, 1994 131-95-2-13

Objective.—Patients with cerebral palsy who undergo selective dorsal rhizotomy for lower limb spasticity present a pain management problem after surgery because of muscle spasms. Pain management in such patients was examined.

Methods.—Selective dorsal rhizotomy was performed on 55 patients, aged 3–22 years. Spastic diplegia was present in 43 patients, and spastic quadriplegia was present in 12. All patients were treated with morphine.

Fifty received initial morphine infusions of 20 μg/kg/hr; the dose was increased as required. Pain management was assessed by nurses.

Results.—Although 1 patient required a maximum infusion rate of 60 μg/kg/hr, the other 49 achieved analgesia with doses of 20–40 μg/kg/hr. Fourteen patients received bolus doses on 2 or more occasions, and 10 received bolus doses on 1 occasion. Four patients used pain-controlled analgesia. One patient required epidural morphine for analgesia, and 6 needed IV ketorolac in addition to morphine. Benzodiazepine was administered to control muscle spasms.

Conclusion.—The combination of morphine infusions and administration of benzodiazepine, with adjunctive administration of ketorolac, was effective in controlling postoperative pain and muscle spasms in patients undergoing selective dorsal rhizotomy.

▶ The authors describe a promising approach to a very difficult postoperative pain problem.—B.S. Shapiro, M.D.

A Comparison of Wound Instillation and Caudal Block for Analgesia Following Pediatric Inguinal Herniorrhaphy

Conroy JM, Othersen HB Jr, Dorman BH, Gottesman JD, Wallace CT, Brahen NH (Med Univ of South Carolina, Charleston)
J Pediatr Surg 28:565–567, 1993 131-95-2–14

Objective.—Regional anesthesia provides effective relief of pain after pediatric inguinal hernia repair. Caudal block and wound instillation were compared regarding total operating room time, emergence time, postoperative relief of pain, and requirement for supplemental analgesics after pediatric inguinal herniorrhapy.

Study Design.—Seventy children, aged 2 months to 10 years, who were undergoing bilateral inguinal repair randomly received either caudal block with .25% bupivacaine, wound instillation with .25% bupivacaine, or no local anesthetic (control). Postoperative pain was assessed using a 10-point objective pain scale.

Outcome.—Caudal analgesia significantly decreased emergence times, minimized pain-related behaviors after surgery, and significantly reduced narcotic to maintain normal hemodynamics, compared with wound instillation or no local anesthetic. Operating room time did not differ significantly among groups. Time to discharge from day surgery was not examined, but all children met the age-related criteria for discharge of the day-surgery unit. No late complications occurred within 24 hours after discharge.

Conclusion.—Perioperative analgesic blocks result in quicker awakening, a more comfortable course after surgery, and potentially earlier discharge from same-day surgery.

▶ This is a nice study, but we need to know more about the clinical course over the first and second postoperative days.—B.S. Shapiro, M.D.

Neonatal Pain

Pain Management in Canadian Level 3 Neonatal Intensive Care Units

Fernandez CV, Rees EP (Izaak Walton Killam Children's Hosp, Halifax, NS, Canada; Dalhousie Univ, Halifax, NS, Canada)

Can Med Assoc J 150:499–504, 1994 131-95-2–15

Background.—It is now accepted that neonates experience pain that may be extreme in intensity. In addition to the humanitarian aspect of pain relief, attenuation of the stress response with adequate pain management is thought to affect outcome. To determine methods of pain management in neonates, a survey was sent to the head nurses of virtually all Canadian level 3 neonatal ICUs (NICUs).

Methods.—A questionnaire of 36 items that assessed pain management in level 3 NICUs was sent to head nurses; 87% responded. A Likert 5 point scale was used to answer questions that concerned methods of treating postoperative, procedural, and disease-related pain in neonates. To correlate the results of the survey, 109 charts of patients who had received an anesthetic in the preceding year were reviewed.

Results.—Ninety-three percent of NICUs that treated cardiac surgery patients reported using a continuous infusion of narcotics almost always. After major surgery, 88% treated with opiates, but 35% did not use narcotics after minor surgery. These findings correlated with information derived from chart review. If an opiate was found inadequate for pain relief, 75% of respondents sedated the patient; 60% would increase the infusion rate of the opiate. Although local anesthetics were often used for placement of a chest tube, they were not commonly used for such procedures as central line insertion (45%) or a lumbar puncture (79% rarely or never used anesthetics). Intubation was accomplished without sedation or anesthesia in 75% of NICUs. For disease-related pain of nonsurgical origin, use of opiates was rare. Use of opiates was stopped with a weaning program that was often prescribed.

Recommendations.—Pain management practices that are used in neonates but are considered unacceptable in older children and adults were revealed. Several guidelines are suggested: neonates should be sedated before intubation; plans for use of analgesics, including weaning and managing breakthrough pain, need development; alternatives should be studied; pain assessment tools should be developed; and physicians and nurses should be better educated about relief of pain in this patient population.

▶ Once again, we have progressed but still have a long way to go. We should be aghast that infants in many nurseries are still not receiving adequate analgesia for minor surgery, that 1 nursery does not use opioids after major surgery, that many nurseries even occasionally use sedation rather than analgesia, and that invasive procedures are performed without analgesia or sedation. I am optimistic that clinical care will continue to improve as a result of the efforts of many clinicians.—B.S. Shapiro, M.D.

Changing Attitudes and Practices Regarding Local Analgesia for Newborn Circumcision

Ryan CA, Finer NN (Royal Alexandra Hosp, Edmonton, Alta, Canada; Univ of Alberta, Edmonton, Canada)

Pediatrics 94:230–233, 1994 131-95-2–16

Background.—Physiologic and behavioral changes have conclusively demonstrated that newborn infants who are undergoing circumcision experience pain. Nevertheless, neonatal circumcisions continue to be performed without benefit of analgesia in most institutions. Routine use of local or regional anesthesia during circumcision was encouraged among physicians from various subspecialties.

Methods.—A wide range of awareness and educational programs were conducted at the newborn nurseries of the Women's Pavilion, Royal Alexandra Hospital, Edmonton, Canada. These programs included posters, newsletters, presentations at grand rounds, video recordings, and practical demonstrations of local anesthesia to the prepuce and dorsal penile nerve block. Physicians who perform newborn circumcisions were targeted. An audit of physician practice was conducted during a 1-month period 12 months after program initiation.

Results.—Only 1 physician used local analgesia for circumcision before the educational program was introduced. At 12-month follow-up, 46 circumcisions had been performed by 22 physicians, each of whom completed 1-6 procedures. Of these 22, 16 physicians used either local anesthesia to the prepuce or dorsal penile nerve block in 19 and 13 patients, respectively. Overall, local analgesia was used in 66% of all circumcisions. Six physicians did not use any form of analgesia during 16 circumcisions.

Conclusions.—This simple educational program has led to a marked change in attitudes and practice regarding local analgesia for neonatal circumcision. Repeated education and practical demonstrations may result in the use of local or regional anesthesia for all newborn circumcisions performed at the institution studied, as well as at other facilities.

▶ This is a cheering testimonial to the efficacy of a targeted and carefully designed educational program in producing change in clinical practice.—B.S. Shapiro, M.D.

Acetaminophen Analgesia in Neonatal Circumcision: The Effect on Pain

Howard CR, Howard FM, Weitzman ML (Univ of Rochester, New York)

Pediatrics 93:641–646, 1994 131-95-2–17

Background.—An estimated 86% of newborn boys in the United States undergo circumcision. Although it has been believed that pain associated with neonatal circumcision is insignificant, neurophysiologic and clinical evidence show that neonates are capable of mature pain perception, even at relatively immature gestational ages. Whether use of acetaminophen can mitigate intraoperative and postoperative pain in neonates undergoing this procedure was studied. This agent has a wide margin of safety and is metabolized and excreted efficiently by newborns.

Patients and Methods.—Forty-four healthy, full-term neonates were included in a prospective, randomized, double-blind, placebo-controlled study. Two hours before undergoing Gomco circumcision, 23 neonates received acetaminophen (15 mg/kg per dose, .15 mL/kg per dose), whereas the remaining 21 were given placebo (.15 mL/kg per dose). The doses were repeated every 6 hours over 24 hours. During the intraoperative period, patients were monitored for changes in heart and respiratory rates and crying time. A standardized postoperative comfort scoring system was used to evaluate postoperative pain at 30, 60, and 90 minutes, and at 2, 6, and 24 hours. Feeding behavior was also evaluated before and after circumcision via nursing observation.

Results.—Significant increases in heart and respiratory rate and crying time were noted for neonates in each group. No clinically significant between-group differences were observed. In addition, no significant between-group differences were noted in postoperative comfort scores until the 6-hour assessment. At that time, a significantly improved score was seen in the acetaminophen group. Feeding behavior declined in breast- and bottlefed infants in both groups. Acetaminophen did not seem to affect this deterioration.

Conclusion.—Neonates experience severe and persistent pain when circumcised. Acetaminophen does not lessen either the intraoperative or immediate postoperative pain caused by this procedure. It may provide some relief, however, immediately after the procedure. Safe and easily administered anesthetic agents need to be identified and used in neonates who are undergoing circumcision.

▶ I do not know of any (sane) adult who would consent to circumcision with acetaminophen as the only analgesic intervention. We already know that circumcision is associated with severe pain. I find it difficult to accept both the use of acetaminophen as the only intervention and the use of a control group that received no analgesic. It is reasonable to use acetaminophen for circumcision pain after the procedure, in a manner similar to that advised for immunization, *in addition to* local analgesia.—B.S. Shapiro, M.D.

Pain Sensitivity and Temperament in Extremely Low-Birth-Weight Premature Toddlers and Preterm and Full-Term Controls

Grunau RVE, Whitfield MF, Petrie JH (Univ of British Columbia, Vancouver, Canada)

Pain 58:341–346, 1994 131-95-2-18

Background.—Possible long-term consequences of neonatal pain is a new issue. High-technology medical care of extremely low-birth-weight infants involves repeated procedures that are potentially painful and may later affect a child's reaction to pain. Early pain experience is one of several factors in the ontogeny of pain expression; the development of pain behavior reflects developmental, familial, and cultural differences. Differences in sensitivity to pain between toddlers who were extremely low-birth-weight infants and toddlers who were full-birth-weight infants were investigated.

Methods.—Toddlers who were extremely low-birth-weight infants were divided into 2 groups: 49 with a birth weight of 480–800 g and 75 with a birth weight of 801–1,000 g. A control group of toddlers was also divided into 2 groups: 42 who were preterm with a birth weight of 1,500–2,499 g and 29 with a birth weight of more than 2,500 g. When the toddlers were 18 months old, the parents' ratings of their children's sensitivity to pain were examined and related to the child's temperament and the parenting style.

Results.—Parents rated the toddlers who were extremely low-birth-weight infants as significantly lower in pain sensitivity than the control toddlers. Relationships between child temperament and pain sensitivity ratings varied systematically across groups. In toddlers with a birth weight of more than 2,500 g (full birth weight), child temperament was strongly related to pain sensitivity ratings. In toddlers with a birth weight of 1,500–2,499 g (preterm) and of 801–1,000 g, child temperament was moderately related to pain sensitivity ratings. In toddlers with a birth weight of less than 801 g, child temperament was not related to pain sensitivity ratings. Ratings of pain sensitivity were not mediated by parenting style.

Conclusions.—Toddlers with a birth weight of less than 801–1,000 g were rated by their parents as significantly less sensitive to pain. Boys were rated as less sensitive than girls. Ratings were significantly associated with temperament, except for toddlers with a birth weight of less than 801 g. These results relate to parents' perceptions of their children's pain and may reveal more about the parent than the child.

► It is not surprising that children exposed to a barrage of unpredictable and recurrent painful stimuli as infants would have perturbations in their responses to various somatic sensations. The authors emphasize that their findings do not establish a causal link, as there are many disruptions of normal caretaking, environment, sensation, and attachment in the neonatal ICU. It is reasonable to speculate, however, that when most externally mediated sensations are noxious rather than soothing, some protective mechanism would be necessary. Unfortunately, abnormally low sensitivity to pain may interfere with the development of appropriate self-care behaviors.—B.S. Shapiro, M.D.

Physiological Responses of Premature Infants to a Painful Stimulus
Stevens BJ, Johnston CC (Univ of Toronto; McGill Univ, Montreal)
Nurs Res 43:226–231, 1994 131-95-2–19

Background.—There currently is much research addressing the pain responses of full-term newborn infants to painful stimuli, but there is significantly less research addressing the pain responses of premature infants. The physiologic responses of premature infants to painful stimuli were studied, and the effect of the infant's behavioral state and severity of illness on these responses was determined.

Methods.—One hundred thirty-eight premature infants, between 32 and 34 weeks' gestational age and 5 days old or younger, underwent a routine heel stick procedure. Heart rate, oxygen saturation, and intracranial pressure were recorded. The procedure included warming, stick, and squeeze.

Results.—Between the baseline and stick and the baseline and squeeze phases, there were significant increases in maximum heart rate and intracranial pressure. Between the baseline and stick and the baseline and squeeze phases, there were significant decreases in minimum oxygen saturation. The only significant difference in variability of heart rate and of oxygen saturation occurred between the baseline and warming phases. There were significant differences in the physiologic responses in the 4 infant states of quiet sleep, active sleep, quiet awake, and active awake between baseline and warming. Severity of illness did not influence physiologic responses.

Conclusions.—Preterm infants exhibited physiologic responses to a heel stick procedure. These responses support their ability to respond to a tissue-damaging stimulus, although physiologic responses are not unique to pain or nociception.

► Painful experiences in premature infants must be taken seriously on a number of counts, including immediate physiologic effects, immediate suffering, and long-term emotional effects and suffering. The increase in intracranial pressure seen in this study is consistent with previous data and is of concern with regard to deleterious physiologic effects.—B.S. Shapiro, M.D.

Factors That Influence the Behavioral Pain Responses of Premature Infants

Stevens BJ, Johnston CC, Horton L (Univ of Toronto; McGill Univ, Montreal; Royal Victoria Hosp, Montreal)

Pain 59:101–109, 1994 131-95-2–20

Background.—Although the physiologic and behavioral responses of premature infants to pain have been described, few studies have addressed factors influencing the behavioral responses. The behavioral responses of premature infants to acute pain and the influences of various factors, including behavioral state and severity of illness, were evaluated.

Methods.—One hundred twenty-four premature infants were observed before, during, and after a routine heel lance procedure. Recordings of the infants' facial activity and cries were systematically analyzed. The influence of 2 contextual variables, severity of illness and behavioral state, was examined using the Physiologic Stability Index and an observational rating system.

Results.—There were significant changes in facial activity between baseline and the stick phase of the heel lance procedure. Analysis of the infants' cries showed that fundamental frequency, harmonic structure, and peak spectral energy of the cry were also significantly increased during the stick phase. The facial activity variables were significantly influenced by the infants' behavioral state; infants in the active-awake state showed significantly more vertical mouth stretch and taut tongue than those in any other behavioral state. The acoustic cry variables were modified by severity of illness; severely ill infants showed significantly higher peak fundamental frequency, shorter cry duration, and longer latency to cry than healthy or mildly ill infants. The covariates of sex, weight, and gestational age did not significantly influence the behavioral responses.

Conclusions.—Factors such as behavioral state and severity of illness can have a significant influence on the behavioral responses of premature infants to a tissue-damaging stimulus. These findings may help improve assessment of the infant's response to potentially painful or noxious procedures. Better assessment of these responses will, in turn, lead to better pain management and reduced risk to the infant's integrity and health.

▶ This article is a contribution to the literature on pain assessment in neonates.—B.S. Shapiro, M.D.

Plasma Fentanyl Levels in Infants Undergoing Extracorporeal Membrane Oxygenation

Leuschen MP, Willett LD, Hoie EB, Bolam DL, Bussey ME, Goodrich PD,

Zach TL, Nelson RM Jr (Creighton Univ–Univ of Nebraska, Omaha)
J Thorac Cardiovasc Surg 105:885–891, 1993 131-95-2–21

Background.—Infants who are undergoing extracorporeal membrane oxygenation (ECMO) therapy may routinely receive the synthetic narcotic fentanyl. The relationships between the dose of fentanyl and both the levels of plasma and the clinical status were analyzed at specific time points during fentanyl analgesia in infants undergoing ECMO.

Patients and Methods.—Twelve infants who were undergoing ECMO received a fentanyl bolus of 5–10 μg/kg, after which infusions at 1–6.3 μg/kg/hr were given. On average, 11 plasma samples were obtained per infant, and the level of fentanyl was measured via radioimmunoassay.

Results.—Eight infants without a primary diagnosis of congenital diaphragmatic hernia survived with fairly short courses on ECMO (less than 7 days). Tolerance to fentanyl did not develop in any infants in this group, and all were maintained with an infusion rate of less than 5 μg/kg/hr throughout. The remaining 4 infants with congenital diaphragmatic hernia had longer ECMO runs; 3 did not survive. Their plasma levels of fentanyl were consistently higher; although the infusion rates were higher early on ECMO, they did not exceed 7μg/kg/hr. In fact, decreased rates were observed after 5 days on ECMO. Lorazepam was given in addition to fentanyl in 5 infants for at least 1 sampling time. Infused doses of fentanyl and levels of plasma were higher in the infants with congenital diaphragmatic hernia who did not survive and were not given lorazepam. An association between decreased clearance of fentanyl and renal dysfunction was noted.

Conclusions.—A bolus of fentanyl, followed by fairly low doses of this agent, provides satisfactory analgesia for infants receiving ECMO. This is particularly evident when fentanyl is supplemented with IV lorazepam.

▶ This article is an addition to the sparse literature on opioids in neonates. Assessment is a problem in this study, as the authors do not state how they decided when analgesia was adequate and when sedation was required.—B.S. Shapiro, M.D.

Sedation With Nasal Ketamine and Midazolam for Cryotherapy in Retinopathy of Prematurity

Louon A, Lithander J, Reddy VG, Gupta A (Sultan Quaboos Univ Hosp, Muscat, Sultanate of Oman)
Br J Ophthalmol 77:529–530, 1993 131-95-2–22

Background.—Anesthesia for short, noninvasive ophthalmic procedures remains a challenge. Nasal administration of anesthetic drugs has provided a noninvasive, pain-free method with a rapid onset of sedation.

Case Report.—Girl, 44 days, who weighed 1.3 kg, was sedated with nasal ketamine and midazolam during cryotherapy for retinopathy of prematurity. The total dose of midazolam was .9 mg, and the total dose of ketamine was 8 mg. Within 4 minutes, the infant was properly sedated. During the 12-minute procedure the pulse rate remained between 140 and 150, and oxygen saturation remained in the range of 94%, with no episode of apnea or bradycardia. The operating conditions were excellent. The postoperative period was uneventful, except for a brief episode of bradycardia that was resolved by bag ventilation.

Conclusions.—Sedation with nasal ketamine and midazolam is safe and efficient for short, noninvasive ophthalmic procedures. This technique requires skillful supervision and adequate monitoring. Larger series are warranted to define its safety and reliability further.

▶ A promising approach.—B.S. Shapiro, M.D.

Procedural Pain

Caring for Children During Procedures: A Review of the Literature

Brennan A (Mem Univ of Newfoundland, St John's, Canada)

Pediatr Nurs 20:451–458, 1994 131-95-2-23

Introduction.—The child care literature contains many suggestions, directives, and "helpful hints" that can help nurses care for children during procedures. At present, however, a long list of recommendations must be reviewed to identify effective interventions. Therefore, the recommended strategies must be examined in terms of their foci. In addition, whether these interventions have been tested in practice must be determined.

Discussion.—Many recommended strategies, including individualization of care, communication, control and allowing choices, clarification of expectations and limit setting, and parent participation, are based in theory. These strategies are directed toward nursing care and appear to be practical and reasonable. However, they have largely been untested, and their efficacy thus remains unknown. Conversely, several interventions for hospitalization and procedure preparation, including hospital tours, books, and films; stress immunization and desensitization; the teaching of coping strategies; and stress-point intervention, have been proposed on the basis of research and clinical testing. Study results have supported the incorporation of specific strategies into practice, but the role and activities of the nurse during these interventions were generally ignored. There are 2 important implications associated with these findings. First, recommended interventions must be tested, particularly across different procedures and age groups. Testing should include purposeful clinical use of interventions and formal studies. Second, the role and activities of nurses assisting children through procedures must be documented so that such interventions can be evaluated.

Conclusions.—Although inroads are being made with respect to documentation of nursing care during procedures, those strategies that can best help children through procedures currently remain undefined. Further studies of actual nursing care and the relative effectiveness of specific interventions are needed to facilitate less stressful and more effective procedures for children, parents, and nurses alike.

▶ An excellent and thoughtful review of the current state of the art.—B.S. Shapiro, M.D.

Primary and Secondary Control Among Children Undergoing Medical Procedures: Adjustment as a Function of Coping Style

Weisz JR, McCabe MA, Dennig MD (Univ of California, Los Angeles; Children's Hosp Natl Med Ctr, Washington, DC)

J Consult Clin Psychol 62:324–332, 1994 131-95-2–24

Objective.—There have been numerous studies on control-related coping strategies of adults and children who are undergoing painful medical procedures. The coping strategies of children in low-controllability situations were examined and classified as primary coping control (modifying conditions), secondary coping control (modifying one's own responses), or relinquished control (no attempt to cope).

Methods.—In 33 children, aged 5–12 years, with acute lymphocytic leukemia, coping skills were assessed in 4 areas: overnight hospital stay, bone marrow aspiration (BMA) or lumbar puncture (LP), vomiting, and loss of hair. On the basis of their own scores and those of the observer and the parents, the children were classified as belonging to the primary control, relinquished control, or secondary control groups.

Results.—Overall, there were no significant age or gender effects in coping skills. The secondary control group had lower levels of distress than the other 3 groups and significantly lower levels than the primary or relinquished groups. These findings were consistent among self-rated, parental, and observer scores. Secondary coping skills may not be the most appropriate response to the more controllable aspects of treatment for leukemia.

Conclusions.—Larger studies need to be conducted on coping style and adjustment. Ways need to be found to assess the coping skills of children without relying only on what the children themselves say. A consistent coding method for responses needs to be developed. Methods also need to be developed for evaluating coping skills in situations with multiple complex traumatic stressors.

▶ In this contribution to the literature about coping, the authors point out that one of the inherent problems in such studies is that coping is, in actuality, multifaceted. Thus, although studies of isolated aspects of coping increase our understanding, the act of coping cannot be reduced to single aspects.—B.S. Shapiro, M.D.

Blowing Away Shot Pain: A Technique for Pain Management During Immunization

French GM, Painter EC, Coury DL (Ohio State Univ, Columbus)
Pediatrics 93:384–388, 1994 131-95-2–25

Purpose.—Fear of injections is widespread among children. Although several different interventions to reduce pain and anxiety associated with immunizations have been described, many children do not receive any such intervention. The effectiveness of a quick, simple active distraction technique to reduce pain and distress was evaluated in young children who were receiving routine injections.

Methods.—One hundred forty-nine children, aged 4–7 years, who were receiving diphtheria, pertussis, and tetanus immunization, were included. The children were randomized into control and intervention groups. Children in the control group were told what to expect and that it was okay to cry. Those in the experimental group were taught to blow out air repeatedly during the injection, as if they were blowing bubbles. Visual analogue scale scores were obtained from the children, parents, and nurses. The children's level of distress was analyzed objectively from videotape recordings.

Results.—Children in the intervention group had significantly fewer pain behaviors than those in the control group. They also had a trend toward lower reported pain scores on the visual analogue scale. The objective distress scores correlated well with the parents' and nurses' visual analogue scale scores, which were not significantly different from each other.

Conclusions.—The active distraction technique described is useful in helping young children cope with the pain of immunizations. The intervention is simple, quick, and free, and it is well accepted by children, parents, and nurses.

▶ The authors point out the possibility that the decrease in observed behavioral distress without a statistically significant change in the visual analogue score may reflect a change of behavior without a decrease of suffering. The important questions deal with whether the children can incorporate the technique into a range of coping skills, and whether the use of the technique enhances self-efficacy. If the technique is incorporated and self-efficacy is enhanced, this effect may be reflected by decreases in the visual analogue score in subsequent procedures. I agree with the authors that this technique is easily incorporated by a busy clinic.—B.S. Shapiro, M.D.

Emergency Department Analgesic Use in Pediatric Trauma Victims With Fractures

Friedland LR, Kulick RM (Univ of Cincinnati, Ohio)

Ann Emerg Med 23:203–207, 1994 131-95-2–26

Introduction.—Fractures are an important cause of acute pain in the emergency department. Fracture-related pain is commonly undertreated in both adults and children. There have been no studies of use of analgesics in victims of multiple trauma seen in the emergency department. Frequency of analgesic use in children seen in the emergency department with presumably painful fractures who are also at risk of associated multiple injuries was studied. Identification of factors that could distinguish which patients should receive analgesics were also sought.

Methods.—The cases of 433 injured children who met trauma team activation criteria over an 18-month period were studied retrospectively. One hundred twenty-one of these children had fractures of the pelvis, long bones, ankle, wrist, or clavicle. Endotracheal intubation was required in 22 children, who were excluded from the evaluation. For the 99 remaining children, 46 of whom had multisystem injuries, trauma registry data relevant to the study question were reviewed.

Findings.—Fifty-three percent of children received analgesics, all of which were narcotics. Analgesics were given in only 62% of children without multisystem injuries. The initial trauma scores and vital signs suggested a mild to moderate level of injury in patients who did and in those who did not receive analgesics. The 2 groups were not significantly different in terms of age, sex, race, mechanism of injury, vehicle speed, height of fall, time to arrival at the emergency department, transport method, prehospital analgesics, or mortality. Neither were there any differences in Injury Severity Score, initial vital signs, Glasgow Coma Scale score, Trauma Score, and Pediatric Trauma Score. Analgesics were given in 59% of children with associated internal injuries to the chest or abdomen, compared with 62% of those with isolated fractures. Children with associated head injury were half as likely to receive analgesics as those with isolated fractures.

Conclusions.—A low level of analgesic use in the emergency department in mildly to moderately injured children with presumably painful fractures who are at risk of associated multisystem injury was documented. Head injury was the only specific factor that distinguished patients who did receive analgesics from those who did not. Further studies are needed to determine whether more of these patients should receive analgesics in the emergency department after their initial evaluation.

► It would be interesting to know whether some of the variability in the use of analgesics was associated with prescribing styles of the physicians in charge at the time.—B.S. Shapiro, M.D.

Age-Related Response to Lidocaine-Prilocaine (EMLA) Emulsion and Effect of Music Distraction on the Pain of Intravenous Cannulation

Arts SE, Abu-Saad HH, Champion GD, Crawford MR, Fisher RJ, Juniper KH, Ziegler JB (State Univ of Limburg, Maastricht, The Netherlands; Prince of Wales Children's Hosp, Randwick, Australia; Prince of Wales Hosp, Randwick, Australia)

Pediatrics 93:797–801, 1994 131-95-2–27

Objective.—The efficacy of a local anesthetic cream was compared with that of music distraction for reducing pain from preoperative IV cannulation in children. The effects of age, gender, needle size, previous experience with venipuncture, or previous levels of anxiety on reported and observed pain were also examined.

Methods.—One hundred eighty children who were undergoing surgery with the use of general anesthesia were enrolled. Sixty children were recruited in each of 3 age groups: 4–6 years, 7–11 years, and 12–16 years. Within each age group, 20 children were randomly assigned to local application of an eutectic mixture of lidocaine-prilocaine (EMLA), 20 to placebo emulsion, and 20 to music via earphones. The children were asked to rate severity of pain on the faces pain scale and with a visual analogue toy. Behavioral reactions to insertion of the needle were rated on a global behavioral assessment scale by an investigator.

Results.—Pain scores after application of EMLA were significantly lower than those recorded after placebo or with music distraction. Regardless of type of intervention, younger children reported higher pain scores and displayed more pain-related behaviors than older children. However, EMLA nearly eliminated all pain-related behaviors in the youngest age group. When the data were adjusted for the effects of EMLA cream, cannula type, gender, previous experience with venipuncture, or previous level of anxiety did not significantly affect pain scores.

Conclusions.—The topical application of EMLA cream effectively prevents or reduces pain from preoperative IV cannulation in children. Young children experience the greatest benefit.

▶ This study, along with others, emphasizes that there is no reason not to use EMLA cream, particularly for infants and children. Perhaps music distraction is more effective when combined with the use of EMLA cream.—B.S. Shapiro, M.D.

The Cold Pressor Test in Children: Methodological Aspects and the Analgesic Effect of Intraoral Sucrose

Miller A, Barr RG, Young SN (McGill Univ, Montreal; Montreal Children's Hosp Research Inst)

Pain 56:175–183, 1994 131-95-2–28

Background.—Oral administration has been shown to calm crying newborns, but whether a sweet taste affects the response of older children to pain is in question. The analgesic effects of sucrose on the cold pressor test (CPT) were investigated in prepubertal children. The validity of the CPT, which determines the first experience of pain (threshold) and the removal from the pain source (tolerance), was also evaluated.

Methods.—Forty-four children, aged 8–11 years, were each tested with a 24% sucrose solution or spring water placed in their mouth, 2 days apart. The children were randomly assigned to receive either the water or the sucrose first. They were divided into 4 groups. Two groups were identified as stimulus-change (change) groups: one received sucrose on day 1 followed by water on day 2, and the other received water on day 1 followed by sucrose on day 2. Two groups were labeled repeat-stimulus groups (repeat): one received sucrose both days, and the other received water both days. The children placed 1 forearm in water warmed at 37°C for 2 minutes; the designated solution was placed in the mouth .5 minutes before the arm was removed from the water bath; the arm was then plunged into water at 10°C. The children were asked to indicate their pain threshold, which was defined as the first time they felt uncomfortable in the cold water, by raising the nonimmersed arm. Their tolerance was defined as the time when their pain in the cold water forced them to remove the arm. Both times were recorded with stopwatches. A visual analogue scale was administered to measure pain subjectively.

Results.—The threshold was longer in 19 children in change groups when they received sucrose. Discomfort was first reported 4.6 seconds later when in the sucrose condition than when in the water condition. There was no effect of the treatment for tolerance to pain. Threshold times were related in children in the change groups, but not in those in the repeat groups. Questionable threshold and visual analogue scale data occurred frequently.

Discussion.—The prolonged threshold response of 35% indicates that oral sucrose may modify the response to pain in prepubertal children. At 10°C, numbness soon replaces pain, which may have contributed to the varied data collected in this study. Because younger children displayed inconsistent threshold responses, CPT studies must be designed carefully to achieve valid research results in pediatrics.

▶ We need to know more about the use of sucrose as an analgesic. In the meantime, it should not be used as substitute for known and effective interventions. The danger is that health care professionals afflicted with opiophobia may rush for a substitution.—B.S. Shapiro, M.D.

Intranasal Versed: The Future of Pediatric Conscious Sedation

Adrian ER (Univ of Iowa Hosp and Clinics, Iowa City)

Pediatr Nurs 20:287–292, 1994 131-95-2–29

Background.—Conscious sedation for children who were undergoing procedures outside the operating room was described. Consciousness was depressed while reflexes persist, and the patient could maintain a patent airway independently and respond to verbal commands. The nurses' role in monitoring the child undergoing conscious sedation was presented. Focus was placed on intranasal administration of midazolam.

Management.—Traditional drugs for conscious sedation include chloral hydrate, 25–100 mg/kg, to a maximum dose of 2 gm given orally or rectally. In hypnotic doses, cardiorespiratory effects are few, but CNS depression must be monitored. Meperidine, promethazine, and chlorpromazine given intramuscularly to a maximum dose of 2 mg/1 mg/1 mg is another traditional approach. Significant respiratory effect can occur, and the child should be monitored closely for at least 8 hours. Pentobarbital sodium given orally, rectally, or intravenously at 2–4 mg/kg to a maximum dose of 120 mg can cause respiratory depression and hypotension.

Midazolam, a short-acting benzodiazepine drug, can be given parentally, as well as through nasal, rectal, and sublingual routes. Ranges for dosing are .035–.2 mg/kg intravenously, .4–.8 mg/kg orally, and .3–.5 mg/kg rectally. Early reports of significant respiratory depression with this drug were probably associated with overdosing.

Intranasal midazolam is given in a dose of .2–.3 mg/kg. Effectiveness intranasally is measured on a sedation scale. Sedation usually lasts 30–60 minutes. Sedation reversal can be achieved with flumazenil, a competitive receptor antagonist, within 1–2 minutes. Doses are not well established for this drug in children.

Nursing implications include having a positive pressure oxygen delivery system and emergency resuscitation equipment available. Every 5–15 minutes, the nurse should assess and record vital signs, respiratory status, and level of consciousness. During the procedure, pulse and blood pressure monitors should be used. After the procedure, assessments should be made every 15 minutes.

Conclusions.—Intranasal midazolam may provide sufficient sedation for diagnostic procedures in which more traditional pharmacologic approaches resulted in significant side effects. Flumazenil can reverse the effects of midazolam quickly; however, little information is available on its use in children.

▶ Intranasal midazolam appears to be effective and safe when proper monitoring is provided. An important caveat is that midazolam and other anxiolytics have no effect on pain and should not be used alone when significant pain is expected. Otherwise, children are sedated and in pain and cannot communicate the pain by words or behavior. Unfortunately, not all clinicians distinguish between sedation and analgesia.—B.S. Shapiro, M.D.

Comparison of Rectal Midazolam and Diazepam for Premedication in Pediatric Dental Patients

Roelofse JA, van der Bijl P (Univ of Stellenbosch, Tygerberg, South Africa)

J Oral Maxillofac Surg 51:525–529, 1993 131-95-2-30

Objective.—Rectally administered midazolam was compared with diazepam as premedication for dental procedures in pediatric patients in a double-blind, randomized trial.

Treatment.—Ninety children, aged 2–7 years, who required dental extraction while under general anesthesia were studied. The patients received either midazolam, .35 mg/kg; diazepam, .70 mg/kg; or placebo rectally 30 minutes before induction of general anesthesia.

Outcome.—All patients accepted the procedure involving rectal administration well. However, mask acceptance and improvement in anxiety and sedation were significantly better for both the midazolam and diazepam groups compared with the placebo group, but they were better for the midazolam group compared with the diazepam group. Only minor adverse effects were noted, but agitation/excitement/disinhibitory reaction was observed more frequently in the diazepam group than in the midazolam group. Both systolic and diastolic blood pressure and heart rate fell significantly in the midazolam group, compared with premedication values, but these changes had probably little clinical significance.

Conclusion.—Both rectal midazolam and diazepam are effective premedication in pediatric dental patients, but midazolam is more efficacious regarding mask acceptance, improvement in anxiety and sedation, and adverse emotional reactions.

▶ This is applicable to other clinical situations in which anxiolysis or sedation is needed.—B.S. Shapiro, M.D.

Pain Associated With Chronic Illness

Cognitive Coping Strategies of Children With Chronic Illness

Olson AL, Johansen SG, Powers LE, Pope JB, Klein RB (Dartmouth Med School, Lebanon, NH)

J Dev Behav Pediatr 14:217–223, 1993 131-95-2-31

Background.—Studies have often focused on the extra burden of illness and its care in children with chronic illness. Little has been said, however, on how these children cope in response to the stress created by these problems. Many studies suggest negative outcomes of chronic illness, but successful adaptation may occur when children respond to the additional stresses of their illness. The process of coping involves cognitive appraisal of a stressor and of response options.

Study Design.—In a cross-sectional study, 175 children from special summer camps for juvenile arthritis, asthma, or diabetes and 145 healthy school children completed questionnaires evaluating cognitive strategies for coping and trait anxiety. Spontaneous responses to common painful and stressful events, including pain of dental injection, giving a talk before the class, and a recent personally stressful event, were categorized into coping or catastrophizing ideation.

Findings.—Sixty-six percent of children with chronic illness and 64% of healthy children reported coping as their predominant cognitive strategy. The percentage of children who use coping increased with age in both groups and was not related to anxiety traits. The individual strategies used were similar for both groups and involved positive self-talk more frequently for coping and focusing on negative affect or fear for catastrophizing response. Children with chronic illness performed similarly, regardless of the severity of disease. In fact, children with severe juvenile rheumatoid arthritis reported higher rates of cognitive coping. The highest proportion of coping was found for the personal stressful event, and adolescents with chronic illness were more than twice as likely as healthy teens to offer more complex coping responses. Children with chronic illness offered coping strategies more often than did healthy children in response to venipuncture but not to dental injection.

Conclusion.—Children with chronic illnesses respond spontaneously with cognitive coping strategies to common painful and stressful events as often as do healthy children, and this expression increases with age. Identifying and using effective cognitions to cope with stressful events is an important skill that children with chronic illness learn to adopt successfully.

▶ This study highlights the strengths of children in the face of adversity. Appreciating and understanding these strengths are crucial in designing intervention programs.—B.S. Shapiro, M.D.

Predictors of Coping With Pain in Mothers and Their Children With Sickle Cell Syndrome

Sharpe JN, Brown RT, Thompson NJ, Eckman J (Emory Univ, Atlanta, Ga)

J Am Acad Child Adolesc Psychiatry 33:1246–1255, 1994 131-95-2–32

Background.—Sickle cell syndrome is a chronic, hereditary condition that affects 1 of 400–500 blacks in the United States. Pain is one of the most frequent symptoms of sickle cell syndrome, and affected individuals may experience 5–7 episodes of pain per year. Although the duration, frequency, and severity of these pain episodes vary considerably, the rate of pain is an important index of severity of disease. Predictors of strategies used by children with sickle cell disease and by their mothers in coping with their children's pain were examined.

Methods.—In 55 mother and child pairs, severity of disease, socioeconomic status, child adjustment and adaptive behavior, maternal psychopathology, and family functioning were examined. The children were aged 3–16 years and were studied while they were asymptomatic and not experiencing pain. Mothers and children reported their pain coping strategies on the Coping Strategies Inventory.

Results.—Family adaptability was associated with the mother's use of engagement coping strategies for managing her child's pain. Internalizing behavioral symptoms in the child, as well as pessimism and negative thinking, were associated with the mother's use of disengagement coping strategies. Mothers who used more active strategies for coping with their children's pain were more likely to use techniques to prevent and manage their children's pain effectively.

Conclusions.—Coping strategies were not predicted by severity of disease, which suggests that psychosocial factors are important in adapting to chronic illness in children and that severity of disease may not necessarily indicate families at risk for adjustment difficulties.

▶ This excellent study indicates the relevance of psychosocial variables to coping, regardless of severity of disease, and highlights the importance of a family systems approach in designing interventions for children and families at high risk of psychosocial dysfunction. The effects of severity of disease might only be evident by examining a population dichotomized to children with very high and low frequencies of pain. As discussed by the authors, however, the results are consistent with those of other studies that have examined the relationship between coping and severity of disease in children with other chronic illnesses.—B.S. Shapiro, M.D.

Death From a Morphine Infusion During a Sickle Cell Crisis
Gerber N, Apseloff G (Ohio State Univ, Columbus)
J Pediatr 123:322–325, 1993 131-95-2-33

Introduction.—The case of an adolescent boy who died during a vaso-occlusive cell crisis after continuous high-dose infusion of morphine was presented.

Case Report.—Boy, 15 years, with hemoglobin SS was seen in vaso-occlusive sickle cell crisis. Intravenous infusion of morphine was started initially at a dose of .5 mg/hr and supplemented with 3 mg given intravenously. The dose was gradually increased to 6 mg/hr on the first hospital day. Although the patient had a decreasing respiratory rate and slept during 22 of 24 nursing evaluations, morphine infusion was continued. On day 3, the patient sustained a cardiopulmonary arrest after receiving a total of 298 mg of morphine; he died on day 4, after a second cardiopulmonary arrest. Laboratory results indicated significant hepatic and renal impairment. Autopsy revealed massive gastrointestinal hemorrhage and multiple organ infarcts.

Discussion.—During a vaso-occlusive sickle cell crisis, high-dose IV narcotic therapy should not be continued when there is evidence of drug excess. The respiratory depression in therapeutic doses of narcotics may cause significant respiratory acidosis and hypoxemia, enhancing polymerization of hemoglobin SS that promotes sickling and vaso-occlusion. In this patient, accumulation of the potent metabolite morphine-6-glucuronide with renal failure may have resulted in further respiratory depression, progressive sickling, and worsening vaso-occlusion with infarcts. When IV narcotics are used during a sickle cell crisis, pharmacokinetically based patient-controlled analgesia appears to the best method.

▶ There is no doubt that opioids, whether administered by infusion, intermittent parenteral injection, or orally, can result in significant respiratory compromise and death if doses are inappropriately high and/or administration is not monitored effectively. In this patient, there were numerous symptoms and signs that the dose of opioid was inappropriately high. However, that inappropriately dosed and monitored administration of morphine can result in death does not mean that morphine and other opioids, when used responsibly according to published guidelines, should not be used in the doses necessary to assuage sickle cell–related pain safely and effectively.

The etiology of the massive gastrointestinal hemorrhage is not evident. Certainly, it could have been secondary to widespread intravascular sickling and infarction. However, data supporting the authors' recommendation for ketorolac as an alternative for opioids are not presented in this report. Ketorolac and other nonsteroidal anti-inflammatory drugs may be associated with gastritis and ulceration and, by themselves, may not provide adequate relief of pain.—B.S. Shapiro, M.D.

High-Dose Intravenous Methylprednisolone Therapy for Pain in Children and Adolescents With Sickle Cell Disease

Griffin TC, McIntire D, Buchanan GR (Univ of Texas, Dallas; Children's Med Ctr, Dallas)

N Engl J Med 330:733–737, 1994 131-95-2–34

Introduction.—Vaso-occlusive crises, which are acute painful episodes, are the most common complication of sickle cell disease and a frequent reason for visiting the emergency department. Because many features of the episodes resemble those of inflammatory processes (fever, local swelling, erythema, leukocytosis, elevated sedimentation rate), the use of high doses of steroid early in the course of a vaso-occlusive crisis might lessen the severity and duration of pain.

Study Plan.—Thirty-six patients, aged younger than 21 years, with sickle cell disease had a total of 56 acute episodes of severe pain. The diagnosis was sickle cell anemia in 27 patients, sickle cell–hemoglobin C disease in 7, and sickle cell–β^+-thalassemia in 2. In a double-blind design, the patients were randomized to receive either an infusion of methylprednisolone, 15 mg/kg up to 1 g, or a saline placebo when hospitalized and again after 24 hours. The patients also received morphine intravenously, followed by acetaminophen with codeine.

Results.—Patients who received placebo required inpatient analgesia for a significantly longer time than those given steroid. The same difference was apparent after excluding 7 episodes complicated by chest syndrome. After therapy was discontinued, those who received methylprednisolone had recurrent pain episodes more often than placebo patients, but they experienced no adverse effects of the drug.

Conclusion.—Duration of severe pain was reduced in children and adolescents with sickle cell disease who received short-course, high-dose methylprednisolone.

► This is a promising treatment that requires further study of long-term efficacy and side effects and assessment over repeated episodes.—B.S. Shapiro, M.D.

Epidural Analgesia in the Management of Severe Vaso-Occlusive Sickle Cell Crisis

Yaster M, Tobin JR, Billett C, Casella JF, Dover G (Johns Hopkins Hosp, Baltimore, Md)

Pediatrics 93:310–315, 1994 131-95-2–35

Objective.—Whether continuous epidural analgesia could effectively treat the pain of vaso-occlusive crisis in children with sickle cell disease who were unresponsive to conventional analgesic therapy was investigated retrospectively.

Treatment.—Nine children during 11 painful vaso-occlusive crises were treated with continuous epidural infusion of lidocaine (5 mg/mL) at 1.5 mg/kg/hr. If pain returned, fentanyl (.5–1.5 μg/kg/hr) was added or bupivacaine (.2–.4 mg/kg/hr) was substituted for lidocaine. All patients had severe pain that was unresponsive to high-dose systemic opioids, nonsteroidal anti-inflammatory drugs, and adjunctive measures. Pain on a numerical scale from 0 to 10 (0 = no pain; 10 = worst pain) and oxygen saturation were monitored.

Outcome.—Analgesia was immediate, with pain scores decreasing from 9 to 1 within 15 minutes in 8 of 9 patients. Analgesia was continuously effective in 9 of 11 crises and dramatically improved arterial oxygen saturation from 91% to 99% in 7 of 9 patients. Plasma levels of lidocaine ranged from 1.1 to 4.6 mg/L, and dose-related toxicity did not occur. Five patients had tachyphylaxis to lidocaine and required either the addition of fentanyl or substitution of bupivacaine for lidocaine to maintain analgesia for 2–5 days. Catheters remained in place for 1.5–5 days. One patient became acutely hypotensive secondary to high sympathetic blockade (T-4) but responded to IV fluids and epinephrine. There were 4 catheter-related complications: 1 inadvertent dural puncture occurred during insertion of the catheter, 1 catheter fell out, 1 catheter was placed incorrectly, and 1 was removed for fever. Epidural analgesia was not associated with sedation, respiratory depression, or limitation of movement. All epidural catheters were cultured on removal, and none showed any bacteriologic growth.

Conclusion.—This study represents the first documented successful use of epidural analgesia in the management of severe vaso-occlusive crises in children with sickle cell disease. Continuous epidural analgesia with local anesthetics, alone or in combination with fentanyl, treats the pain of sickle cell vaso-occlusive crises effectively and safely without causing sedation, respiratory depression, or significant limitation on ambulation. Further, early treatment of the painful crisis with this technique improves oxygenation, a critical factor in the evolution of further sickling. Until more information is known, epidural analgesia should be administered using very conservative infusion rates and should be limited to patients for whom conventional therapy has failed.

▶ Some very severe painful episodes are difficult to treat effectively and safely using parenteral opioids. In these cases, epidural analgesia is a promising alternative. The cautions of the authors are well taken. Further investigation of efficacy and side effects is necessary. Sickle cell–related pain is often recurrent over the lifetime of the individual, and long-term management of the pain and coping with the illness must be considered when designing interventions for the acute episode.—B.S. Shapiro, M.D.

A Comparison of Child and Parent Ratings of Disability and Pain in Juvenile Chronic Arthritis

Doherty E, Yanni G, Conroy RM, Bresnihan B (St Vincent's Hosp, Dublin; Royal College of Surgeons in Ireland, Dublin)

J Rheumatol 20:1563–1566, 1993 131-95-2–36

Background.—The Childhood Health Assessment Questionnaire (Child-HAQ), completed by the child's parent, represents the parent's opinion of the child's level of disability and pain. Using the recently introduced standardized measures of child disability and pain, parents' and children's assessments of chronic physical disease were compared.

Methods.—The Child-HAQ was used for 20 children, aged 8–16 years, with juvenile chronic arthritis and their mothers. Pain was assessed using a visual analogue scale.

Results.—The median child's disability score was .75, and the median mother's disability score was .375. The child's and mother's median pain scores were both .1. There was a high level of agreement between the child's and mother's assessment of disability. In contrast, there was no correlation between their assessment of pain. Mothers' ratings of disability and pain correlate highly with each other and also correlated significantly with contact with health professionals and school attendance. In contrast, none of the children's own assessments correlated with any of these items, nor did their ratings of disability and pain correlate with each other. Further, qualitative analysis of the children's feelings toward arthritis suggested negative attitudes in the child. In 5 of these 6 children with negative attitudes, there was mother-child disagreement on pain ratings, and most mothers rated the children's pain less severely.

Implication.—Parents of children with juvenile chronic arthritis give accurate information regarding disability but not regarding pain. Children apparently view their disability and pain as separate, whereas mothers interpret them to be related, casting doubt on the validity of measuring a child's pain by questioning the parent.

▶ This fascinating study reinforces the principle of interviewing both the child and the parents, especially for such subjective symptoms as pain and depression. Further study of the relationship between pain and disability, as viewed from the patients' experiences, would be informative.—B.S. Shapiro, M.D.

Chronic Pain Unrelated to Chronic Disease

Early Pain Experience, Child and Family Factors, as Precursors of Somatization: A Prospective Study of Extremely Premature and Full-term Children

Grunau RVE, Whitfield MF, Petrie JH, Fryer EL (BC Children's Hosp, Vancouver, Canada; Univ of British Columbia, Vancouver, Canada)

Pain 56:353–359, 1994 131-95-2–37

Purpose.—Investigations of the causes of recurrent pain and somatization in children without any medical problems have been inconclusive. Whether pain experienced in infancy has a role in the development of childhood somatization was investigated.

Methods.—Thirty-six preterm, extremely low-birth-weight (ELBW) children and 36 full-term children with normal birth weights underwent psychological assessment at ages 3 and 4½ years. Mother-child interaction was rated immediately after psychometric testing at the 3-year visit, and mothers completed detailed questionnaires at both visits. Somatization scores were calculated from a 30-item survey. Extremely low-birth-weight children were studied because they had experienced prolonged hospitalization and undergone repeated medical interventions in infancy.

Results.—At age 4½, ELBW children had significantly higher rates of somatic complaints of unknown origin than full-term children, even though there was no significant difference in the rate of actual medical problems between the 2 groups. The mothers' behaviors as rated during observation of mother-child interaction when the children were 3 years old did not differ significantly between the 2 groups. However, the combination of family relations, neonatal ICU experience, poor maternal sensitivity to child cues, and child avoidance of touch or holding at age 3 was predictive of somatization scores at age 4½. A comparison of ELBW children with normal somatization scores and ELBW children with clinically significant somatization confirmed the importance of maternal involvement. Child personality traits such as anxiety and depression were not related to somatization.

Conclusions.—The repeated procedures that ELBW infants endure during prolonged care in a neonatal ICU appear to contribute to the later development of abnormal responses to pain and other somatic events.

▶ Clinicians who deal with either hospitalized neonates, extremely premature children, or children and adolescents with chronic pain should read this polished and thoughtful study in its entirety. Pain in hospitalized, extremely premature neonates must be viewed within the entire context of the effects of hospitalization on infant development and parent-child relationships. Patterns of somatization or aversion to touch do not develop in all children. Empathic attunement of the parents and teaching children to respond appropriately to their somatic cues may aid normal development. Vigorous treatment of pain in the neonatal ICU, in and of itself, is necessary but inadequate when viewed within the total context of barriers to development experienced by the hospitalized premature infant.—B.S. Shapiro, M.D.

Headache Characteristics Among High School and University Students

Montgomery GT (Univ of Texas, Edinburg)
Headache 34:247–256, 1994 131-95-2–38

Objective.—Adolescents and young adults are thought to be at high risk for headache, and females are believed to have more headaches than males. Whether university students have more frequent and severe headaches than do high school students was determined. In addition, whether female students have more headaches than male students was investigated. Also examined were the causes of headache, trends, and coping mechanisms.

Methods.—Questionnaires were completed by 283 female and 254 male high school students (mean age, 16 years) and 205 female and 95 male university students (mean age, 21 years).

Results.—The frequency and severity of headaches were significantly higher and the duration of headaches was significantly longer for female students than for male students. The university students reported significantly more severe headaches than did high school students. Female students reported significantly higher headache characteristic scores in 5 of 6 categories, and university students had significantly higher headache characteristic scores in 4 of 6 factors. Female and university students also reported higher scores in 4 of 6 factors of headache antecedents. Under coping strategies, the university students scored significantly higher with 1 factor only.

Conclusions.—Although factor analysis is useful in providing valuable diagnostic information, the sample size must be large and questions need to be standardized to facilitate comparison. The relationships between headaches and student age and sex were similar to those found in other studies.

Prevalence of Headache and Migraine in Schoolchildren

Abu-Arefeh I, Russell G (Royal Aberdeen Children's Hosp, Scotland)

BMJ 309:765–769, 1994 131-95-2–39

Objective.—Although there have been studies of the prevalence and causes of headache in adult and pediatric hospital patients, little data are available on nonhospitalized schoolchildren. The rate of migraine headache in schoolchildren was determined using International Headache Society (IHS) criteria.

Methods.—A total of 2,165 children, aged 5 to 15 years, in Aberdeen, Scotland, were sent a questionnaire. From the 1,907 questionnaires returned, 240 children with severe recurrent headache were selected and interviewed along with their parents. After neurologic examination, the headache was classified as migraine if it met IHS criteria, as migraine-like if it met IHS criteria but lasted less than 2 hours, and as tension headache if it had no associated migraine symptoms but recurred daily for at least 10 days. A specific diagnosis, such as sinusitis or poor eyesight was determined in some children, and nonspecific headache was diagnosed when the above categories did not apply.

Results.—The prevalence rates for migraine were 10.6%; for migraine-like headache, .7%; for tension headache, .9%; for specific diagnosis, .2%; and for nonspecific headache, 1.3%. The percentage of girls and boys with migraine was approximately equal, although migraine was more common in girls older than 12 years of age and in boys younger than 12. Girls had a higher incidence of migraine with aura. Children with migraine missed significantly more days of school than did children without migraine. There was a higher, although not significant, incidence of asthma and family breakdown in children with asthma.

Conclusion.—Migraine is a common cause of activity-restricting headache in schoolchildren, and the incidence may have increased in the past 30 years.

Sociodemographic Differences in the Prevalence of Self-Reported Headache in Icelandic School-Children

Kristjánsdóttir G, Wahlberg V (Univ of Iceland, Reykjavik; Nordic School of Public Health, Göteborg, Sweden)

Headache 33:376–380, 1993 131-95-2–40

Objective.—The prevalence of headache experiences in relation to sociodemographic background was studied in a random sample of 2,400 Icelandic school children, aged 11–12 years and 15–16 years.

Methods.—The study was part of a larger investigation of self-reported pain in schoolchildren. Questionnaires were completed by 2,140 children, for a response rate of 89.2%. Headache was defined as a self-reported painful experience.

Findings.—Overall, the prevalence of "at least monthly" headache was 51.4% and "at least weekly headache" was 21.9%. The prevalence of headache was significantly higher among younger children and among girls. The gender difference was related to the markedly lower prevalence in older than younger boys. There were no gender differences in the younger group. Social class was not significantly related to headache but did interact with gender; there was a significantly higher prevalence of frequent headache among lower class girls. The frequency of headache correlated strongly with the use of medications in the past months to relieve headache. Children with frequent headache took pain medications but were much less likely to consult school health professionals, particularly physicians.

Summary.—The high overall prevalence of frequent headache among schoolchildren was similar to that reported in earlier studies. The prevalence of headache varied with age, gender, and social class and was particularly high among young and lower-class girls. The high prevalence of frequent headache, coupled with the low use of school health services, should be of great concern. The relationship between headache and drug use in children also must be addressed.

▶ There are a lot of articles on the incidence of headaches. The question of interactions between gender and social class is briefly discussed in this study by Kristjánsdóttir and Wahlberg. One can question whether the incidence of headaches has increased over the years or whether the differences lie in study methodology or demand characteristics.—B.S. Shapiro, M.D.

Cluster Headaches in Childhood

D'Cruz OF (Univ of North Carolina, Chapel Hill)

Clin Pediatr 33:241–242, 1994 131-95-2–41

Background.—Cluster headaches, although uncommon in the first decade of life, have typical initial features in children. Appropriate diagnosis and treatment can be achieved once a thorough history is taken. The clinical features and treatment of cluster headaches in children were described based on 2 case histories.

Case 1.—Boy, 8 years, reported sharp headaches in the right temporal region. These headaches were accompanied by lacrimation, nasal congestion, photophobia, and nausea. The duration of headaches was 10 minutes to 1 hour. There were normal findings on general and neurologic examinations, as well as ears, nose, and throat and dental evaluations. Results of sinus radiographs and an MRI scan of the head were also normal. After trial treatments with propranolol, amitriptyline, and biofeedback, the headaches were successfully controlled with indomethacin, 25 mg twice daily.

Case 2.—Girl, 10 years, experienced headaches since the age of 7½ years. Headaches were sharp and located in the left temporal region. They were accompanied by lacrimation and nasal congestion. Episodes lasted 1–2 hours, 3–6 times per week. Occasional throbbing headaches with nausea and dizziness were also reported. Family history was positive for migraines. No other related findings were noted on the general or neurologic examinations. Indomethacin, 25 mg twice daily, controlled the headaches successfully.

Discussion.—Cluster headaches occur most frequently in males. Family history may be negative. Headaches are recurrent, severe, and unilateral. They are located in the periorbital and temporal region and are accompanied by ophthalmic and nasal symptoms. The duration can vary from 15 to 180 minutes, and there may be periods of remission. Successful treatments of cluster headaches include verapamil and aspirin, although the risk of Reye's syndrome and gastrointestinal side effects may limit the use of aspirin in children. Indomethacin and aspirin both inhibit prostaglandin synthesis. The effect of verapamil may result from stabilizing vascular tone. Hematopoietic side effects with indomethacin must be monitored. Cluster headaches are rare but severe and occur daily. They are also unresponsive to treatments used for migraine. Accurate diagnosis assists in early appropriate treatment.

▶ Clinicians who treat children with headaches need to be familiar with the varying presentations associated with cluster headaches, because the interventions are often different from those used for children with other kinds of headaches.—B.S. Shapiro, M.D.

Prevalence and Persistence of Stomach Ache and Headache Among Children: Follow-Up of a Cohort of Norwegian Children From 4 to 10 Years of Age

Borge AIH, Nordhagen R, Moe B, Botten G, Bakketeig LS (Natl Inst of Public Health, Oslo, Norway)

Acta Paediatr 83:433–437, 1994 131-95-2–42

Purpose.—Few studies have examined whether preschool children who complain of stomach ache or headache eventually outgrow these complaints. In a longitudinal study, a group of children was followed for 6 years to determine the outcome of somatic complaints first reported by parents when their child was 4 years of age.

Methods.—One hundred thirty-six children born in 1981 and with permanent residence in a rural town outside of Oslo were included. The first interview took place at the child's regular preschool health examination. Interviews with mothers were conducted by a trained health nurse who collected information on the various somatic symptoms about which the child complained. Six years later, when the child was 10 years of age, parents as well as teachers were interviewed to determine how often the child complained of headache or stomach ache.

Results.—Complete data sets were available for 129 children. At age 4 years, 24.3% of children had infrequent complaints of stomach ache only, 6.6% had frequent complaints of stomach ache only, 1.5% had infrequent complaints of headache only, and 4.4% had infrequent complaints of headache and stomach ache. By the time the children were 10 years of age, 14.7% had infrequent complaints of stomach ache only and 5.1% had frequent stomach ache. Headache only occurred frequently in 5.9% and infrequently in 8.1%. Stomach ache co-occurred with headache frequently in 14.7% and infrequently in 5.9%. Among the 88 children who never complained at age 4 years, 67% remained free of pain 6 years later, whereas 33% had experienced the onset of stomach ache. Children with somatic complaints at age 4 years were almost 3 times more likely to have complaints at age 10 than those without complaints at age 4.

Conclusions.—Complaints of stomach ache were common in preschool children but complaints of headache were not. The overall prevalence of stomach ache and headache increased over time, and early complaints tended to persist.

▶ The persistence of somatic symptoms in this group of children is striking but not surprising, given other research data and common clinical experience. The efficacy of anticipatory guidance aimed at family and child reactions and coping efforts is speculative. We do not know whether early intervention might prevent later development of pain problems and other symptoms that interfere significantly with function and mood.

A problem of this study, as discussed by the authors, is that only parent and teacher reports were used. Based on the report by Doherty and colleagues (Abstract 131-95-2–36), which showed the divergence between child and parent assessment of rheumatoid arthritis, we must view the data with some skepticism. Depending on family milieu, temperament, and cultural expectations, children may or may not report their symptoms.—B.S. Shapiro, M.D.

Preliminary Findings on Increased Muscle Tension and Tenderness, and Recurrent Abdominal Pain in Children: A Clinical Study

Alfvén G (Huddinge Hosp, Sweden)

Acta Paediatr 82:400–403, 1993 131-95-2–43

Background.—Recurrent abdominal pain of "nonorganic origin" is a common problem in children; however, the origin of the pain remains unexplained. Recurrent nonorganic abdominal pain may be directly related to a stress-induced increase in tension and tenderness in the abdominal muscles and part of a more generally increased tension, noted particularly in the shoulder-neck-cephalic muscles. Whether nonorganic recurrent abdominal pain is of muscular origin was investigated.

Methods.—A subjective quantification of muscle tone and tenderness in the abdominal wall and other muscle groups was undertaken in 15 boys and 12 girls with recurrent abdominal pain that persisted for 1–60 months. All had a typical history of recurrent abdominal pain located mainly around the navel, in the epigastrium, or both; psychosocial difficulties coinciding with the onset of such events as divorce; and no signs of organic disease. A control group of 16 children was also studied.

Findings.—All children with recurrent nonorganic abdominal pain exhibited tense and tender abdominal muscles, primarily in the umbilical area. In addition, these children displayed a typical pattern of muscular tension and tenderness in other muscles, including the shoulder and cephalic muscles and lateral insertions of the great pectoris and the subclavius. Tension headache, "tension" chest pains, and more generalized symptoms, such as loss of appetite and disturbed bowel function, were also common in these children.

Implication.—Recurrent abdominal pain of nonorganic origin is probably only a part-phenomenon of a broader complex of reactions of CNS origin that consists of stress-induced tension and attacks of pain in different muscle groups, especially in the abdominal, galea, and thoracic muscles, and vegetative symptoms. This reaction may be a phylogenetic remnant of a biologically old primeval protective reflex.

▶ There are many methodological problems in this study, but the findings make sense based on our knowledge of the mechanisms of pain. I wish more data were reported on the blinded differentiation of children with and without recurrent abdominal pain on the basis of the physical examination. Hopefully, the observations will be useful to clinicians and to researchers in the generation of hypotheses to be tested. I have examined many children with recurrent abdominal pain who have tenderness in various muscle groups. The finding of abdominal muscle tenderness, especially if palpation reproduces the pain, is useful in demonstrating psychophysiologic interactions and in reassuring children and their families. It makes sense that even if alterations in gastrointestinal motility, along with attributional and temperamental factors, are primarily associated with the pain, the surrounding muscle groups would become activated, resulting in a worsening of the pain. It is often easy for patients and families to understand the relationship between stress and muscles.—B.S. Shapiro, M.D.

Back Pain in School Children: A Study Among 1,178 Pupils

Troussier B, Davoine P, de Gaudemaris R, Fauconnier J, Phelip X (Univ Hosp of Grenoble, France)

Scand J Rehabil Med 26:143–146, 1994 131-95-2–44

Objective.—Back pain afflicts approximately 80% of the population in industrialized countries and has a prevalence of 7% to 49% in children. Studies in children, however, have used differing methodologies, making it difficult to compare results. The incidence and risk factors relating to back pain were compared.

Methods.—A total of 1,178 students, aged 6–20 years, of relatively high social class returned questionnaires relating to back pain.

Results.—The prevalence of back pain was 51.2% with significantly more girls than boys reporting pain. The incidence of back pain increased with age for both boys and girls. Pain was most common in the lumbar region, thoracic area, and lumbar and leg region. Time spent watching television, smoking, and the position used to carry school bags were contributing factors.

Conclusion.—Multivariate analysis showed a correlation between back pain and female sex, age, previous back injury, volleyball, and time spent watching television. The incidence of back pain, particularly low back and leg pain, in children is similar to that found in other studies and increases with age for both girls and boys older than 12 years of age.

Non-Specific Low-Back Pain Among Schoolchildren: A Field Survey With Analysis of Some Associated Factors

Balagué F, Nordin M, Skovron ML, Dutoit G, Yee A, Waldburger M (Cantonal Hosp, Fribourg, Switzerland; Hosp for Joint Disease, New York)

J Spinal Disord 7:374–379, 1994 131-95-2–45

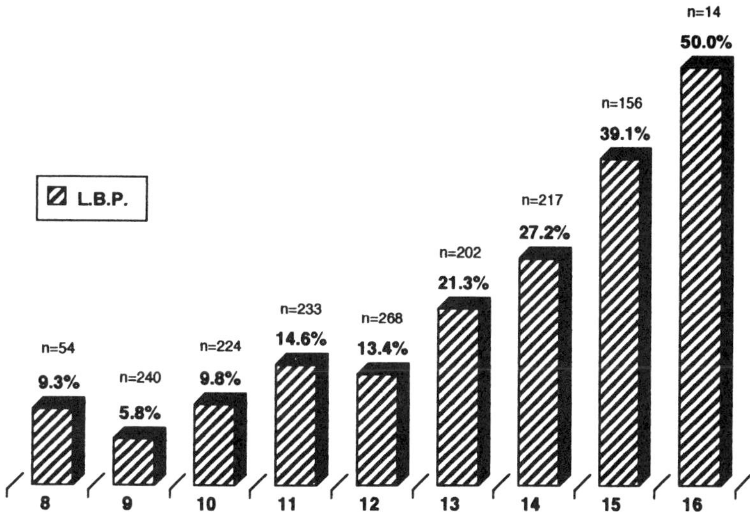

Fig 2–1.—Lifetime prevalence of low back pain (*LBP*) by age (years) in 1,716 children (1,608 valid answers). (Courtesy of Balagué F, Nordin M, Skovron ML, et al: *J Spinal Disord* 7:374–379, 1994.)

Background.—Low back pain (LBP) is thought to be uncommon in individuals younger than 20 years of age. Values for lifetime prevalence of back trouble in children and adolescents, however, reportedly range from 7% to 63%. Associations between LBP and social factors were investigated.

Methods and Findings.—A total of 1,755 children, aged 8–16 years, were surveyed using a 15-item, self-administered questionnaire; 1,716 (97.7%) completed the questionnaire. Approximately 34% of children reported having had at least 1 episode of spinal pain. Of those, 66.8% reported LBP (Fig 2–1). Twelve percent had had back pain in the previous week, and 6% said they had had to refrain from some normal daily activities because of back pain. The risk for LBP among children, after controlling for age and gender, was significantly increased by parental history of treated LBP, competitive sports activity, and time spent watching television.

Conclusions.—A history of nonspecific LBP was common in these children. The condition was significantly associated with age and female gender, positive parental history of LBP treatment, a high frequency of sports activities, and amount of time spent watching television. Reports of recent disabling LBP are relatively uncommon.

▶ So much for the aphorism that back pain in children and adolescents is usually associated with either disease or significant anatomical alterations. It makes sense that LBP would not suddenly arise, unannounced, after age 20. One would suspect that the antecedents of back pain in some adults lie in childhood risk factors. This is yet another reason to advise against excessive television watching and for moderate activity.—B.S. Shapiro, M.D.

Reflex Sympathetic Dystrophy in Children: An Orthopedic Perspective

Stanton RP, Malcolm JR, Wesdock KA, Singsen BH (Alfred I duPont Inst, Wilmington, Del)

Orthopedics 16:773–780, 1993 131-95-2–46

Objectives.—Reflex sympathetic dystrophy (RSD) is described infrequently in children. Diagnostic criteria for RSD in pediatric patients were defined, and a prospective treatment protocol was initiated.

Study Design.—The records of 24 girls and 12 boys (mean age, 13.4 years) with 49 episodes of RSD were reviewed. The minimum diagnostic criteria for RSD included pain out of proportion to the inciting event and evidence of dysfunction of the neurovascular system as shown by 3 or more of the following: dependent edema, dependent rubor, mottling of skin, hypersensitivity of skin to light touch, skin temperature changes, altered perspiration, and changes in patterns of hair growth.

Findings.—The mean time from onset of pain to diagnosis was 9.2 months, and many patients saw multiple physicians before RSD was recognized. At presentation, 61% of children had "severe" pain, and at least 75% had changes in skin color, swelling, hyperesthesia, abnormal skin temperatures, muscle weakness, and decreased range of motion. Radiographs showed osteopenia in 40%. In 24 patients, bone scans showed increased uptake in 46%, decreased uptake in 25%, and normal findings in 29%. In 23 children with psychological evaluations, 83% had some type of significant emotional dysfunction.

Treatment and Outcome.—Intensive physical therapy appeared to be the most effective treatment. Analgesics, anti-inflammatory medications, local injections, and regional blockades were not effective. The average time to complete resumption of age-appropriate physical activities was 9 months in 25 patients with documented resolution. Twelve patients had recurrences, and 11 had persistent limitations of physical activity.

Summary.—The minimal diagnostic criteria for pediatric RSD should include pain out of proportion to the inciting event and documented dysfunction of the neurovascular system. Resumption of age-appropriate activities can usually be achieved with an inpatient diagnostic and rehabilitation program for treating chronic pain, including orthopedics, rheumatology, psychology, and twice-daily physical therapy.

▶ Although this study is based on retrospective data, it is truly an excellent review and discussion of RSD and its treatment. Unfortunately, diagnosis is often delayed, and the resultant anxiety, confusing and sometimes pejorative explanations, and visits to multiple specialists contribute to the biomedically based explanatory model so frequently observed in patients and families. Education of primary practitioners and specialists in a biopsychosocial approach to symptoms might help prevent the iatrogenic contribution to the difficulties encountered in treatment. I recommend full reading of this article.—B.S. Shapiro, M.D.

Meralgia Paresthetica in Children

Edelson R, Stevens P (Pediatric Orthopedic Assoc, Salt Lake City, Utah)
J Bone Joint Surg (Am) 76–A:993–999, 1994 131-95-2–47

Background.—Although meralgia paresthetica is considered rare among pediatric patients, experience over the past decade has suggested that this condition is much more common in children than previously reported. However, the lesion is frequently unrecognized or misdiagnosed. Experience with chronic meralgia paresthetica in children since 1985 was reported.

Patients and Findings.—The records of 20 children and young adults, aged 20 years or younger, were reviewed. All patients had meralgia paresthetica, with bilateral involvement noted in 10 patients. Thus, a total of 30 lesions were evaluated. Open decompression of the lateral femoral cutaneous nerve was eventually used to treat 24 lesions, 21 of which were followed for at least 2 years. The initial complaint was severe pain that led to marked restriction of activities. Palpation of the nerve reproduced the pain, and a trial injection of Xylocaine (lidocaine) always resulted in temporary relief of symptoms. The average age at onset of symptoms was 10 years (range, 1–17 years). The diagnosis was initially missed in 10 patients, all of whom subsequently had to undergo multiple and unnecessary diagnostic tests. The average duration of symptoms before patients were first assessed was 24 months (range, 2–84 months). The average length of follow-up after the 21 surgeries was 38 months (range, 25–60 months). Excellent results, including compete relief of pain and no limitation of activity, were obtained in 14 of 21 operations. Good results, with occasional pain but no limitation of sports or other activities, were achieved in 5 patients, and fair results were noted in 2, with pain that interfered with sport activities, but not walking.

Conclusions.—Meralgia paresthetica occurs more frequently in children than has been suspected. This condition should therefore be considered in the differential diagnosis of children with hip and thigh pain. The diagnosis can be made on the basis of clinical examination and verified by the injection of a local anesthetic. Multiple unnecessary and costly diagnostic tests can therefore be avoided. Operative decompression can provide satisfactory results in patients with severe meralgia paresthetica, but surgery need not be performed in those with mild pain, unless there is progression.

▶ This is a diagnosis to keep in mind.—B.S. Shapiro, M.D.

3 Oncology

Introduction

The publication last year of the *Cancer Pain Guidelines* by the Agency for Health Care Policy and Research represented an important statement for medical practice and the patient with cancer. The *Guidelines* clearly indicate that cancer-related pain should be and can be adequately treated. The principles of cancer pain management have also received widespread support from a number of medial societies and other organizations. The *Guidelines* therefore establish in writing that the relief of cancer-related pain is considered a priority in oncologic care by the National Institutes of Health.

Intended to provide a reference for care, the principles of cancer pain management and therapeutic recommendations are included in the *Guidelines.* However, several publications continue to show that cancer-related pain is undertreated. Health care professionals still need education in the principles of cancer pain management. Control of cancer-related pain, as documented through the vital signs and other areas of the medical record, is an aspect of care now being incorporated into quality assurance evaluations. Reviews that indicate less-than-optimal management of cancer-related pain can then effect changes in medical practice. Many of the articles included in this chapter address issues related to the incidence of unrelieved cancer pain and quality of life. Despite the publication of and publicity surrounding the *Guidelines,* barriers continue to be encountered in the treatment of cancer-related pain, and the impact of unrelieved pain on patients and families remains profound.

Other issues exist beyond the continued need to educate health care professionals so that they can apply established treatments for cancer-related pain and the cancer. In addition to ethical considerations and standards of care, cost-benefit analyses must also be performed. The socioeconomics of treating cancer-related pain need to be addressed so that the indications for interventional therapy can be clarified. Cost-benefit analyses will need to include factors like prognosis, the degree and durability of benefit, and the cost for subsequent treatment. Delineating specific indications for specific therapies will provide the most efficient use of limited health care dollars, because ineffective therapy is the most wasteful financial and personal expenditure. Established and developing analgesic, interventional, and antineoplastic therapies are important to allow continued improvement in the control of cancer pain.

The specialty of Cancer Pain and Symptom Management continues to emerge. Recognition of its importance, through the publication of the *Guidelines* and other efforts, has increased research into the pathophysiology of cancer pain, allowed optimization of established therapies and development of new therapies, and has increased experience in the management of cancer pain. As the specialty expands and quality assurance issues gain greater prominence, it is anticipated that more health care professionals will apply the principles used to treat cancer-related pain. It is hoped that future studies will demonstrate that the *Guidelines*, and the efforts of those who support the principles of cancer pain management, have resulted in a significant improvement in treatment of cancer-related pain.

Nora A. Janjan, M.D.

Incidence

Pain In Ovarian Cancer Patients: Prevalence, Characteristics, and Associated Symptoms

Portenoy RK, Kornblith AB, Wong G, Vlamis V, Lepore JM, Loseth DB, Hakes T, Foley KM, Hoskins WJ (Memorial Sloan-Kettering Cancer Ctr, New York)
Cancer 74:907–915, 1994 131-95-3–1

Introduction.—The investigation of pain in patients with ovarian cancer has been largely anecdotal. Thus, the prevalence, characteristics and impact of pain, as well as other symptoms, are relatively unknown. An increased understanding of pain can improve clinical management and the quality of life in these patients.

Methods.—A total of 151 patients (111 inpatients) undergoing treatment in a cancer center participated in the study. Several questionnaires were distributed, including a comprehensive pain survey, the Rand Mental Health Inventory, the Functional Living Index-Cancer, the Karnofsky Performance Status scale, and the Memorial Symptom Assessment Scale.

Results.—The patients averaged 55 years of age, and 82% had stage III or IV disease. Active disease was present in 69% of the patients. Pain preceded the onset or recurrence of disease in 62%. Persistent or frequent pain was noted in approximately half the patients during the 2 weeks before therapy (Table 1). The pain was localized to the abdominopelvic region (80%) and interfered with selected activities, mood, work, and overall enjoyment of life in 60% to 70% of patients (Table 2). Performance status and the extent of the tumor were the main predictors of pain that interfered with function.

Conclusions.—Pain interfered with activities of daily living in 40% of the patients. Pain substantially affected function in one half to two thirds of these patients. A stereotypic pain syndrome in the abdominopelvic region preceded the diagnosis or recurrence of the disease.

TABLE 1.—Characteristics of Pain Associated With Ovarian Cancer (n = 63)

Duration of worst or only pain			
Median	2 wk		
Range	<1–756 wk		
Pain severity "in general"		Pain severity "at its worst"	
VAS*		VAS*	
Mean (SD)	48.1 (21.4) mm	Mean (SD)	66.7 (24.9) mm
Median	47.5 mm	Median	69.5 mm
Range	7–100 mm	Range	3–100 mm
VRS†		VRS†	
Mean (SD)	4.9 (1.5)	Mean	6.5 (1.3)
Median	5.0	Median	7.0
Range	2–8	Range	3–8
Frequency of any pain		Frequency of worst pain	
Almost constantly	25 (40%)	Almost constantly	13 (21%)
Frequently	17 (27%)	Frequently	21 (33%)
Intermittently	15 (24%)	Intermittently	15 (24%)
Occasionally	4 (6%)	Occasionally	8 (13%)
Rarely	2 (3%)	Rarely	6 (10%)
Site of worst or only pain		Quality of worst or only pain	
Abdomen	32 (51%)	Sharp	14 (22%)
Lower back	9 (14%)	Aching	16 (25%)
Pelvis	6 (10%)	Pressing/squeezing	9 (14%)
Rectal/genital	3 (5%)	Crampy	8 (13%)
Shoulder/upper back	3 (5%)	Radiating	8 (13%)
Leg	2 (3%)	Other	8 (13%)
Other	8 (13%)		

* VAS represents a 100-mm visual analogue scale anchored by "no pain" at one end and "worst possible pain" at the other end.
† VRS represents an 8-point verbal rating scale, where 5 corresponds to "moderate," 6 corresponds to "strong," 7 corresponds to "severe," and 8 corresponds to "excruciating."
(Courtesy of Portenoy RK, Kornblith AB, Wong G, et al: *Cancer* 74:907–915, 1994.)

▶ This thorough evaluation of pain and symptoms in patients undergoing treatment for ovarian cancer effectively documents the significance of pain. Although the location of the tumor was in the abdominopelvic region, the symptoms in these patients were localized to the site of disease; pain was associated with advanced disease in the majority of patients. Validating the importance of pain descriptors, these patients consistently reported moderate-to-severe symptoms that were characterized as a frequent-to-constant aching or cramping abdominal pain. Despite the presence of these symptoms and the fact that 75% of the population was composed of inpatients,

TABLE 2.—Pain Interference With Function (n = 63)

	No. (%) of patients reporting moderate or greater pain-related interference
Activity	43 (68)
Mood	39 (62)
Walking	35 (56)
Work	39 (62)
Social relations	21 (33)
Sleep	33 (52)
Life enjoyment	38 (61)

(Courtesy of Portenoy RK, Kornblith AB, Wong G, et al: *Cancer* 74:907–915, 1994.)

the Karnofsky Performance Status (KPS) was 80 or greater in 80% of the patients studied. The KPS (P < .0001) and the extent of tumor (P =.02) proved to be the most significant predictors of the severity of pain on multiple linear regression analysis. More important, 90% of the patients were able to achieve moderate-to-complete relief of pain with analgesics.

Symptoms, including pain, continue to be a sensitive marker of disease activity in patients with cancer. This activity includes cancers that more frequently arise in, or secondarily invade, viscera. Pain related to visceral involvement can also be effectively managed in the majority of patients.—N.A. Janjan, M.D.

Pain Characteristics of Advanced Lung Cancer Patients Referred to a Palliative Care Service

Mercadante S, Armata M, Salvaggio L (Buccheri La Ferla Hospital FBF, Palermo, Italy; Pain Relief and Palliative Care, SAMOT, Palermo, Italy)

Pain 59:141–145, 1994 131-95-3–2

Background.—Lung cancer, the most common of all cancers, accounts for one fourth of all cancer deaths in the United States. In most patients, the disease is so advanced that treatment focuses on their symptoms, particularly pain. Because there are few data on the topic of pain, patients with lung cancer were followed up until death for information on the prevalence, characteristics, and location of pain.

Methods.—Sixty consecutive patients with advanced lung cancer were studied. The pain mechanisms were categorized on the basis of history, physical examination, anatomical site, primary tumor and distant metastases, and other tests. The treatment was evaluated periodically by using the Opioid Escalation Index (OEI) and the Effective Analgesic Score (EAS). A nurse determined the visual analogue scale (VAS). Three classes of responses were identified: good (slow increase in the EAS); mild (low VAS, but a rapid increase in the EAS or OEI); and ineffective (high VAS).

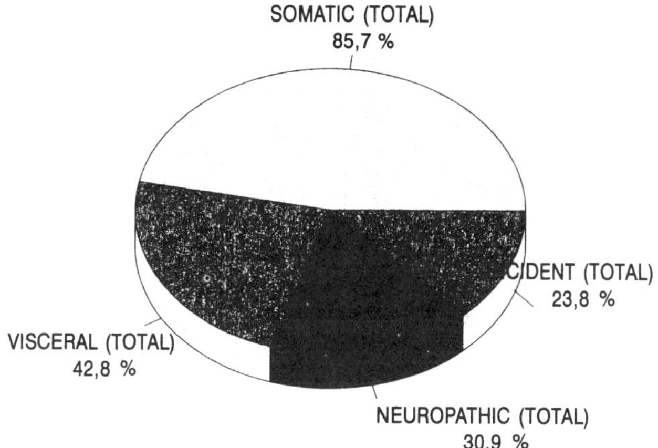

Fig 3–1.—Pain mechanisms. (Courtesy of Mercadante S, Armata M, Salvaggio L: *Pain* 59:141–145, 1994.)

Findings.—Complete data were obtained on 52 patients. The average period of observation was 51 days, and 46 of the patients (88%) experienced pain. The principal sites of metastases, in descending order of occurence, were chest wall, brain, nodes, pleura, and liver. The pain was localized to the chest, legs/lumbar, abdomen/arms and head. The pain mechanisms were differentiated as somatic, visceral, neuropathic, and incident (Fig 3–1). The EASs for 8 weeks before death are shown in Figure 3–2. Pain relief was good in 24 patients, mild in 12, and poor in 6.

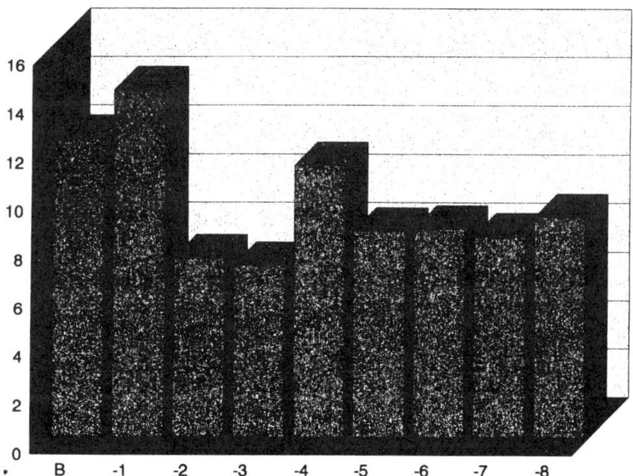

Fig 3–2.—Mean effective analgesic scores for 40 patients from referral to 1 day before death. The values are expressed as mean ± standard deviation. *B* represents the score 1 day before death; −1, 1 week before death; −2, 2 weeks before death; −3, 3 weeks before death, etc. (Courtesy of Mercadante S, Armata M, Salvaggio L: *Pain* 59:141–145, 1994.)

Comment.—Pain in patients with lung cancer was similar in prevalence to pain in the general cancer population, with the chest being the most common site. Incident pain seemed to influence the outcome of using recognized treatments. The picture will be more complete with data on the characteristics of opioid-resistant and responsive pain for each cancer syndrome.

▶ This report correlates the symptoms and effectiveness of analgesic therapy with disease extension. Because the majority of patients with lung cancer have locally advanced disease, the prevalence of pain in more than 90% of these patients is significant. Most patients have complex pain presentations, including somatic, visceral, and neuropathic types. Although neuropathic pain was identified in 31% of the cases, 86% of patients also experienced somatic pain. As stated in other reports, only 40% of the patients had adequate management of cancer-related pain; however, adequacy of pain management was not influenced by the type of pain. Given the frequency of lung cancer, optimization of pain management is not only achievable, despite the complex nature of the pain syndromes, but it is also imperative.—N.A. Janjan, M.D.

Hodgkin Disease of the Spine Presenting As Alcohol-Related Pain: A Case Report and Review of the Literature

Callahan BC, Coe R, Place HM (Fitzsimons Army Med Ctr, Aurora, Colo; DeWitt Army Community Hosp, Fort Belvoir, Va)

J Bone Joint Surg (Am) 76–A:119–121, 1994 131-95-3–3

Objective.—A patient with an unusual, alcohol-related pain in the back secondary to Hodgkin's disease was studied.

Case Report.—Woman, 29, complained of a 4-month history of dull, aching, low-back pain radiating to the anterior part of the right thigh. Pain was associated with ingestion of a small amount of alcohol. Magnetic resonance imaging of the lumbar spine revealed an infiltrative lesion of the second lumbar vertebral body, with extension into the pedicles; a Craig-needle biopsy specimen was consistent with Hodgkin's lymphoma of the nodular sclerosing type. Complete remission was achieved with chemotherapy, and the pain in the back disappeared completely.

Discussion.—A neoplasm should be considered in the differential diagnosis of pain in the back, particularly when pain is precipitated by the ingestion of alcohol. In an evaluation of 1,060 patients with cancer, Brewin noted alcohol-related pain in 31% of the patients with Hodgkin's disease. Atkinson et al. noted that 7% of 506 patients with Hodgkin's disease had pain after the ingestion of alcohol, including 20% with osseous involvement. Alcohol-induced pain in Hodgkin's disease often involves female patients and is associated with unfavorable prognostic factors (e.g., systemic symptoms, stage II disease with involvement of multiple sites, or stage III or IV disease). Nodular sclerosis is the predominant histologic type of Hodgkin's disease in patients with alcohol-induced pain.

▶ This case report demonstrates the importance of evaluating pain as a symptom of an underlying medical problem. Although the patient in this case report had a low overall risk for a malignancy, the history of alcohol-related pain is typical for Hodgkin's disease. Bony metastases, however, are rare in Hodgkin's disease, even when there is extensive mediastinal involvement. Despite the unusual presentation, this case report emphasizes that pain should be diagnostically evaluated to determine its etiology and the necessary treatment.—N.A. Janjan, M.D.

Patient-Related Barriers to Management of Cancer Pain in Puerto Rico

Ward SE, Hernandez L (Univ of Wisconsin, Madison; Univ of Puerto Rico, San Juan)

Pain 58:233–238, 1994 131-95-3-4

Background.—Hispanics reportedly receive less medication for their pain than do non-Hispanic Caucasians. In studies of non-Hispanic Caucasians, patients with more concerns about reporting pain and using analgesics tend to use less-than-adequate medication. Both the extent to which Puerto Ricans with cancer have concerns about analgesia and the relationship between these concerns and the adequacy of pain medication used were examined.

Methods.—Demographic data are given for the 263 ambulatory oncology patients older than 21 years who completed the questionnaires (Table 1). The instruments used included the Barriers Questionnaire (BQ-PR), which measures 8 concerns: fear of addiction, fear of developing tolerance, belief in the inevitability of pain with cancer, belief that side effects may outweigh advantages, belief that good patients do not complain, worry that physician will be distracted from treating the disease, belief that increased pain indicates disease progression, and fear of injection (0 = do not agree at all, 5 = agree very much). The Brief Pain Inventory (BPI) allows self-assessment of pain severity and the extent to which pain interferes with activity (0 = no pain, 10 = worst imaginable pain). The Pain Management Index (PMI) compares the most efficacious analgesic *actually used* to the level of reported pain.

Results.—Descriptive information given regarding the severity of pain was analyzed via the BPI (Table 2). The BQ-PR study showed that 90% of participants had at least some agreement with each of the 8 listed concerns; tolerance and disease progression factors were most heavily regarded. All mean scores were near the scale midpoint. Inverse relationships between education and income level and BQ-PR scores were sig-

TABLE 1.—Demographic Information (n = 263)

	n	%
Marital status		
Married	160	(61%)
Widowed	42	(16%)
Separated/divorced	33	(13%)
Single	27	(10%)
Income		
<$5000	132	(50%)
5–9000	85	(32%)
10–14,000	20	(8%)
15–24,000	15	(6%)
>$25,000	10	(4%)
Religion		
Catholic	172	(65%)
Evangelical	33	(13%)
Pentecostal	18	(7%)
Baptist	11	(4%)
No religion	4	(1.5%)
Other	25	(9.5%)
Education		
<8th grade	98	(37%)
Completed 8th grade	22	(8%)
Some high school	45	(17%)
High school graduate	46	(18%)
Some college	21	(8%)
College grad	21	(8%)
Missing data	10	(4%)

(Courtesy of Ward SE, Hernandez L: *Pain* 58:233–238, 1994.)

nificant. Of patients who had cancer-related pain on the day of questioning, those using adequate analgesic medication had lower BQ-PR scores.

Conclusion.—Although a high level of concern exists among Hispanics, particularly those of low socioeconomic status, regarding analgesic use, we do not know if these concerns contribute to the fact that Hispanics receive less adequate management of pain than do non-Hispanics. Because a large percentage of patients in pain were using analgesics that were not effective, the assessment and prescribing behavior of health care professionals should be examined along with patient compliance. Improvement of clinical management of cancer-related pain in Puerto Rico should include educational efforts to address patients' concerns.

▶ Cultural factors influence both the patient and physician, and they have been shown to affect the adequacy of cancer pain management. Patients with cancer in Puerto Rico were evaluated to determine possible factors in

TABLE 2.—Mean (SD) Pain Severity and Interference With Life

Scale	Full sample (n = 263)		Subsample (n = 70)†	
	Mean	SD	Mean	SD
Interference	2.83	2.90	4.60	2.79
Worst pain	3.76	3.56	5.89	3.15
Least pain	2.34	2.61	3.60	2.65
Average pain	2.60	2.76	4.49	2.84
Now pain	2.24	2.90	3.96	3.26

Note: Range for these scales is 0–10.
* Persons reporting cancer pain on the day they completed the questionnaire.
(Courtesy of Ward SE, Hernandez L: *Pain* 58:233-238, 1994.)

the Hispanic culture that might affect the treatment of cancer-related pain. This study identified 3 important barriers to the management of cancer pain. First, 90% of patients expressed concern about the use of analgesics. It is important that patients with cancer who had pain described greater concerns about use of analgesics than did patients who were prescribed adequate analgesics and had achieved control of their cancer-related pain. Second, socioeconomic status significantly influenced attitudes about cancer pain management. Third, these findings are consistent with those from previous studies. Although these barriers exist for all cultural and socioeconomic levels, they are less profound in higher socioeconomic levels and in non-Hispanic Caucasian populations. Informing patients, their families, and society is as critical as the education of health care professionals in overcoming barriers to the control of cancer-related pain.—N.A. Janjan, M.D.

Subacute Sensory Neuropathy Associated With Hodgkin's Disease

Plante-Bordeneuve V, Baudrimont M, Gorin NC, Gherardi RK (Inst of Neurology, London; Hôpital Saint-Antoine, Paris; Hôpital Henri Mondor, Créteil, France)

J Neurol Sci 121:155–158, 1994 131-95-3-5

Introduction.—Only .1% to 2% of the patients with malignant lymphomas experience peripheral neuropathies, which are most rare in patients with Hodgkin's disease (HD). Two patients with subacute predominantly sensory neuropathy were recently treated for HD, and their neuropathy was relieved as well.

Case 1.—Woman, 55, was found to have stage IVB nodular-sclerosis HD. After receiving chemotherapy, she achieved complete remission. Three years after the initial diagnosis, she complained of progressive bilateral toe numbness, paresthesia in her left hand, and difficulty in walking. She had lost pinprick sensation in all 4 limbs, toe-joint position sense, pallesthesia to the hips, limb tendon reflexes, and had leg weakness. Electrophysiologic examination suggested axonal neuropathy. A lumbar magnetic resonance imaging examination revealed an enlarged prevertebral lymph node, which was removed. Histologic examination confirmed a relapse of HD. With chemotherapy, bone marrow transplantation, and the withdrawal of steroid therapy, her neurologic function returned to normal.

Case 2.—Woman, 40, reported paresthesia in the first 3 fingers of each hand and in the toes, as well as intermittent facial paresthesia. Electrophysiologic examination suggested axonal neuropathy. After 6 months, a mediastinal lymph node biopsy revealed stage IIA nodular sclerosing HD and hyperplasia suggestive of Castleman's disease. The symptoms resolved after tumor resection without steroid therapy. With chemotherapy, transient distal paresthesia returned, associated with vincristine therapy. A gait disorder and facial paralysis developed, which were associated with a herpes zoster infection. She was treated with acyclovir and prednisone and all symptoms resolved.

Discussion.—In both patients, the symptoms of sensory neuropathy and areflexia improved after the tumor was removed. The clinical findings in these patients and the responsiveness of the symptoms to treatment of the underlying tumor suggest that these patients experienced a variant of an HD-associated inflammatory demyelinating polyneuropathy and not a true paraneoplastic sensory ganglionitis.

▶ This article demonstrates the diagnostic sensitivity of pain in malignancy. These 2 case reports describe clinical presentations that are typical for subacute sensory neuropathy associated with Hodgkin's disease. This inflammatory demyelinating polyneuropathy represents another sensitive marker of disease activity. Pain is an important symptom that should be diagnostically evaluated in patients with cancer.—N.A. Janjan, M.D.

Pain and Its Treatment in Outpatients With Metastatic Cancer

Cleeland CS, Gonin R, Hatfield AK, Edmonson JH, Blum RH, Stewart JA, Pandya KJ (Univ of Wisconsin, Madison; Dana-Farber Cancer Inst, Boston; Carle Cancer Ctr, Urbana, Ill; et al)

N Engl J Med 330:592–596, 1994 131-95-3-6

Background.—Pain in patients with cancer, even when treated, is often severe enough to impair functioning. Both patients and health care providers agree that pain is frequently managed poorly. The proportion of patients with cancer who have moderate-to-severe pain, the adequacy of the treatment administered, and the characteristics of patients at the greatest risk of undermedication with analgesic drugs were determined.

Methods.—Fifty-four centers contributed data on a total of 1,308 outpatients with metastatic cancer. The patients rated their pain severity in the preceding week, the degree of pain-related functional impairment, and the degree of relief provided by analgesic agents. Physicians also provided data on the causes of pain, described the pain treatment, and gave their estimations of the relative severity and impact of pain on the patient's ability to function.

Findings.—Sixty-seven percent of the patients said they had experienced pain or taken analgesics daily during the preceding week. Thirty-six percent had functional impairments caused by pain. Forty-two percent of patients with pain did not receive adequate analgesic treatment. Patients treated at centers serving mostly minority populations were 3 times more likely to have insufficient pain management than patients treated elsewhere. A discrepancy between patient and physician in judging the severity of pain predicted insufficient pain management. Other factors predicting insufficient pain treatment included physician assessment that the pain was not attributed to cancer, better performance status, age of 70 years of more, and female gender. Patients with less adequate analgesia had less relief and greater functional impairment.

Conclusions.—Many patients with cancer have considerable pain and receive inadequate analgesia, despite published guidelines for pain management. Most of the patients with pain in this series had pain that was severe enough to impair functioning.

▶ The significance of this report is the continued failure to adequately treat cancer-related pain, even in facilities affiliated with a National Cancer Institute Oncology Study Group. Treatment strategies, and the medical and ethical imperatives involved in cancer pain management, were championed more than 10 years ago by the World Health Organization. Recently, these principles were reinforced by the publication of *Cancer Pain Guidelines*, produced by the Agency for Health Care Policy and Research for the management of cancer-related pain. Evaluations like these demonstrate the continued need for education to overcome knowledge deficits and attitudinal barriers that obstruct the adequate treatment of pain caused by cancer. Such studies not only document the inadequacy of cancer pain management but, also, provide the information needed to affect change in clinical practice through the mechanisms of professional education and quality assurance.—N.A. Janjan, M.D.

Socioeconomics

Cost Issues Related to Pain Management: Report From the Cancer Pain Panel of the Agency for Health Care Policy and Research

Ferrell BR, Griffith H (City of Hope Natl Med Ctr, Duarte, Calif; Office of Disease Prevention and Health Promotion, Washington, DC)

J Pain Symptom Manage 9:221–234, 1994 131-95-3-7

Background.—During the past 10 years, the clinical problem of unrelieved pain has received increased attention, with emphasis placed on both cancer and acute postoperative pain. The previously neglected areas of pain assessment, pharmacologic treatment, and the knowledge and attitudes of health care providers have been addressed by various organizations, including the World Health Organization, the National Cancer Institute, and the American Pain Society, among others. However, health policy issues associated with pain, such as areas of cost, access to care, regulatory perspectives, and ethical and legal issues, have also been overlooked. The Agency for Health Care Policy and Research (AHCPR) has developed a 13-point framework in an attempt to begin examining costs associated with pain. These 13 areas of cost analysis were described, as were directions for further health policy research related to pain management.

Discussion.—The AHCPR framework was designed to isolate specific cost issues, identify what is known in these areas, and address implications for future research. Included within this framework are the following issues involving the cost of oral medications; parenteral and spinal analgesics; personnel; surgical and anesthetic procedures; radiation therapy; unrelieved pain at home; nondrug interventions; various types of care settings; morbidity; justification of services; reimbursement biases; conflict of interest; and indirect costs to patients and families. At present, most areas of cost associated with pain are unsupported by research. However, treatment advances for acute and chronic pain should be based on both clinical standards of care and cost data to provide maximum benefits and minimal harm to the patient and the global health care system. The AHCPR framework has helped identify areas of cost analysis essential to exploring pain management within a cost-constrained system.

Conclusions.—Patterns of practice must consider costs as well as overall outcomes for patients, family caregivers, and the health care system. The best care is provided when standards are set and guidelines such as those devised by the AHCPR provide a basis for practice.

▶ Socioeconomic changes are greatly influencing medical care. These factors also must be evaluated in cancer pain management to ensure that palliation is achieved in the most cost-effective manner. The most important factors involve treatment-related morbidity, the efficiency and degree of pain relief, and functional outcome. Cost evaluations should give a higher relative value to efficiency and efficacy of therapy when overall factor analysis is performed. Although palliation represents noncurative therapy, the ethical responsibility to relieve suffering mandates the need for optimal cancer pain management. Analyses of cost-effectiveness should critically evaluate patterns of care for specific clinical presentations. As in other disciplines, treatment must be justified by outcome because the most wasteful expenditure of health care and personal resources is ineffective therapy.—N.A. Janjan, M.D.

Minnesota Population Cancer Risk

Kennedy BJ, Bushhouse SA, Bender AP (Univ of Minnesota, Minneapolis; Minnesota Cancer Surveillance System, Minneapolis; Minnesota Dept of Health, Minneapolis)

Cancer 73:724–729, 1994 131-95-3–8

Background.—The Minnesota Cancer Surveillance System (MCSS) was established in 1988. The aim of this system was to provide timely and accurate data on newly diagnosed cancers among state residents. Between 1988 and 1990, more than 62% of reported cancers had occurred in individuals older than 65 years of age, and 72% of the cancer-related deaths were within this age group. The impact of cancer incidence on the rapidly growing older population and the accumulative lifetime risk of cancer pose a significant health care problem for patients with cancer in the coming years. Population cancer risk (PCR) was determined as a measure of the number of cancers that will occur in the lifetime of 1,000 individuals.

Methods.—Nearly 98.6% of all cancer diagnoses among Minnesota residents are reported by pathologists to the MCSS. Statistical methods were used to estimate the total number of cancers that will be diagnosed in the lifetime of 1,000 individuals, based on the Minnesota cancer and life expectancy rates reported from 1988 to 1990.

Results.—New cancers were diagnosed in 53,729 residents. Estimates of the total number of cancers expected in the lifetime of 1,000 individuals born today include 494 malignancies in males, and 430 malignancies in females. In males and females, the total number of prostate and breast cancers, respectively, exceeds the total number expected for lung, colon, and rectal cancers. The overall PCR is 459 cancers per 1,000 lifetimes, or 45,900 cancers per 100,000 lifetimes. By the year 2020, cancer will develop in more than 100,000 living Minnesota residents.

Conclusions.—Because a significantly greater proportion of our population is reaching the age where the risk of cancer is greatest, further knowledge of geriatric cancer care will be required. In addition, the need for facilities will become major public health, bioethical, economic, and social issues.

▶ This represents an important socioeconomic study of the future demands for health care, as indicated by population-based, projected risks for cancer. As a greater proportion of our population reaches the age of highest risk for cancer, the health care system will need to be prepared to meet these demands for cancer therapy. Proportionate needs for health care will also change because the cancer incidence will be relatively greater as the risk of cardiovascular disease continues to decrease. As changes in the health care system evolve, projections of the incidence of cancer within the population must be considered in decisions that affect allocation of resources and availability of care.—N.A. Janjan, M.D.

The Economics of Dying: The Illusion of Cost Savings at the End of Life

Emanuel EJ, Emanuel LL (Dana-Farber Cancer Inst, Boston; Harvard Med School, Boston)

N Engl J Med 330:540–544, 1994 131-95-3-9

Background.—Advance directives and hospice care have been proposed as means for decreasing medical costs at the end of life. Numerous survey results indicate that Americans do not wish to be kept alive if they receive diagnoses of irreversible diseases. Thus, it is argued that if physicians would eliminate the use of high-technology interventions at the end of life, patient autonomy would be respected and tens of billions of dollars could be saved. The persistent interest in saving money at the end of life via advance directives and hospice care makes it essential to determine how much money might realistically be saved.

Discussion.—At present, the cost savings that could be realized through the wider use of advance directives, hospice care, and curtailment of futile care have not been extensively studied. However, the available information indicates that such cost savings are not likely to be substantial. At most, the amount that could be saved by decreasing aggressive, life-sustaining interventions is 3.3% of total national care expenditures. In 1993, this savings would have amounted to $29.7 billion of the $900 billion allocated for health care. This savings, however, would not curb the rate of growth of health care spending, and this amount represents only a fraction of the increase caused by inflation in health care costs. Additionally, less than $50 to $90 billion are needed to cover the uninsured population. There remain many good reasons to fund hospice care, use advance directives, and use less aggressive life-sustaining treatments at the end of life, even though substantial savings in health care costs are not likely. These reasons include respect for patient wishes, reduction of pain and suffering, and the administration of compassionate and dignified care at the end of life. Cutting the amount spent on life-sustaining interventions to reduce overall health care costs is probably futile.

Conclusions.—At present, options for obtaining substantial savings in health care costs appear to be confined to major changes in the financing and delivery of care that require difficult choices in the allocation of services. Regardless of what type of reform in the health care system is chosen, it should be understood that advance directives and less aggressive care at the end of life will not solve the financial difficulties associated with the current health care system.

▶ This significant article supports the treatment of cancer-related pain through cost-benefit analysis. The study emphasizes the principles of hospice care that place great importance on maintaining patient dignity through the process of dying. In addition to the ethical considerations in terminal care are the issues of burgeoning health care costs in the United States. This analysis indicates that the cost of terminal care represents a small fraction of the overall cost for health care in this country. To have a significant impact on the increasing cost of medical therapy, other aspects of the health care delivery system should be considered for cost reductions. Terminal care, which provides relief of suffering, is cost-effective and provides the ethical administration of medical care.—N.A. Janjan, M.D.

Are Health-Care Reimbursement Policies a Barrier to Acute and Cancer Pain Management?
Joranson DE (Univ of Wisconsin, Madison)
J Pain Symptom Manage 9:244–253, 1994 131-95-3–10

Background.—Failure to relieve acute postoperative or cancer pain has been reported in one half or more of the patients in the United States. Whether reimbursement factors act as barriers to acute and cancer pain management was determined through a review of United States health care policy and recent literature.

Discussion.—Although systematic outcome research is minimal, the available evidence indicates that lack of coverage and uneven reimbursement policies for health care, including prescription drugs, medical equipment, and professional services, limits access to acute and cancer pain management for millions of citizens. This is particularly noteworthy in poor, elderly, and minority populations. Although low-income individuals eligible for Medicaid have access to health care services, some states have restrictions that inhibit appropriate medication use and encourage more costly forms of pain therapy. A review of Medicare reimbursement policies also showed that more expensive and intensive forms of pain management may be favored. Private health insurance coverage for pain-related services and products varies. Some plans do not cover outpatient pain medications; those that do may be limited by co-payments, deductibles, exclusions, and caps. Mail-order pharmacies, used by some plans, may restrict the amount of opioids dispensed to patients, despite the amount ordered by a physician and deemed medically necessary. For patients with cancer in particular, the amount of analgesics needed may vary significantly with the often rapid changes in clinical status. In HMO plans, restrictive drug benefits are common, although they are infrequently disclosed in advertising materials. This hampers consumer ability to make an informed decision concerning coverage. At present, there are certain programs that assist the medically indigent to obtain outpatient prescription drug coverage. Both the Pharmaceutical Manufacturers Association and the United States Senate have compiled directories of indigent patient program initiatives sponsored by various companies. The American Cancer Society and certain patient care facilities, such as New York's Cancer Care, Inc., are other referral sources for indigent cancer patients. Participation in these programs is currently unknown, although it is probably quite limited.

Conclusions.—Pain management is receiving increased attention in the public sphere. Accordingly, reimbursement for acute and cancer pain management should be reviewed and addressed in current efforts to reform national health care policy.

▶ The reimbursement policies for pain management are reviewed, and the significance of these policies are analyzed. Unless these issues are addressed, necessary medications and procedures will not be available to a large segment of patients. Restrictive reimbursement policies may prove to be the most significant of the barriers to controlling pain. Efforts to educate health care professionals in pain management may be undermined by restrictive reimbursement policies that do not allow the health care professional to provide adequate pain management. Inadequate therapy still retains cost at no benefit to the patient. Additionally, the physician becomes liable for prescribing inadequate therapy. Economic issues are critical to patients and health care professionals in these times of health system reform. These issues must be evaluated and reported so that care, including pain management, is not compromised.—N.A. Janjan, M.D.

Quality of Life

Pain Measurement in Cancer Patients: A Comparison of Six Methods

De Conno F, Caraceni A, Gamba A, Mariani L, Abbattista A, Brunelli C, La Mura A, Ventafridda V (Natl Cancer Inst of Milan, Italy; San Gerardo Hosp, Monza, Italy)

Pain 57:161–166, 1994 131-95-3–11

Introduction.—Pain is a complex personal experience involving neurophysiologic and psychological mechanisms, with its perception and expression affected by cultural and other variables. Several tools, however, have been successful in objectively quantifying the subjective experience of pain. Six different pain-intensity scales were evaluated in a group of patients with chronic cancer pain.

Methods.—The patient group included 28 men and 25 women with a mean age of 53.9 years. All had been given a diagnosis of a definite cancer pain syndrome. Pain was evaluated by a trained nurse using 5 instruments: a vertical visual analogue scale (VAS) ranging from extremes of "no pain" to "the worst pain imaginable"; an 11-point numerical rating scale (NRS) of 0–13; a 6-level verbal rating scale (VRS); the Italian Pain Questionnaire (PRI), a version of the McGill Pain Questionnaire; and the Integrated Pain Score (IPS), a measure that combines intensity and duration of pain. These scales were administered before and at least 2 days after a change in pain treatment. A pain relief scale (IRS) with 5 categories (0%, < 50%, 50%, > 50%, and 100%) was administered at the second evaluation. Principal factor analysis (PFA) was used to assess the relative and concurrent validity of the 5 pain intensity measures and the degree of association of changes in these 5 measures with the IRS score.

Results and Conclusion.—The 6 scales were used by the patients with chronic cancer pain as though they were measuring a single underlying construct. A single factor clearly emerged from PFA, indicating that a change in these measures could be interpreted clinically. The IPS was found to be a reliable instrument for quantifying pain in the patient with cancer. Logistic regression analysis demonstrated VAS, NRS, and VRS to be more strongly associated with IRS than with PRI and IPS. Quantification of cancer pain is important for determining how analgesic drugs work and in optimizing clinical analgesia.

▶ In the literature on pain, a variety of instruments are noted to be used to quantify pain. This abstract represents an ambitious study that directly compares 5 different pain-intensity scales, including the VAS, the NRS, a VRS, a version of the McGill Pain Questionnaire, and a newly developed IPS. The IRS, administered only after completion of therapy, was correlated with the pain intensity scales listed above. The following, as summarized by the authors, characterizes salient differences among these scales. The VAS, NRS, and VRS require the patient to determine the average amount of pain experienced. The IPS allows patients to relate variable levels of pain throughout the day. The McGill Pain Questionnaire requires a forced rather than a free choice of descriptors and places greater emphasis on the sensorial dimension. A high degree of association among variables was observed on multifactorial analysis. However, the IRS was most closely associated with the VAS, NRS, and VRS scales on logistic regression. The authors emphasize that the choice of pain measurement scales in research should match the design of the study, the clinical aim, or both. Comparative evaluation of these pain assessment scales should continue to determine further the aspects of pain that are best measured by each of these methods.—N.A. Janjan, M.D.

Concerns About Reporting Pain and Using Analgesics: A Comparison of Persons With and Without Cancer

Ward S, Gatwood J (Univ of Wisconsin, Madison; Meriter Hosp, Madison, Wis)

Cancer Nurs 17:200–206, 1994 131-95-3–12

Background.—A majority of patients with advanced disease, malignant or benign, have moderate-to-severe pain. Many of them may not be adequately treated because they are reluctant to report pain or to use analgesics. Patients may be concerned about addiction, or they may hold a fatalistic belief that pain is an unavoidable result of cancer. Concern about side effects or a belief that the physician may be deterred from taking curative measures also may preclude adequate treatment of pain.

Objective and Methods.—The Barriers Questionnaire (BQ) is designed to determine the extent to which patients hold these beliefs about pain associated with disease. Forty individuals from community groups and 53 clinic patients with cancer, ranging from 20 to 79 years of age, completed the BQ as well as single-item measures of hesitance in reporting pain and using analgesics. The BQ was administered twice at an interval of 1 week.

Findings.—Responses to the BQ could not be related to either age or educational level. The only significant gender difference involved higher fatalism scores in men. Total BQ scores did not differ between research subjects with or without cancer, and there were no impressive differences in subscale scores. Responses to the BQ remained quite stable over time, with a correlation coefficient of .9. On retesting, respondents who said they hesitated to report pain had relatively high BQ scores.

Conclusions.—Interventions designed to overcome barriers to effective pain management should be examined in both community and patients settings. The BQ is a reliable measure of beliefs about disease-related pain.

▶ A number of factors have been recognized that prevent patients from reporting the pain they experience. These factors include 1) fatalism that nothing can or will be done about the pain; 2) fears of drug addiction; 3) concerns about side effects resulting from the use of analgesic agents; 4) concerns about alienating the medical staff by complaining; 5) concerns that the evaluation or treatment of the pain will interfere with treatment of the cancer; 6) denial—pain represents progression of the disease; 7) concerns about tolerance—saving the analgesics for when they are really needed; and 8) fears about injection of analgesics.

This study compared the survey responses of patients with cancer with those of adults who had never been given a diagnosis of cancer. The most significant finding was the consistent concern about reporting or treating pain, even after the diagnosis of cancer. These data indicate that the general population has significant and unwavering concerns about the treatment of cancer-related pain.

Consideration should be given to the reason that patients with cancer do not alter their perspective on the management of cancer-related pain. Two underlying issues may encompass the listed factors and contribute to the failure of cancer patients to change their attitudes about cancer pain management. The first involves hope. Patients maintain hope that their disease is being actively treated and controlled; anticipating that they will be cured, patients do not wish to be rendered incompetent or addicted to drugs once cured. The second factor relates to the desire to maintain independence. Requiring therapy for pain and having increased dependence on the medical staff result in a further loss of autonomy and increase the perception of dysfunction. Other studies have indicated that only when the clinical condition is acknowledged as hopeless do physicians prescribe—and patients with cancer accept—opioid analgesics. Addressing the concerns about cancer pain management and emphasizing pain control as an integral part of cancer therapy may relieve silent suffering and significantly improve the quality of life of cancer patients.—N.A. Janjan, M.D.

Symptom Control in Terminally Ill Patients With Malignant Bowel Obstruction (MBO)

Fainsinger RL, Spachynski K, Hanson J, Bruera E (Univ of Alberta, Edmonton, Canada)

J Pain Symptom Manage 9:12–18, 1994 131-95-3-13

Objective.—Prolonged conservative management using nasogastric suction and IV fluids for malignant bowel obstruction (MBO) does not provide significant palliation. Previous reports have outlined an approach to MBO that focuses on the main distressing symptoms, of pain, nausea, and vomiting. Based on these reports and clinical experience, a basic approach to the management of MBO on the Palliative Care Unit was outlined.

Patients.—In a review of 100 consecutive patients who died while in the Unit, 15 who required medical management for bowel obstruction were identified. Their mean length of stay was 25 days, compared with 31 days for the overall patient group; symptomatic MBO was treated for a mean of 18 days. Twelve had previous abdominal surgery, and 5 had palliative surgery for bowel obstruction. Ten of the 15, who were not candidates for surgery, died with complete bowel obstruction. Patients were treated with opioids, median dose equivalent of 64 mg/day; dexamethasone, median dose of 40 mg/day; and various drugs for nausea. Percutaneous gastrostomy was used in 4 patients. Seven patients became delirious and were managed with haloperidol. Hydration with hypodermoclysis was performed in all patients.

Conclusions.—For patients with MBO, intensive medical management can yield good symptomatic control without the need for IV lines and with minimal need for nasogastric tubes. Management includes high doses of corticosteroids, the use of percutaneous gastrostomy, and hydration by hypodermoclysis. Further studies are needed to define the value of somatostatin analogues in these patients.

▶ Malignant bowel obstruction can cause significant suffering, and, often, patients are not candidates for surgery. Adequate medical management, then, is imperative. Morphine and corticosteroids are important in the management of abdominal pain. This report emphasizes that percutaneous gastrostomy tubes are preferable to nasogastric tubes, which are poorly tolerated, are sometimes difficult to place, and often fall out or become blocked. The electrolyte abnormalities associated with MBO were also studied. Hyponatremia was the most common abnormality and was a poor prognostic factor. Symptom control, as assessed by a visual analogue scale in this study, can be achieved in MBO with adequate medical management.—N.A. Janjan, M.D.

Pain in Hospitalized Patients With AIDS: Analgesic and Psychotropic Medications

Lebovits AH, Smith G, Maignan M, Lefkowitz M (State Univ of New York, Brooklyn; Harbor Univ of Calif at Los Angeles Med Ctr, Torrence)

Clin J Pain 10:156–161, 1994 131-95-3–14

Background.—Recent findings indicate that pain can alter human immune function. Accordingly, increased attention has been given to the prevalence and management of pain in patients with AIDS. The use of analgesic and psychotropic medication in patients with AIDS was assessed, and whether previous findings of a high prevalence of pain in patients with AIDS who were hospitalized could be duplicated was determined. In addition, other factors related to pain were investigated, including death during hospital stay, IV drug use, and length of hospital stay.

Patients and Methods.—The medical records of 139 patients with AIDS were randomly selected from 909 hospital admissions occurring during a 12-month period. The mean patient age was 35.7 years, and the median time from diagnosis to admission was 7.5 months. Records were systematically reviewed for pain notations, prescription of analgesic and psychotropic medication, disease characteristics, and patient demographics.

Results.—At least 1 note of nonprocedural pain was found in 61% of the records. A non-narcotic agent, the most common of which was acetaminophen, was prescribed for 68% of the patients with pain. Narcotic agents were given to 44% of the patients. Analgesics and psychotropic medication, particularly a sedative-hypnotic, were significantly more likely to be given to patients with, as opposed to those without, pain. Aside from length of hospital stay, no significant associations between pain and factors such as IV drug abuse were noted. Although most of the previous study findings were replicated, the rate of prescribed psychotropic medications and acetaminophen was substantially increased in the present investigation.

Conclusions.—Although pain is a frequent problem in hospitalized patients with AIDS, narcotics and antidepressants appear to be underprescribed. Further education pertaining to pain management in patients with AIDS may facilitate a more aggressive treatment approach.

▶ Pain is a common problem in patients with cancer, and this study shows that it is also as prevalent among patients with AIDS who are hospitalized. More than 60% of patients reported pain, but only 84% of these patients received an analgesic. Of the patients who received an analgesic, 44% were prescribed a narcotic to treat their pain. Factors such as IV drug abuse did not predict for pain, but the length of hospital stay was associated with the level of pain. The types and locations of pain that were documented included the chest (21%); headache (17%); abdomen (12%); oral cavity (10%); musculoskeletal/generalized aching (20%); and low back pain (5%). Pain can be a significant issue in patients with AIDS, given the wide-ranging sequelae of the disease, including infection, mucositis, and malignancy. This report documents the frequency and type of pain experienced by patients with AIDS, and the authors conclude that pain in this patient group is also undertreated.—N.A. Janjan, M.D.

The Ethics of Pain Management for Cancer Patients: Case Studies and Analysis

Hammes BJ, Cain JM (Lutheran Hosp-La Crosse, Wisconsin; Univ of Washington, Seattle)

J Pain Symptom Manage 9:166–170, 1994 131-95-3–15

Introduction.—The fear of pain often turns into reality for patients with cancer, many of whom do not obtain adequate pain relief. A treatment approach must be designed that encompasses the needs of the patient and family while preserving moral values. Despite attempts at establishing guidelines for pain management, it is often difficult to apply ethical standards to individual cases. Two such cases were presented for a discussion of the ethical issues raised.

Case Report 1.—Woman, 54, is receiving hospice care at home for metastatic carcinoma of the pancreas. Only palliative care is now possible. She is taking 210 mg of controlled-release morphine every 4 hours, but this treatment is inadequate. The pain is particularly severe when she has to be moved. Her family fears than an increase in morphine might hasten her death.

Case Report 2.—Man, 40, has end-stage metastatic adenocarcinoma of the stomach and is undergoing terminal care in the oncology unit of a hospital. He is receiving an IV morphine infusion at 1 mg/hr with orders to titrate between 1 and 8 mg. By day 6, the infusion rate is increased to 110 mg/hr, but the patient is often awake and anxious. The patient's family, the attending physician, and the nursing staff are now in conflict regarding pain management. The physician increases the dose of morphine in response to the family's desire that the patient be kept somnolent; the nurses object to the increase, believing that pain was controlled at a lower dose and a higher dose may compromise his respiratory drive. The patient had asked that his family make treatment decisions.

Discussion.—In both cases, the goal of treatment must be comfort care. It should be assumed that patients want their pain managed, although some patients may accept some pain to remain awake. The risk of an earlier death in these 2 patients can be justified, because pain management is essential for comfort. In case 1, the patient's request for more complete pain management is legitimate. Factors to optimize pain control, like administrating the morphine more closely to the times when she is moved, may be beneficial. Families also need to understand that changes in pain management are consistent with medical goals. In the second case, the nurses' concerns must be considered. If the patient does have adequate pain control, he should not be given additional morphine at the family's request. The family's suffering when the patient is awake cannot justify changes in comfort care, even given their designated role for treatment decisions. The conflict might be resolved by providing the family with emotional support. Both cases demonstrate the multidimensional aspects of cancer pain management to control both the physiologic pain and emotional suffering of the patient and his/her loved ones.

▶ Treatment of cancer-related pain involves decisions as individual as the clinical presentation. The wishes of patients and family members must be considered, as well as the clinical judgment of the involved health care providers. Ethical issues can arise from differences in perspective that are generally resolved with communication. Often, what is desired by the patient and family may not be based on knowledge of possible outcomes or the potential toxicities of available therapeutic options. Health care providers must also remain objective yet understand their own feelings about the goals of comfort care. In this report are included 2 cases that provide a vehicle for discussion of these and other issues involved in the management of cancer-related pain.—N.A. Janjan, M.D.

Management of Bowel Obstruction in Advanced Cancer Patients

Ripamonti C (Natl Cancer Inst, Milan, Italy)
J Pain Symptom Manage 9:193–200, 1994 131-95-3–16

Introduction.—Bowel obstruction is a frequent and clinically consequential complication of primary or metastatic disease within the peritoneal cavity. It is similarly frequent in patients with colorectal and ovarian cancers (Table 1). Considerable time may elapse before the diagnosis is made (Table 2).

Causes and Diagnosis.—The most prevalent causes of bowel obstruction are extrinsic luminal occlusion resulting from an enlarging primary or recurrent tumor, mesenteric masses, surgical adhesions or postradiation fibrosis; intraluminal occlusion from a polypoid lesion or infiltration of intestinal muscle; or an intestinal motility disorder (pseudo-obstruction). Benign causes are responsible for varying proportions of cases (Table 3). Obstruction is rarely acute in patients with advanced cancer. Intestinal colic, abdominal pain, and vomiting are the most common manifestations. Constipation is a feature of complete obstruction. Abdominal radiography is the initial study for suspected bowl obstruction.

Management.—Surgical treatment either is not always responsible or does not always relieve symptoms in patients with advanced cancer. Prolonged nasogastric suction and IV fluids are not recommended for patients with inoperable conditions. Percutaneous gastrostomy is preferable, although it requires a brief hospital stay. A wide range of analgesic,

TABLE 1.—Incidence of Bowel Obstruction in Patients With Cancer

Authors	Primary cancer	%
Castaldo et al.	Ovary	5.5
Tunca et al.	Ovary	25
Solomon et al.	Ovary	14.7
Baines et al.	Colorectal	10*
Baines et al.	Miscellaneous	3*
Phillips et al.	Large bowel	16
Kyllonen	Colon	24
Kyllonen	Rectum	4.4
Soo et al.	Gynecologic	5
Lund et al.	Ovary	14
Beattie et al.	Ovary	42*
Steiner	Various	6

* Advanced cancer.
(Courtesy of Ripamonti C: *J Pain Symptom Manage* 9:193-200, 1994.)

anticholinergic, and antiemetic drugs is used to control symptoms of obstruction (Table 4). Steroids have been recommended for reducing peritumoral inflammatory edema, but controlled clinical trials have not been done. The role of total parenteral nutrition in this setting remains controversial.

▶ Bowel obstruction can cause severe intractable symptoms that debilitate patients with cancer and are distressing for those who take care of them. Obstruction can result in dehydration, malnutrition, and severe pain. Effective management of bowel obstruction in these patients is important because the survival rate after surgery ranges from 3 to 7 months, and surgical interven-

TABLE 2.—Time from Cancer Diagnosis to Obstruction

Authors	Primary cancer	Stage	Months
Tunca et al.	Ovary	All	8.3 median
Rubin et al.	Ovary	All	29.0 mean
Beattie et al.	Ovary	All	13.1 mean
Spears et al.	Colorectal	—	19.0 median
Turnbull et al.	Carcinomatosis	Advanced	15.0 median
Aabo et al.	Abdominal-pelvic	Advanced	18.0 median

(Courtesy of Ripamonti C: *J Pain Symptom Manage* 9:193-200, 1994.)

TABLE 3.—Rate of Bowel Obstruction Resulting From Benign Causes in Patients With Advanced Cancer

Authors	No. patients	Primary cancer	Benign causes (%)
Soo et al.	64	Gynecologic	34.0
Clarke-Pearson et al.	49	Ovary	6.1
Tunca et al.	127	Ovary	9.4
Gallick et al.	50	Various	26.0
Osteen et al.	66	Various	31.8
Spears et al.	62	Colorectal	48.0
Aabo et al.	41	Various	12.0
Annest and Jolly	34	Various	3.0

(Courtesy of: Ripamonti C: *J Pain Symptom Manage* 9:193–200, 1994.)

tion often is not possible. Relief of symptoms, however, can be accomplished with other therapies. Pharmacologic treatment can relieve intestinal colic in 68% of patients, and 90% will have relief of continuous pain as a result of tumor mass effect and abdominal distention. Nausea and vomiting are more difficult to control with pharmacotherapy, and in patients with these symptoms, surgical decompression should be performed when possible. Bowel obstruction resulting from cancer causes significant morbidity and requires interdisciplinary involvement to provide symptom relief.—N.A. Janjan, M.D.

TABLE 4.—Pharmacologic Therapy for Colicky Pain

1. Hyoscine butylbromide starting with 40–60 mg/day up to 380 mg/day.
2. Hyoscine hydrobromide 0.8-2.0 mg/day subcutaneously.
3. Hyoscine hydrobromide 0.3–0.6 mg sublingually as needed.
4. Loperamide 2 mg four times daily.
5. Morphine subcutaneously starting with 2.5 mg/hr increasing the dose until relief is achieved.
6. Transdermal scopolamine 1.5–3 mg every 3 days.
7. Celiac plexus block with alcohol.

Note: With all therapies, treatment with gastrokinetic antiemetic agents such as metoclopramide and domperidone and stimulant laxative should be discontinued.

(Courtesy of Ripamonti C: *J Pain Symptom Manage* 9:193–200, 1994.)

Quality of Life of Patients With Prostate Cancer and Their Spouses: The Value of a Data Base in Clinical Care

Kornblith AB, Herr HW, Ofman US, Scher HI, Holland JC (Mem Sloan-Kettering Cancer Ctr, New York)

Cancer 73:2791–2802, 1994 131-95-3–17

Background.—The quality of life of men with prostate cancer has not been studied extensively compared with that for patients with neoplasms at other sites. The nature and extent of problems experienced by patients and their spouses in adapting to a diagnosis of prostate cancer were examined.

Methods.—A 58-item questionnaire for patients and a 35-item questionnaire for spouses/partners assessing the 4 basic dimensions of quality of life (physical symptoms, physical functioning, general and cancer-specific psychological distress, and social functioning) were distributed to a sample of patients with prostate cancer who attended a health education lecture series.

Results.—One hundred seventy-two patients and 83 spouses/partners completed the questionnaire. Patients most often reported the following problems that moderately or severely affected their lives: limited ability to have erections (78%), decreased sexual enjoyment (74%), decreased sexual interest (58%), tiredness (38%), need to rest (31%), increased frequency of urination (38%), difficulty controlling urine (25%), worrying (29%), and trouble sleeping (29%). Spouses reported problems including: decreased sexual enjoyment (49%), decreased sexual interest (41%), tiredness (56%), need to rest (33%), worrying (56%), tenseness (35%), trouble sleeping (37%), and depression (25%). The problems of pain, lack of energy, frequency of urination, and decreased sexual interest were significantly correlated with other patient and spouse quality-of-life scales. Significantly, greater psychological distress was reported by spouses than patients. Those patients experiencing adaptation problems were significantly more likely to have advanced-stage disease and to have received surgical or medical hormonal treatments. Hormonal therapy alone, of all the medical treatment and demographic variables, was found to be the only significant predictor of quality of life: those receiving hormone therapy had a significantly worse quality of life.

Conclusions.—These early data indicate that it would be possible to illuminate the key psychosocial issues for men with prostate cancer. Such understanding would lead to more effective treatment for these men and their loved ones.

▶ Prostate cancer, like breast cancer, has a high overall incidence and is treated by surgical removal of the gland, radiotherapy, and systemic therapies that can affect hormonal regulation. Although a large body of data exists regarding the impact of breast cancer on the quality of life, little data are available on the impact of these therapies in prostate cancer for both the patient and spouse. This report documents significant problems with sexual functioning and other physical symptoms like pain and difficulty with urination. Unlike breast cancer, in which sexual functioning is affected by body image, for prostate cancer, the difficulties with sexual functioning after treatment are more physiologic. Significant quality-of-life issues for patients with prostate cancer and their spouses are identified, and these issues require further study to determine the specific medical and psychological interventions necessary to improve function and the quality of life.—N.A. Janjan, M.D.

Analgesic Therapy

Withdrawal Symptoms During Therapy With Transdermal Fentanyl (Fentanyl TTS)?

Zenz M, Donner D, Strumpf M (Univ Hosp Bergmannsheil, Bochum, Germany)

J Pain Symptom Manage 9:54–55, 1994 131-95-3–18

Introduction.—Transdermally administered fentanyl is a new approach to treating chronic pain that provides serum drug levels that ensure constant analgesia for 72 hours. Several clinical studies have shown that the fentanyl transdermal therapeutic system (TTS) effectively relieves chronic cancer pain. The withdrawal symptoms that developed in 2 patients shortly after they were switched from sustained-release morphine to fentanyl TTS were discussed.

Case Report.—Woman, 29, was receiving 200 mg of sustained-release morphine 3 times daily for pain caused by metastatic ovarian cancer. She also was taking metamizole, domperidone, diazepam, and metoclopramide. The morphine was discontinued and converted to fentanyl TTS in a dose of 6 mg/day. Pain relief was initially unchanged, but within 24 hours, the patient described feeling restless and had a crawling sensation in her extremities, which later became painful. Her heart rate and blood pressure both increased. The symptoms were relieved by IV morphine, returned after a few hours, and then decreased during the next 2 days. The patient did not seek morphine. Clonidine was given orally for 2 weeks, and the dose of fentanyl TTS was increased to 8.4 mg/day as the malignancy progressed. The patient died after receiving fentanyl TTS for 4 months, which had provided continued pain relief.

Discussion.—Both this patient and another, a woman with relapsed colon cancer, gained good pain relief after being switched from sustained-release morphine to fentanyl TTS, but clinical signs of opioid withdrawal soon developed that were not accompanied by drug-seeking behavior. The symptoms are attributed to opioid withdrawal secondary to physical dependence after long-term morphine administration.

▶ The relatively long interval before a steady state of drug level is reached with transdermal delivery systems is emphasized in this report. When transdermal analgesics are initiated in patients who are already taking analgesics by other routes, the pharmacokinetics of the 2 agents must be considered to ensure uninterrupted relief of pain and to reduce the risk for physical withdrawal. These clinical examples demonstrate the need to closely monitor symptoms that occur with changes in prescribed analgesics.—N.A. Janjan, M.D.

Tolerability of Ketorolac Administered Via Continuous Subcutaneous Infusion for Cancer Pain: A Preliminary Report

De Conno F, Zecca E, Martini C, Ripamonti C, Caraceni A, Saita L (Natl Cancer Inst, Milan, Italy)

J Pain Symptom Manage 9:119–121, 1994 131-95-3–19

Objective.—The local and systemic tolerability of tromethamine ketorolac administered continuously by the subcutaneous route was evaluated for control of the pain of advanced malignancy. This new agent is a nonopioid analgesic free of effects on the CNS.

Methods.—The patients were 5 men and 5 women with a mean age of 56 years. All had somatic and visceral pain, and 5 had bone pain. Ketorolac was administered by continuous infusion at a starting dose of 90 mg/day. During the week of treatment, patients were assessed daily for the presence or absence of pain. The Integrated Pain Score, based on severity and duration of pain, was completed daily by the patients. Nine symptoms were recorded on a 4-point scale at baseline and after the week of ketorolac therapy.

Results.—None of the patients experienced inflammatory reactions or burning at the site of drug injection. Seven of 10, however, showed mild local bleeding and required repositioning of the needle. All patients reported acceptable pain control and expressed a favorable judgment of the test treatment. The only side effects appeared to be an increase in xerostomia and sweating, which increased in 3 patients.

Conclusion.—Continuous subcutaneous delivery of analgesics with a syringe driver or pump can be useful in patients with cancer pain. Nonsteroidal anti-inflammatory drugs such as ketorolac are not commonly administered by this method, but findings in this small group of patients suggest that subcutaneous infusion of such agents may be an alternative to other forms of parenteral drug administration. Additional information will be needed on the bioavailability of ketorolac after subcutaneous administration and the frequency of bleeding at the injection site.

▶ The availability of active agents in cancer pain management continues to expand. Experience continues to demonstrate that infusional palmidronate is an important therapeutic option in patients with refractory bone pain. Infusional ketorolac, a nonsteroidal anti-inflammatory agent, also has been shown to be highly effective in controlling cancer-related pain, including somatic and visceral pain; half of the patients studied had bone pain. Although its effects do not include antineoplastic properties, ketorolac may be a significant alternative to other analgesics. Specifically, the side effects of nausea, sedation, and constipation that are associated with opioid analgesics can be avoided with the administration of ketorolac. Toxicities, such as bleeding, that are associated with nonsteroidal anti-inflammatory agents must also be closely evaluated. With further experience, ketorolac may prove to be an important infusional agent in palliating cancer-related pain, particularly in patients who do not tolerate opioid analgesics.—N.A. Janjan, M.D.

Opioid Responsiveness of Cancer Pain Syndromes Caused by Neuropathic or Nociceptive Mechanisms: A Combined Analysis of Controlled, Single-Dose Studies

Cherny NI, Thaler HT, Friedlander-Klar H, Lapin J, Foley KM, Houde R, Portenoy RK (Mem Sloan-Kettering Cancer Ctr, New York; Cornell Med Ctr, New York)

Neurology 44:857–861, 1994 131-95-3–20

Background.—Pain commonly is referred to as "nociceptive" when it is perceived as being commensurate with tissue damage from an identifiable somatic or visceral lesion. "Neuropathic" pain, in contrast, is caused either by disease of or injury to the peripheral or central neural structures. The latter type of pain is thought to be sustained by abnormal somatosensory processing. Whether these types of pain are differentially responsive to opioids remains uncertain.

Objective.—Data from 4 controlled, double-blind, single-graded-dose, relative analgesic potency studies were analyzed to discern the influence of the inferred mechanism of pain on the response to opioid treatment. Morphine or heroin was administered 474 times to 168 patients, most of whom had metastatic or locally advanced tumors. The analgesic response was monitored for 6 hours using visual analogue scales to yield a total pain relief (TOTPAR) score. High or low doses of the drugs were administered orally or intramuscularly. Two clinicians who were experienced in pain disorders classified the cases on the basis of the inferred mechanism of pain.

Results.—Nociceptive pain only was judged to be present in 205 patients, neuropathic pain alone in 49, and mixed pain in 220. After adjusting for the duration of previous opioid treatment, the most recent dosage, and baseline pain intensity, TOTPAR scores were significantly lower for patients having any neuropathic pain component. Patients with nociceptive pain alone had the highest pain relief scores. A significant dose-response relationship was evident in patients with neuropathic pain.

Implications.—Opioid treatment should not be withheld from patients experiencing severe pain solely because of the inferred mechanism of pain production. Patients with neuropathic pain may be less likely to respond, but dose titration trials are needed to learn which patients will benefit most from higer doses of opioid therapy.

▶ The variability in the response to opioids among patients with cancer was evaluated in this single-dose analgesic trial. The analgesic effect of the single dose differed on the basis of the etiology of the pain. Analgesic response was significantly less in patients who had neuropathic pain as any component of their cancer-related pain. Patients who had only nociceptive pain had the best response to the administered dose of analgesics. These data emphasize that cancer pain syndromes are often complex in etiology, resulting in a wide variability of response to analgesics. The second important issue identified is that neuropathic pain does respond to opioid analgesics. Even though higher doses of analgesics are necessary to achieve adequate relief ("titrating to effect") of neuropathic pain, opioid analgesics continue to be important in the management of cancer-related pain.—N.A. Janjan, M.D.

Transdermal Fentanyl in Uncontrolled Cancer Pain: Titration on a Day-to-Day Basis as a Procedure for Safe and Effective Dose Finding—A Pilot Study in 20 Patients

Korte W, Morant R (Kantonsspital, St Gallen, Switzerland)

Support Care Cancer 2:123–127, 1994 131-95-3-21

Introduction.—The continuous fentanyl transdermal therapeutic system (F-TTS) can provide effective pain control in patients experiencing side effects of other analgesics or swallowing difficulties. However, it is recommended that F-TTS be initiated while the patient's pain is already controlled with another agent, such as a short-acting narcotic. The feasibility of initiating F-TTS in patients with poorly controlled cancer pain without using a short-acting narcotic during the titration phase was investigated in a prospective, open, nonrandomized trial.

Methods.—Twenty patients with uncontrolled or poorly controlled cancer pain were treated with F-TTS. Dosing was adjusted daily to achieve adequate pain relief. Morphine was used as rescue medication. The patients recorded their pain levels 3 times a day and at pain peaks using a visual analogue scale (VAS) for 4 weeks. Morphine rescue requirements were recorded, as were side effects and the number of bowel movements.

Results.—Adequate pain control, with VAS scores lower than 35 mm, was achieved within an average of 48 hours, dramatically improving the VAS scores compared with pretreatment pain assessments. The F-TTS doses were increased significantly in the first 2 weeks, but not thereafter. The mean morphine rescue doses decreased dramatically after the first day, then steadily but nonsignificantly from 11 mg/day in the first week to 3 mg/day in the fourth week. There were no severe side effects, although 2 patients experienced dizziness and 1 patient experienced slight hypotension and dyspnea, which disappeared with dose adjustment. One patient had respiratory depression, which may have been associated with concomitant initiation of continuous 5-fluorouracil. Thirteen patients experienced some nausea. Some laxative treatment was necessary in 16 patients, with continuous treatment in 2 patients.

Discussion.—Treatment with F-TTS can be initiated immediately to patients with poorly controlled cancer pain, although morphine is required for rescue medication. Dose titration can be accomplished on a day-to-day basis, which simplifies dose finding. The patients experienced fewer and less severe side effects than expected with conventional opiate therapy, but this finding will require confirmation with controlled clinical trials.

▶ Severe pain is generally managed with immediate-release, short-acting analgesics, and the analgesic is titrated to the dose that results in pain relief. Acute management of severe pain is often performed with IV analgesics to minimize the oral agents' delay in achieving analgesic effect as a result of the time necessary for gastrointestinal absorption. The total dose of analgesic necessary for pain control is determined, and sufficient doses of longer-acting, sustained-released preparations are then administered.

Alternatively, it has been suggested that dose titration can be performed with longer-acting preparations, including transdermal fentanyl. In the past, dose titration has not specifically been evaluated with transdermal fentanyl, because the dose patch is generally administered every 3 days, rather than twice a day with sustained-release morphine, and because of the more-than-12-hour initial delay in absorption before a steady state of analgesic concentration is achieved. This report indicates that dose titration can be efficiently performed with long-acting preparations, such as transdermal fentanyl, to quickly achieve steady-state concentrations while using rescue doses of immediate-release analgesics.—N.A. Janjan, M.D.

A Pilot Study to Assess the Efficacy of Salmon Calcitonin in the Relief of Neuropathic Pain Caused by Extraskeletal Metastases

Kovčin V, Jelić S, Babović N, Tomašević Z (Inst of Oncology and Radiology, Belgrade, Yugoslavia)

Support Care Cancer 2:71–73, 1994 131-95-3–22

Background.—Salmon calcitonin has demonstrated pain-relieving activity, primarily in patients with bone metastases. Further evidence suggests that this agent possesses a central analgesic activity independent of the opiate receptor system and that its pain-relieving effect may be the result of elevated levels of circulating endorphins. If either of these statements are correct, pain-relieving activity should also be apparent in conditions other than painful bone metastases. Thus, the pain-relieving effect of salmon calcitonin was investigated in patients with pain caused by extraskeletal metastases.

Patients and Methods.—Sixteen patients with advanced locoregional and/or metastatic disease who were heavily pretreated and had no possibility of specific anticancer treatment were evaluated. All patients had a poor response to previous drug treatment, including opiate-type analgesics (11 patients) and nonopiate-type analgesics (5 patients). Pain was caused by radicular compression via retroperitoneal metastatic tumor mass or radicular compression in the cervical region via metastatic lymph node conglomerates. All patients received 200 IU of salmon calcitonin in 500 mL of .9% sodium chloride on a daily basis, infused during 60 minutes. The total duration of treatment was 20 days. A 4-grade scale (very good, good, moderate, or poor) of pain relief was used to evaluate treatment efficacy.

Results.—Poor pain relief was noted in 10 patients; 9 of them had been pretreated with opiate-type analgesics. In the remaining patients, moderate, good, and very good pain relief was achieved in 2 patients each. Undifferentiated carcinoma of the nasopharynx was noted in a significant number of responders. One patient with embryonal carcinoma who had been previously treated with daily opiates experienced complete pain relief with total withdrawal from all analgesic drugs. This patient remained pain-free until his death 3 months later. No alterations in calcium and hydroxyproline urinary excretion or in serum alkaline phosphatase, calcium, and phosphorus levels attributable to salmon calcitonin treatment were observed.

Conclusions.—Salmon calcitonin may be beneficial in patients refractory to membrane-stabilizing drugs. The pain relief activity of this agent may depend on tumor type, previous intake of pain-relieving drugs, and the site of metastatic disease.

▶ This report evaluates the mechanism of action of salmon calcitonin. Although it was efficacious in bone metastases, it was unclear whether a secondary mechanism of analgesia was also observed. This trial evaluated the use of calcitonin in neuropathic pain secondary to extraosseous metastases. The drug failed to control pain in 9 of 11 patients who had been previously treated with opiates; 6 of 16 patients, however, reported moderate to very good control of pain.

This pilot study raises questions regarding the possible mechanisms of action of calcitonin, and the authors suggest that factors such as the primary histology, characteristics of disease extension, and previous therapy may have an impact on response. However, this is only a pilot experience, and it requires more controlled trials to determine whether calcitonin does have analgesic activity independent of its action on bony metastases.—N.A. Janjan, M.D.

Comparison of Morphine and Ketorolac for Intravenous Patient-Controlled Analgesia in Posoperative Cancer Patients

Bosek V, Miguel R (University of South Florida, Tampa)

Clin J Pain 10:314–318, 1994 131-95-3–23

Background.—In appropriate doses, nonsteroidal anti-inflammatory drugs may control severe pain. The effectiveness of patient-controlled (PCA) IV ketorolac tromethamine was compared with that of IV-PCA morphine in the treatment of postoperative pain in patients with cancer.

Methods.—After surgery for abdominal or truncal cancer, 70 adults were randomly assigned to receive morphine (1 mg/mL) or ketorolac (5 mg/mL). On arrival at the postanesthesia care unit (PACU), patients were given 2 mL of medication every 5 minutes until analgesia was achieved. If pain continued after 20 mL of the study drug had been administered, IM morphine, .1 mg/kg, was given. At discharge from the PACU, all patients were given an IV-PCA prescription consisting of 1 mL of basal infusion per hr and a 1-mL on-demand bolus, with a lockout interval of 10 minutes. The morphine injections were offered every 6

TABLE 1.—List of Surgical Procedures

	Ketorolac (K)	Morphine (M)
Abdominal		
Hysterectomy	14	11
Exploratory laparotomy	3	6
Gastric resection	1	2
Colon surgery	7	7
Prostatectomy	3	3
Retroperitoneal		
Node dissection	2	1
	30	30
Truncal		
Vulvectomy and groin		
Dissection	4	4
Abdominal wall		
Resection		
Scrotectomy	1	1
Total	35	35

(Courtesy of Bosek V, Miguel R: *Clin J Pain* 10:314–318, 1994.)

TABLE 2.—Visual Analogue Pain Score

	Ketorolac	Morphine
12 h (mm)	67 ± 33	64 ± 30
24 h (mm)	33 ± 27	35 ± 21
36 h (mm)	31 ± 23	31 ± 30
48 h (mm)	23 ± 19	20 ± 18

Note: Values are expressed as mean ± standard deviation.
(Courtesy of Bosek V, Miguel R: *Clin J Pain* 10:314–318, 1994.)

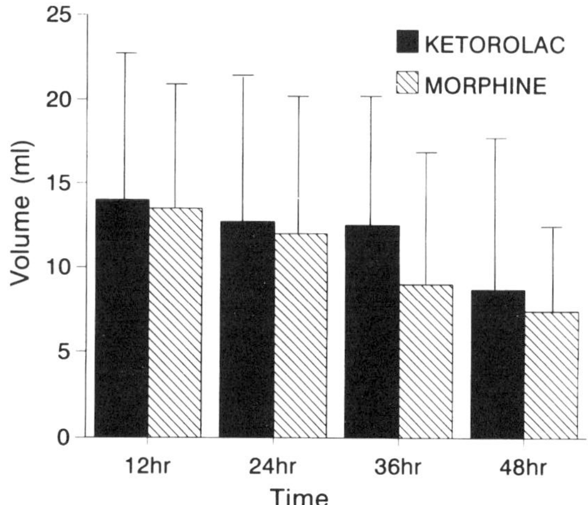

Fig 3–3.—The amount of ketorolac or morphine delivered from an IV patient-controlled system; mean ± standard deviation. (Courtesy of Bosek V, Miguel R: *Clin J Pain* 10:314–318, 1994.)

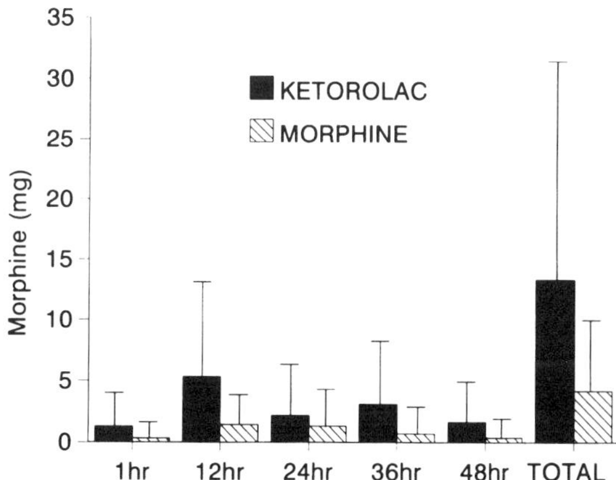

Fig 3–4.—The amount of supplemental IM morphine requested by the patients. Values are expressed as mean ± standard deviation. Statistical significance and difference are expressed at the level of $P \leq .05$. (Courtesy of Bosek V, Miguel R: *Clin J Pain* 10:314–318, 1994.)

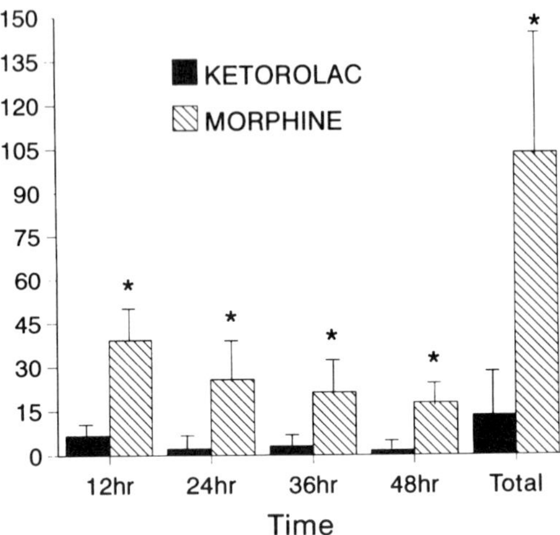

Fig 3–5.—Amount of morphine delivered via PCA or IM. The values are expressed as mean ± standard deviation. *Statistically significant differences expressed at the level of $P \leq .05$. (Courtesy of Bosek V, Miguel R: *Clin J Pain* 10:314–318, 1994.)

hours; the patients could refuse them. Patients were interviewed every 12 hours for 48 hours after discharge from the PACU, with pain and sedation scores being recorded at those times. The medication volumes, and the presence of nausea, vomiting, and pruritis were recorded.

Findings.—The surgical procedures for the 2 groups are listed in Table 1, and the pain scores for the 2 groups, which were comparable, are shown in Table 2. The groups did not differ in the volume of analgesic delivered (Fig 3–3), but the ketorolac group requested more supplemental morphine (Fig 3–4). However, the total dose of morphine (Fig 3–5) and the incidence of side effects (Table 3) were greater in the morphine group.

Conclusions.—The use of IV-PCA ketorolac, with supplemental morphine, resulted in a lower incidence of side effects like nausea, vomiting, and pruritis when compared with morphine administered alone. This combination may reduce potential side effects of each agent and result

TABLE 3.—Incidence of Side Effects

	Ketorolac	Morphine
Nausea	31.4	42.9*
Vomiting	34.3	42.9*
Sedation	28.6	25.7
Pruritus	17.1	40.0*

Note: Values are expressed in percentages.
*$P \leq .05$.
(Courtesy of Bosek V, Miguel R: *Clin J Pain* 10:314–318, 1994.)

in improved relief of pain by targeting different etiologies of postoperative pain.

▶ Ketorolac is an important new agent in the analgesic armamentarium. This and other studies are helping to define its role and associated toxicities in cancer-related pain. The important finding from this study is that ketorolac potentiates the analgesic effects of morphine. Nonsteroidal anti-inflammatory agents (NSAIDS), which act by blocking the prostaglandin cycle, target a different etiology of postoperative pain. Because ketorolac provided additional analgesic effect, the necessary dose of morphine could be reduced, thereby also reducing the toxicities associated with morphine, including nausea and sedation. However, the toxicities of ketorolac and other NSAIDS, including renal insufficiency, gastrointestinal ulceration, and bleeding caused by platelet inhibition, must also be closely monitored, particularly in the postoperative setting. The study demonstrates that NSAIDS are potent adjuvant analgesics when combined with morphine, both in oral and infusional analgesic therapy.—N.A. Janjan, M.D.

Use of Ketorolac by Continuous Subcutaneous Infusion for the Control of Cancer-Related Pain

Myers KG, Trotman IF (Mount Vernon Hosp, Middlesex, England)

Postgrad Med J 70:359–362, 1994 131-95-3–24

Introduction.—Ketorolac tromethamine (Toradol) is a nonsteroidal anti-inflammatory agent with an analgesic action that exceeds its anti-inflammatory effect. It may be administered parenterally, and it has effectively controlled postoperative pain in a variety of settings.

Objective.—Ketorolac was given by continuous subcutaneous infusion to 36 patients, (19 women and 17 men; age range, 19 to 79 years) with advanced malignant disease. All were receiving opioid analgesics, and a majority had serious adverse effects. In all cases, the pain was inadequately controlled by current medication, which most often included oral nonsteroidal anti-inflammatory drugs.

Treatment.—Ketorolac was given in an initial dose of 60 mg in physiologic saline for 24 hours, using a Graseby syringe driver. A majority of patients first received a bolus of 30 mg to determine the likely response. Other nonsteroidal drugs were discontinued. The patients were prescribed oral misoprostol in a dose of 200 μg 3 times daily.

Results.—Twenty-nine patients (80%) were completely relieved of pain within 48 hours after infusion began, and they continued to respond for at least 72 hours. Two other patients responded transiently. More than two thirds of the responders had control of pain after receiving 60 mg of ketorolac every 24 hours. A large majority of patients who responded had bone pain, with or without visceral pain. The infusion continued for an average of 3 weeks. Four patients had gastrointestinal bleeding during treatment.

Conclusion.—Ketorolac, given by continuous subcutaneous infusion, is a useful co-analgesic for patients who have pain from advanced cancer.

▶ This article expands the reported experience with ketorolac in the treatment of cancer-related pain. As in other reports, ketorolac was found to be efficacious in controlling cancer pain but had an associated risk of gastrointestinal bleeding, which occurred in 10% of the patients studied. The development of this infusional nonsteroidal anti-inflammatory agent significantly increases the therapeutic alternatives for the management of cancer-related pain, most specifically in the treatment of pain related to bone metastases. Although this report describes the use of ketorolac as a subcutaneous infusion, it has also been used intravenously. The availability of an infusional route for nonsteroidal anti-inflammatory agents allows for greater flexibility in administration, which may be a significant factor for patients who are unable to take oral medications or when rapid relief of pain is imperative.—N.A. Janjan, M.D.

Comparative Clinical Efficacy and Safety of Immediate Release and Controlled Release Hydromorphone for Chronic Severe Cancer Pain

Hays H, Hagen N, Thirlwell M, Dhaliwal H, Babul N, Harsanyi Z, Darke AC (Misericordia Hosp, Edmonton, Alta, Canada; Univ of Calgary, Alta, Canada; McGill Univ, Montreal; et al)

Cancer 74:1808–1816, 1994 131-95-3–25

Background.—Some patients with chronic, cancer-related pain are unable to take morphine orally because of unmanageable side effects. Hydromorphone, a semisynthetic morphine congener, provides an alternative treatment for patients with pain, but its short half-life makes dosing every 4 hours necessary to maintain an optimal level of analgesia. The clinical efficacy and safety of controlled-release hydromorphone were compared with the effects of immediate-release hydromorphone in 45 patients who had severe, chronic, cancer-related pain.

Methods.—With the use of a double-masked crossover design, these patients were randomized to receive immediate-release hydromorphone at 4-hour intervals for 1 week or controlled-release hydromorphone every 12 hours for 1 week. The pain intensity was estimated by using both a visual analogue scale and the Present Pain Intensity Index of the McGill Pain Questionnaire.

Results.—The mean daily dose of hydromorphone was 76 mg. Neither of the pain assessment measures demonstrated significant differences between the immediate-release and the controlled-release forms of hydromorphone (Tables 1 and 2). The need for rescue analgesia also did

TABLE 1.—Comparison of Clinical Efficacy and Safety Variables by Day of Treatment After Controlled-Release (CR) and Immediate-Release (IR) Hydromorphone

	CR hydromorphone								IR hydromorphone							
Variable	*Day 1*	*Day 2*	*Day 3*	*Day 4*	*Day 5*	*Day 6*	*Day 7*	*Overall*	*Day 1*	*Day 2*	*Day 3*	*Day 4*	*Day 5*	*Day 6*	*Day 7*	*Overall*
Pain intensity VAS (0–100 mm)	19.2	19.0	20.3	17.1	19.2	21.9	17.7	19.4	19.8	19.1	20.7	19.7	18.8	18.7	20.1	19.7
Pain intensity ordinal (0–5)	1.1	1.2	1.2	1.0	1.1	1.3	1.1	1.2	1.2	1.1	1.2	1.2	1.1	1.1	1.2	1.2
Rescue analgesic use (doses/day)	0.7	1.2	1.0	1.0	1.0	1.1	1.3	1.1	0.6	1.0	1.1	1.1	1.1	1.0	1.2	1.0
Sedation VAS (0–100 mm)	20.8	18.8	18.8	16.8	17.3	17.7	17.2	18.6	18.3	18.3	20.9	17.8	17.8	18.9	18.7	18.8
Nausea VAS (0–100 mm)	13.1	11.9	13.1	14.2	13.1	12.4	11.5	12.6	12.1	10.5	12.3	10.2	9.9	10.8	12.3	11.1

Note: The data represent the mean daily score over 4 assessment periods (0700, 1100, 1500, and 1900 hours). The overall score represents the mean overall days and times.
Abbreviation: VAS, visual analogue score.
(Courtesy of Hays H, Hagen N, Thirlwell M, et al: *Cancer* 74:1808–1816, 1994.)

TABLE 2.—Comparison of Clinical Efficacy and Safety Variables by Time of Day After Controlled-Release (CR) and Immediate-Release (IR) Hyromorphone

	CR hydromorphone					IR hydromnorphone				
Variable	*7:00 a.m.*	*11:00 a.m.*	*3:00 p.m.*	*7:00 p.m.*	*Overall*	*7:00 a.m.*	*11:00 a.m.*	*3:00 p.m.*	*7:00 p.m.*	*Overall*
Pain intensity VAS (0–100 mm)	20.9	18.3	18.8	19.0	19.4	19.5	19.6	19.6	19.8	19.7
Pain intensity ordinal (0–5)	1.2	1.1	1.2	1.1	1.2	1.1	1.2	1.2	1.2	1.2
Rescue analgesic use (doses/4 hr)*	1.8	1.3	2.0	1.3	—	1.6	1.5	1.6	1.6	—
Sedation VAS (0–100 mm)	19.3	17.5	18.3	18.7	18.6	20.0	17.2	18.1	20.1	18.8
Nausea VAS (0–100 mm)	11.0	13.2	13.0	13.7	12.6	10.3	10.5	11.7	11.8	11.1

Notes: The data represent the mean score by time of day over 7 days. The overall score represents the mean over all days and times.
*Total over 7 days.
Abbreviation: VAS, visual analogue score.
(Courtesy of Hays H, Hagen N, Thirlwell M, et al: *Cancer* 74:1808–1816, 1994.)

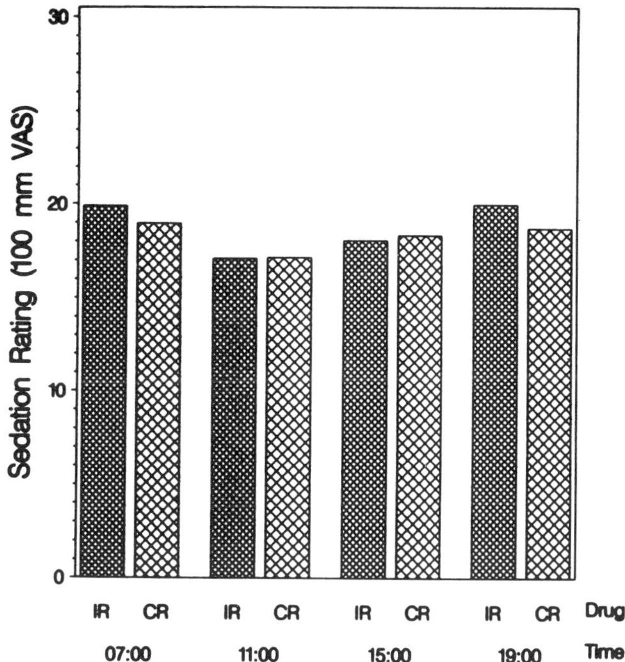

not differ significantly with the form of opioid used. Among patients who expressed a preference, more preferred the controlled-release form. Similar degrees of sedation were produced by the 2 dose forms (Fig 3–6), and the nausea scores did not differ significantly (Fig 3–7).

Conclusion.—Treatment with controlled-release hydromorphone at 12-hour intervals is a highly effective approach to relieving chronic, severe, cancer-induced pain.

▶ Occasionally, tolerance does not develop to the side effects of nausea and sedation that occur with the use of morphine sulfate. Hydromorphone represents an effective alternative analgesic, but until now it had the disadvantage of offering only a short-acting preparation. The development of alternative long-acting analgesics provides important flexibility in the management of cancer-related pain.—N.A. Janjan, M.D.

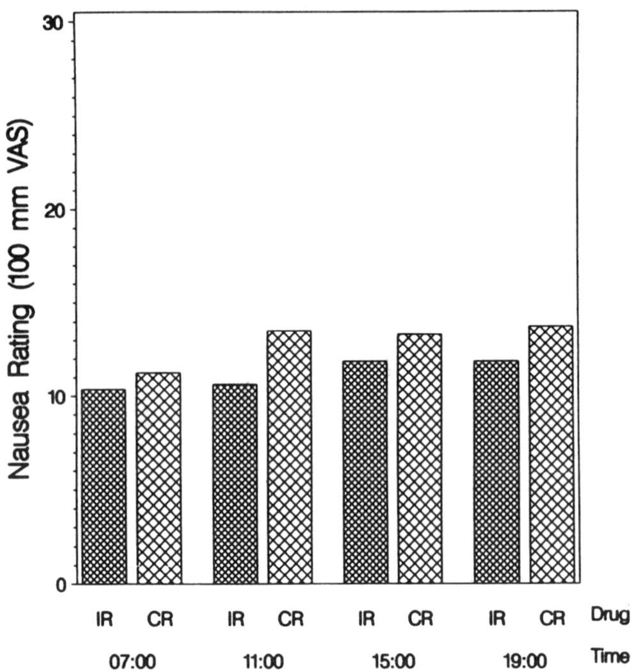

Fig 3–7.—The mean nausea visual analogue score (*VAS*) by time of day after controlled-release (*CR*) hydromorphone and immediate-release (*IR*) hydromorphone. (Courtesy of Hays H, Hagen N, Thirlwell M, et al: *Cancer* 74:1808–1816, 1994.)

Interventional Therapy

Long-Term Intrathecal Morphine and Bupivacaine in Patients With Refractory Cancer Pain: Results From a Morphine:Bupivacaine Dose Regimen of 0.5:4.75 mg/mL

Sjöberg M, Nitescu P, Appelgren L, Curelaru I (Sahlgrenska Hosp, Gothenberg, Sweden)

Anesthesiology 80:284–297, 1994 131-95-3–26

Background.—No clinical data are available on the concentrations and ratios in which intrathecal morphine and bupivacaine should be combined to optimize analgesia and minimize adverse effects. The efficacy and safety of a constant intrathecal infusion of morphine, .5 mg/mL, plus bupivacaine (morphine: bupivacaine ≈1:10), 4.75 mg/mL, in the treatment of refractory cancer pain were assessed.

Methods.—In 53 patients with refractory cancer pain, this intrathecal combination of morphine and bupivacaine was administered, and the dosage was increased, as needed, for 6 months. Patients were also able to use nonopioid analgesics and sedatives as needed. The efficacy of this treatment was measured by scoring the following parameters: pain relief, total opioid daily dosages, total daily nonopioid analgesic and sedative use, patient's sleep pattern, patient's gait pattern and body movements, and adverse effects.

Results.—During the intrathecal period, which was a median of 29 days, the median intrathecal daily dose was 6 mg for morphine and 50 mg for bupivacaine. Compared with prior intrathecal treatment, all patients had acceptable relief of their pain during treatment. The median total daily use of opioids decreased from 120 mg to 10 mg. The use of nonopioid analgesics and sedatives decreased by about one half. The sleep pattern improved significantly, but the gait pattern did not. Urinary retention, paresthesias, and paresis/gait impairment were the most common side effects.

Conclusion.—Intrathecal administration of morphine, .5 mg/mL, plus bupivacaine, 4.75 mg/mL, may significantly relieve cancer pain, although side effects may occur as a result of the bupivacaine.

▶ The authors of this study evaluated the efficacy of a 1:10 ratio of morphine and bupivacaine and compared their results with those of a previous trial that administered a 1:1 ratio of these agents through an epidural catheter. Response and toxicities were evaluated according to the total dose administered. The dose of intrathecal morphine that was necessary to achieve relief of pain increased most rapidly during the first month of intrathecal treatment, and it later plateaued. Side effects, including urinary retention, paresthesias, and gait impairment, were primarily related to the dose of bupivacaine infused. However, the pain relief achieved with the 1:10 ratio of morphine and bupivacaine was better than that achieved with the 1:1 ratio. This conclusion was based on the median total dose of opioids (2.5 times greater with the 1:1 ratio) and the median dose of intrathecal morphine (4 times greater with the 1:1 ratio) that were necessary to achieve relief of pain. The mechanism of action of this synergistic antinociceptive effect involves inhibition of neuronal excitability and selective sensory processing that results in a decrease in the onset and an increase in the duration of analgesia.

This report attempted to evaluate the synergism between these agents based on comparative dose ratios. Although increased toxicity was observed with higher doses of bupivacaine, morphine-related toxicity decreased and the efficacy of therapy was improved. Based on individual clinical characteristics, further optimization of relative dose ratios of these agents may be pursued.—N.A. Janjan, M.D.

Spinal Analgesia in Terminal Care: Risk Versus Benefit

Devulder J, Ghys L, Dhondt W, Rolly G (Univ Hosp Gent, Belgium)

J Pain Symptom Manage 9:75–81, 1994 131-95-3-27

Background.—According to the World Health Organization, oral administration of analgesics is preferred in the early stages of cancer pain treatment. When pain cannot be controlled, however, alternatives must be considered. One alternative is administration of spinal morphine, which may be combined with clonidine, bupivacaine, or other drugs. Complications of this technique are considered to be rare, but the complication rate has not been comprehensively evaluated in this patient subgroup.

Patients.—Ninety-two patients with cancer were treated for 18 months at a pain clinic. Thirteen of these patients were successfully treated until death with intrathecal analgesics. This led to an evaluation of the experience in 33 patients with cancer who were also treated in the past 4 years with intrathecal morphine.

Findings.—Fifty-four of the 92 patients received sufficient pain relief from oral analgesics; 19 needed a subcutaneous infusion of analgesics; and 13 required intrathecal administration of opioid analgesics. Six patients underwent neurodestructive procedures for pain relief. Among the second group of 33 patients, 25 received "good" pain relief with intrathecal analgesics until death, management of pain was difficult only right before death in 7, and in 1 patient, pain remained uncontrolled. Meningitis developed in 3 patients, possibly as a result of a disconnection of the pump tubing system.

Discussion.—Most of the 92 patients attained adequate analgesia with oral or subcutaneous treatment. For the 33 patients who received intrathecal treatment, pain relief was good. However, intrathecal treatment should be used only after oral and subcutaneous drug administration have failed. Although either epidural or intrathecal administration of spinal analgesics is possible, intrathecal administration may be preferred for some patients without previous epidural treatment who may not tolerate a change in systems well if epidural fibrosis occurs, or if epidural therapy becomes less effective and must be discontinued.

▶ Intrathecal therapy is becoming more commonly administered as a means of treating cancer-related pain that is refractory to oral analgesics. The risks of therapy, including meningitis, are recognized, but most patients achieve excellent relief of symptoms throughout the terminal phase of their disease. The dose and combination of analgesics can be individualized to achieve maximum relief of symptoms. Techniques that include the use of pumps also minimize difficulties in the administration of analgesics. Spinal analgesia is an extremely important option for the management of cancer pain that is uncontrolled by other means.—N.A. Janjan, M.D.

Altered Reactivity of Isolated Segmental Lumbar Arteries of Dogs Following Exposure to Ethanol and Phenol

Brown DL, Rorie DK (Mayo Clinic and Found, Rochester, Minn)

Pain 56:139–143, 1994 131-95-3–28

Introduction.—Neurolytic celiac plexus block has provided effective analgesia for patients with pain from cancer of the upper abdominal organs. However, neurologic complications, including paraplegia, have precluded the widespread use of this technique. Paraplegia is thought to result from neurolytic drug-induced spasm of lumbar spinal arteries. To test this hypothesis, the effect of phenol or ethanol on the reactivity of isolated lumbar segmental arteries was investigated.

Methods.—After anesthesia and exsanguination, the segmental arteries of mongrel dogs were severed and placed in oxygenated Krebs-Ringer solution (KRS). Intact arterial rings 3–4 mm in length were formed and suspended in 10-mL organ baths. After a 30-minute rest, the arterial rings were stretched to the optimal point on their length-tension curve; after 45 minutes, norepinephrine at a concentration of 3×10^{-7} M (ED_{50}) was used to cause a control contraction for each ring. After a 45-minute rest in fresh KRS, the contractile response of the rings was allowed to return to baseline. Phenol (1%, 3%, 6%, 7%, 8%, 9%, or 12%) or ethanol (3%, 6%, 10%, 25%, 50%, 75%, or 90%) was then added to the KRS, and the change in resting tension from baseline was calculated. Phentolamine, papaverine, tetrodotoxin, procaine, ketanserin, propranolol, and atropine were subsequently added to identify the mechanism by which phenol and ethanol alter contractile response.

Results.—After exposure to norepinephrine, the mean ($\pm$ standard error of the mean) contractile response of segmental arteries was 116 $\pm$ 3.8 g/100 mg of tissue. The addition of ethanol to KRS resulted in a change in contractile response inversely proportional to the concentration of ethanol; 90% ethanol caused a small and transient contractile response, whereas lower concentrations of 3% and 6% resulted in sustained contractile responses. At 15 minutes after the addition of 3% and 6% ethanol, the resulting contractile responses were 105% and 120%, respectively, of the ED_{50} norepinephrine-induced response. Phenol-induced contractile responses were directly proportional to the concentration, with 1%, 3%, and 6% concentrations producing small, transient responses; 8%, 9%, and 12% phenol resulted in sustained contractile responses that, at 15 minutes, were 105%, 220%, and 200% of norepinephrine-induced responses. Phentolamine, which diminished the norepinephrine-induced response, had no effect on the contractile response produced by 3% ethanol or 9% phenol. Pretreatment with or addition of either ketanserin, propranolol, atropine, papaverine, or tetrodotoxin had no effect on the contractile response induced by ethanol or phenol. Procaine .25% and .5% abolished the response to 3% ethanol. Procaine .5% significantly decreased the contractile response induced by 9% phenol; procaine .25% did not alter the phenol-induced response.

Conclusion.—These results suggest that if human lumbar segmental arteries react similarly to those of a dog, local injection of phenol in concentrations of 8% to 12% may induce spasm when injected near a lumbar artery. These concentrations of phenol are sometimes used clinically in neurolytic celiac plexus block. Because ethanol is used clinically in concentrations greater than 25%, it would need to be injected at a distance from the lumbar artery to achieve a concentration gradient between the injected ethanol and the lumbar artery. However, it is important to note that this study did not measure blood flow; it cannot be determined whether a sustained contraction of the lumbar segmental arteries induced by either phenol or ethanol can lead to ischemia large enough to cause paraplegia.

▶ The pathophysiology of neurologic complications with celiac plexus block was investigated in this experimental setting. Injection of phenol may induce spasm of the vertebral artery; the phenol-induced arterial spasm was directly related to the concentration administered. In contrast, the ethanol-induced spasm was inversely related to the concentration and could be overcome by the infusion of procaine. These responses are not considered to be mediated through sodium channels, or adrenergic, opioid, muscarinic, or serotonin receptors. However, no direct evidence was found to indicate that injection of phenol or alcohol results in vertebral artery spasm sufficient to cause ischemia and paraplegia. The etiology of this rare complication remains indeterminate. Overall, complications are infrequently seen with celiac plexus neurolysis, and this procedure remains an important therapeutic option in the treatment of intractable pain resulting from upper abdominal cancer.—N.A. Janjan, M.D.

Long-Term Intrathecal Infusion of Morphine and Morphine/Bupivacaine Mixtures in the Treatment of Cancer Pain: A Retrospective Analysis of 51 Cases

Van Dongen RTM, Crul BJP, De Bock M (Univ Hosp Nijmegen, The Netherlands)

Pain 55:119–123, 1993 131-95-3–29

Background.—Long-term intrathecal (i.t.) morphine is used in patients with cancer who have inadequate pain relief. Intrathecal morphine plus bupivacaine may be useful in pain syndromes inadequately relieved by i.t. morphine alone.

Study Design.—In a retrospective fashion, the effectiveness of i.t. morphine infusion in 51 patients with cancer pain was studied. Continuous morphine infusion was performed through a tunneled percutaneous catheter inserted between the second and fifth lumbar vertebrae and advanced 3–5 cm in the intrathecal space. Effectiveness of treatment was judged based on patient report and analgesic requirements.

Findings.—Total duration of i.t. treatment was 3,140 days. All patients required a gradual dose increment, with an initial rapid increase in daily dose occurring until day 20. Because of inadequate pain relief with i.t. morphine alone, 17 patients received a combined infusion of morphine and bupivacaine for a total of 1,900 patient days. The mean daily bupivacaine dose was 31 mg (range, 10–100 mg). Ten of the 17 patients with combined i.t. infusion had significant pain relief and 4 had moderate improvement. Three patients with clinical signs of severe mental depression had no adequate pain relief with the morphine/bupivacaine mixture. There were no bupivacaine-induced side effects with a daily dose of less than 30 mg. There were no serious complications, neurologic sequelae, or meningitis.

Conclusion.—Long-term i.t. infusion of morphine through a tunneled catheter can provide adequate pain relief in patients with cancer with an acceptable risk-benefit ratio. Prospective studies are needed to define the effects of long-term i.t. co-administration of local anesthetics, particularly bupivacaine.

▶ This report adds to the body of literature that says cancer-related pain that is uncontrolled by oral analgesics can be effectively managed by intrathecal infusion or analgesics. The infusion can be administered for a long period without significant morbidity. As in the other studies included in this section, bupivacaine was effective in controlling pain in patients who did not respond to intrathecal morphine alone. The side effects related to bupivacaine in this study were also found to be dose related. Clinical experience is consistent with the administration of intrathecal analgesics. Future clinical studies will be necessary to exploit the synergistic effect between morphine and bupivacaine and achieve the most optimal control of cancer-related pain.—N.A. Janjan, M.D.

Intrathecal and Epidural Somatostatin for Patients With Cancer: Analgesic Effects and Postmortem Neuropathologic Investigations of Spinal Cord and Nerve Roots

Mollenholt P, Rawal N, Gordh T Jr, Olsson Y (Örebro Med Ctr Hosp, Sweden; Uppsala Univ, Sweden)

Anesthesiology 81:534–542, 1994 131-95-3–30

Background.—The finding of somatostatin (SST) at several sites in the CNS has supported the existence of a somatostatinergic pain-inhibiting mechanism. In vivo, SST depresses the nociceptive response of dorsal horn neurons. Neurotoxic effects have accompanied the analgesic action of synthetic peptides such as SST, but some species may be less sensitive to these toxic effects than are rats.

Patients.—The analgesic potential of SST, delivered epidurally or intrathecally, was studied in 8 adult patients with pain related to cancer and skeletal metastases (or, in one case, to sarcomatous invasion of the spinal column). The patients had varying combinations of neuropathic and somatic pain, and they had failed to respond well to large doses of opioids.

Treatment.—An epidural or intrathecal block was carried out, and SST was administered in a bolus dose of 250 μg, followed by a continuous infusion of 2 mL/hr (5–60 μg/mL) with the use of a portable pump. The maximum daily dose was 3,000 μg.

Results.—Six of the 8 patients had excellent-to-good relief of pain when given SST. Analgesia began within 10 minutes of the bolus dose. All the patients required increasing doses of SST. Half the patients were able to increase their level of physical activity, and 6 of the 8 had an improved mental status. No patient had a neurologic deficit or respiratory depression that could be ascribed to SST therapy. Neuropathologic changes were observed in the spinal cord in 2 of 5 autopsied patients. Both patients had moderate degenerative changes in some dorsal roots of the cauda equina, and 1 also had slight degenerative changes in the dorsal columns.

Conclusions.—Epidural or intrathecal treatment with SST is an effective means of relieving pain in patients with terminal cancer. The neuropathologic changes seen in 2 of these patients might have resulted from the malignant disease itself or from chemotherapy or radiation therapy.

▶ The number and types of agents available for intrathecal and epidural infusion in the treatment of cancer-related pain continue to expand. This study evaluated the analgesic efficacy of somatostatin and provided neuropathologic correlation. Six of 8 patients with intractable pain achieved good-to-excellent relief of their pain. Demyelination was observed in 3 patients; however, it was unknown whether these neuropathologic changes were related to SST, the tumor, or to the prior antineoplastic therapy, because there had been no clinical evidence of neurologic deficit. Intrathecal and epidural SST should be judiciously considered in cases of uncontrolled pain in patients with a limited prognosis. This experience is important with regard to clinical outcome and the further understanding of the neurologic mechanisms involved in cancer-related pain.—N.A. Janjan, M.D.

Injection of Alcohol into Bone Metastases Under CT Guidance

Gangi A, Kastler B, Klinkert A, Dietemann JL (Univ Hosp of Strasbourg, France)

J Comput Assist Tomogr 18:932–935, 1994 131-95-3–31

Background.—Radiotherapy or chemotherapy is the traditional method of pain management in patients with bone metastases. Although the methods are effective, the techniques require 2–4 weeks. In 25 terminally ill patients with painful osteolytic bone metastases in whom opiate analgesics, radiotherapy, and/or chemotherapy failed, percutaneous injection of ethanol (PIE) was performed under CT guidance.

Methods.—Twenty-seven bone metastases in 25 patients had 39 injections of 3–25 mL of 95% ethanol under CT guidance. The procedure allowed precise positioning of the needle and control of the diffusion of

Patient Data and Results of Alcoholization of Bone Metastases

Case/ sex/ age (years)	Primary	Localization	No. of treatments	Analgesic score
1/M/58	Lung	Vertebra,	1	4
		Hip	1	4
2/M/55	Lung	Vertebra	1	3
3/M/72	Lung	Vertebra	2	2
4/M/60	Lung	Ribs,	1	3
		Vertebra	1	3
5/M/55	Lung	Clavicle	1	3
6/M/63	Lung	Vertebra	2	1
7/F/47	Breast	Hip	3	3
8/M/67	Lung	Hip	2	1
9/M/46	Lung	Ribs	1	4
10/M/42	Lung	Sternum	2	1
11/F/52	Breast	Ribs	1	3
12/M/50	Lung	Hip	1	3
13/F/47	Breast	Vertebra	2	2
14/M/57	Lung	Ribs	2	1
15/M/47	Melanoma	Scapula	2	1
16/F/61	Breast	Vertebra	1	3
17/F/31	Breast	Scapula	2	1
18/M/56	Lung	Humerus	1	2
19/M/61	Lung	Hip	1	3
20/F/52	Breast	Vertebra	1	2
21/F/48	Uterus	Humerus	2	3
22/M/69	Lung	Ribs	1	4
23/F/64	Breast	Vertebra	2	1
24/M/48	Lung	Ribs	1	2
25/M/47	Lung	Hip	1	3

(Courtesy of Gangi A, Kastler B, Kinkert A, et al: *J Comput Assist Tomogr* 18:932–935, 1994.)

the ethanol to minimize complications. A perceptual scale of pain relief (1 = little or no relief; 4 = complete relief) was determined beginning 48 hours after PIE, which was confirmed on physical examination 2 weeks later. The procedure was repeated if there was insufficient relief of pain. Eleven patients had 2 or more treatments (table).

Results.—Within 1–2 days, nearly 75% of the patients reported a reduction in the need for analgesics, as indicated by an analgesic score of 2 or more. The tumor size increased in 5 patients, decreased in 7 patients, and stayed stable in the remaining 15 patients. Duration of pain relief was 10–27 weeks. None of the patients survived more than 6 months. Patients with small metastases, 3–6 cm, had the best results. Low-grade fever occurred in 7 patients within 72 hours.

Comment.—The percutaneous injection of ethanol, under CT guidance, reduces pain and improves the quality of life in patients with painful bone metastases. A larger trial to define the efficacy of the method is necessary.

▶ This report presents another option that can be used to palliate localized bony metastases. Similar to the procedure used for a nerve block to treat neuropathic cancer-related pain, ethanol was infused (under CT guidance) into the affected bone with little related morbidity. The duration of pain relief, achieved in more than 75% of patients, was comparable to that achieved with radiotherapy. Although it is an invasive procedure, localized infusion of ethanol into the bone rapidly achieves palliation of symptoms and is of particular benefit in patients who have persistent pain after conventional therapy. The observed time course for and duration of response also provides insight into the pathophysiology of pain associated with bone metastases.—N.A. Janjan, M.D.

Intrathecal Morphine and Bupivacaine in Advanced Cancer Pain Patients Implanted at Home

Mercadante S (Buccheri La Ferla Hosp, Palermo, Italy)

J Pain Symptom Manage 9:201–207, 1994 131-95-3–32

Background.—Pain resulting from advanced cancer may no longer be controlled by opioids or systemic nonopioid analgesics, and even epidural or intrathecal opioids may be only partially effective if severe nociceptive stimulation is present. Because local anesthesia enhances opioid-induced analgesia, it has been suggested that it be used with epidural or intrathecal opioid treatment.

Series.—Fifteen patients with cancer pain, who previously had received morphine orally or parenterally but whose pain was no longer relieved, were entered in a trial of home-based intrathecal treatment with morphine and bupivacaine. Thirteen patients were implanted with a catheter at home because they were bedridden or had refused admission to the hospital.

Management.—The subarachnoid space was entered with a nylon catheter using a 17-gauge Tuohy needle and a midline approach. Intrathecal treatment began with 1 mg of morphine in a 1-mL volume as needed for 24 hours. Bupivacaine was then added, and both drugs were given continuously. The dose of bupivacaine was initially 12.5 mg and was increased to 25 mg/day before the daily dose of spinal morphine was increased.

Results.—The patients remained at home until they died, 8–25 days after the institution of spinal treatment. The mean survival time was 16 days. The mean final dose of intrathecal morphine was 4.6 mg/day. Pain scores did not increase, and all but 2 of the 15 patients continued to have good pain relief. Although fluid leakage was a problem in 1 case, no pumps malfunctioned, and no patient had clinical evidence of infection.

Conclusions.—Refractory cancer pain may be controlled at home by placing a spinal catheter and administering both morphine and bupivacaine. In this way, patients who are not able or not willing to be hospitalized may remain comfortable during their last days.

▶ For some time, there has been a substantial increase in outpatient therapy. Chemotherapeutic agents are routinely infused through pumps attached to central venous catheters. This report indicates that an intrathecal catheter and infusion can be initiated at the bedside at home with little associated morbidity in patients who refuse hospitalization. Important in home hospice care, this treatment provides an important therapeutic option for patients with advanced cancer and cancer-related pain. However, the most significant obstacles to the implementation of this plan in the United States may be administrative. The availability of time, reimbursement considerations, and potential liability issues that encompass epidural catheter placement in the home may prove overwhelming. Performing this procedure at home, however, provides a cost-effective means of relieving pain in patients with advanced cancer. Socioeconomic issues will need to be delineated to provide this important analgesic option to patients within their homes.—N.A. Janjan, M.D.

The Dilemma of Conversion From Systemic to Epidural Morphine: A Proposed Conversion Tool for Treatment of Cancer Pain

Du Pen SL, Williams AR (Swedish Tumor Inst, Seattle; Univ of Washington, Seattle)

Pain 56:113–118, 1994 131-95-3-33

Introduction.—There is considerable debate about dose equivalencies when switching from systemic to epidural morphine. The difficulty in determining the appropriate starting dose for epidural morphine is further complicated in patients, with cancer who have widely variable analgesic requirements. Extended titration periods may result in unacceptably long periods of unrelieved pain and prolonged hospitalization.

TABLE 1.—Conversion Factor for Pain Severity

0–10 Pain Scale	Conversion Factor
0–4	0
5–6	0.5
7–8	1.0
9–10	1.25

(Courtesy of Du Pen SL, Williams AR: *Pain* 56:113–118, 1994.)

TABLE 2.—Equianalgesic Conversion Chart

Opioid	Equianalgesic dose (mg)	
	Oral	Parenteral
Morphine	30	10
Hydromorphone	7.5	1.5
Oxycodone	30	
Methadone	20	10
Levorphanol	4	2
Fentanyl		0.1
Oxymorphone		1
Meperidine	300	75

(Courtesy of Du Pen SL, Williams AR: *Pain* 56:113–118, 1994.)

Therefore, an individualized epidural morphine conversion tool (IEMCT) was developed to guide the approach when converting from systemic to epidural morphine.

The Model.—Conversion from systemic to epidural morphine therapy should be guided by 4 patient-specific factors: pain severity, age, the previous systemic morphine dose, and the presence or absence of neuropathic pain. In the starting formula, the 24-hour epidural starting dose is one tenth of the previous 24-hour IV dose; this formula is then modified by the 4 patient-specific factors. Pain severity, reported with a verbal 0–10 scale, adds conversion factors of .5 for a pain rating of 5–6, 1 for a 7–8 rating, and 1.25 for 9–10 (Table 1). Because elderly patients are more sensitive to drug therapy, ages 70–80 years add a conversion factor of −.25, and ages older than 80 years add a conversion factor of −.5. Because a tolerance to opioids can develop in patients, the formula must account for the degree of probable tolerance as indicated by the patient's previous systemic dose. A conversion factor of .75 is added for patients taking 100–200 mg of IV morphine per day, 1 is added for an IV dose of 200–500 mg/day, and 1.5 is added for a dose exceeding 500

TABLE 3.—Stepwise Epidural Morphine Dose Adjustment

0–10 Pain scale	Epidural morphine Dose adjustment
0–1 with sedation	−10%
1–3	0
4–6	15%
7–8	25%
9–10	50%

(Courtesy of Du Pen SL, Williams AR: *Pain* 56:113–118, 1994.)

mg/day. When the patient's history suggests neuropathic pain, a conversion factor of .5 is added to the formula. The 24-hour starting dose of epidural morphine is then calculated by multiplying the 24-hour IV morphine dose by the sum of the conversion factors and dividing by 10. If patients are being converted from other opioids or oral morphine, the equianalgesic dose of IV morphine can be calculated with standard charts (Table 2). When the epidural dose is initiated, the systemic opioid should be reduced by as much as 50% daily. The epidural dose should then be adjusted incrementally, with the adjustments dependent on the patient's verbal pain assessments (Table 3).

Conclusion.—This IEMCT can effectively guide an accurate calculation of each patient's required starting epidural morphine dose. Accurate conversion from either oral or parenteral opioids can be accomplished easily with relatively uncomplicated clinical observation. The tool increases the efficiency of both dose titration and pain relief.

▶ Epidural analgesia is being used with increased frequency in the treatment of cancer-related pain. However, the necessary dose of epidural opioids is often difficult to predict based on the dose of oral analgesics that the patient was prescribed before placement of the epidural catheter. The level of pain control that is achieved with the oral analgesics must also be considered, because an increase in the opioid dose may be required. The article also discusses other factors, such as age and the presence of neuropathic pain, that can affect the efficacy of epidural opioids. These factors were incorporated into a formula that converts the oral analgesic to the dose of morphine that will be necessary in epidural administration. With validation, this tool could prove important and allow more efficient titration of epidural analgesics to accomplish rapid control of cancer-related pain.—N.A. Janjan, M.D.

A Comparison of Epidural Catheters With or Without Subcutaneous Injection Ports for Treatment of Cancer Pain

de Jong PC, Kansen PJ (Dr. Daniel den Hoed Cancer Ctr, Rotterdam, The Netherlands)

Anesth Analg 78:94–100, 1994 131-95-3–34

Objective.—The use of epidural analgesia for treatment of cancer pain has associated problems. The complications associated with the use of epidural catheters for treatment of such pain were analyzed.

Methods.—Patients received either percutaneous or subcutaneous injection ports. Morphine was the most commonly used opioid. Sufentanil was used in 10% of the patients. Bupivacaine was added for all patients receiving continuous infusion. Clonidine was used in 6 patients. Dislodgement, infections, leakage, and occlusion were recorded.

Results.—A total of 149 patients received 250 catheters; 198 of these were percutaneous, including 41 that were tunneled, and 52 were subcutaneous. Approximately 21% of percutaneous catheters became dislodged. No subcutaneous injection ports became dislodged. About 14% of catheters in both groups became infected. However, the percutaneous (nonport) group had an infection incidence twice that of the subcutaneous (port) group when the rate of infection was indexed to the parameter of time (1,000 catheter-days). Leakage and occlusion incidents were significantly more common in the subcutaneous port group. There was no significant difference in the incidence of pain on injection between the 2 groups.

Conclusion.—The complication rate for epidural catheters, including catheter dislodgement and early infections, was lower for catheters equipped with injection ports.

▶ The goal of cancer pain management is to relieve symptoms as quickly as possible with the fewest possible side effects. Potential toxicities of analgesic therapy are to be anticipated and prevented when possible. As with any procedure, risk exists in the placement of epidural catheters for the control of severe cancer-related pain. The variety of options that are available for epidural catheter placement, and the morbidity related to each technique, are reviewed in this article. This represents an important experience that assists in the selection of the type of epidural catheter used to palliate intractable cancer pain.—N.A. Janjan, M.D.

Bone Metastases

High-Dose Intravenous Pamidronate for Metastatic Bone Pain

Purohit OP, Anthony C, Radstone CR, Owen J, Coleman RE (Weston Park Hosp NHS Trust, Sheffield, England)
Br J Cancer 70:554–558, 1994 131-95-3–35

Background.—Many patients with advanced cancer and bone metastases experience only partial and temporary relief from pain with standard treatments. Bisphosphonates, however, inhibit osteoclast activity and have been effective in relieving pain and promoting bone healing when given intravenously. The benefits of IV pamidronate, administered in a

TABLE 1.—Previous Treatments

Tumour type	*Radiotherapy*	*Endocrine*	*Cytotoxic*	*Strontium-89*	*Clodronate*
Breast	22	21	10	0	1
Prostate	5	5	0	2	1
Other*	7	1	2	0	0
Total	34	27	12	2	2

* Two Ewing's sarcoma, 1 melanoma, 1 non-small-cell lung cancer, 1 bladder, 1 kidney, 1 unknown primary.
(Courtesy of Purohit OP, Anthony C, Radstone CR, et al: *Br J Cancer* 70:554–558, 1994.)

TABLE 2.—Subjective Response to Treatment

Tumour type	*Responders (>20% reduction)*	*No change (0–20% reduction)*	*Progression (increase in pain)*
Breast	15 (68%)	7 (32%)	0
Prostate	3 (60%)	2 (40%)	0
Other*	2 (29%)	5 (71%)	0
Total	20 (59%)	14 (41%)	0

* Two Ewing's sarcoma, 1 melanoma, 1 non-small-cell lung cancer, 1 bladder, 1 kidney, 1 unknown primary.
(Courtesy of Purohit OP, Anthony C, Radstone CR, et al: *Br J Cancer* 70:554–558, 1994.)

single high dose, were examined in 34 patients with painful bone metastases. Previous IV treatment with the bisphosphonates used small, repeated doses.

Patients and Methods.—Twenty-two of the 34 patients had breast cancer. All had progressing, symptomatic bone metastases and had undergone radiotherapy to various sites. Some had received endocrine treatment, chemotherapy, strontium 89, or oral clodronate (Table 1). All were given a single IV infusion of pamidronate (120 mg in 1 L of .9% normal saline). Patients were seen every 2 weeks for 8 weeks, then monthly, and evaluated for the effect of pamidronate on pain, mobility, analgesic consumption, and quality of life (QOL). They were asked to complete a pain questionnaire and standardized measures of mobility and QOL.

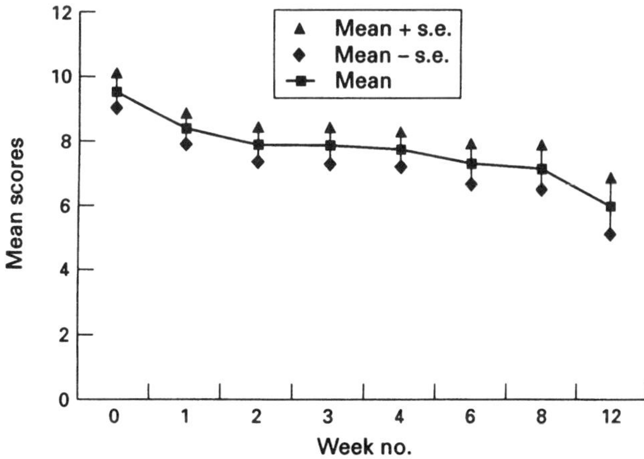

Fig 3–8.—Changes in pain score. Values are means ± standard error (*s.e.*). Pain score was calculated by combining the individual scores for pain, analgesic consumption, and World Health Organization performance status. (Courtesy of Purohit OP, Anthony C, Radstone CR, et al: *Br J Cancer* 70:554–558, 1994.)

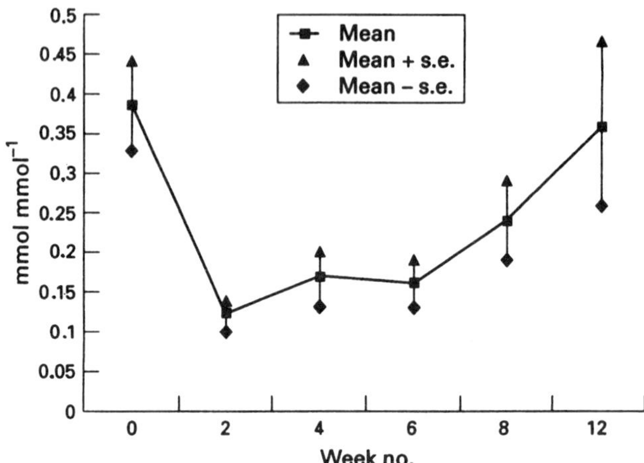

Fig 3–9.—Changes in urinary calcium excretion expressed as a molar ratio of urinary calcium to urinary creatinine. Values are means ± standard error (*s.e.*). (Courtesy of Purohit OP, Anthony C, Radstone CR, et al: *Br J Cancer* 70:554–558, 1994.)

Results.—The single treatment with IV pamidronate brought about a response in 20 patients (59%), including 15 (68%) of those with breast cancer (Table 2). Response was defined as a more than 20% reduction from baseline in the symptom score (Fig 3–8), a composite of pain, analgesic use, and QOL. The median duration of symptomatic response was 12 weeks. Pamidronate treatment was generally well tolerated, and no patient experienced symptomatic hypocalcemia. Urinary calcium excretion, as expected, decreased significantly after treatment (Fig 3–9). Twenty-one patients were re-treated with IV pamidronate. Eight of 15 who were responders to the initial treatment again showed a reduction in pain score of more than 20%, whereas the 6 nonresponders again failed to respond.

Conclusion.—In this open phase II study of high-dose IV pamidronate, a large proportion of patients with metastatic bone pain obtained symptomatic relief for a median duration of 12 weeks. It was not clear why some patients failed to respond, because symptomatic relief appeared to be unrelated to tumor type, type of bone metastases, or previous systemic treatment.

▶ Persistent pain after localized irradiation and cytotoxic endocrine therapies for bone metastases can respond to other therapeutic interventions, such as pamidronate. In this study of 34 patients, 23 had severe-to-intolerable pain, 13 were taking more than 100 mg of morphine sulfate daily, and 19 were confined to bed for more than half the day. Despite the severity of these symptoms, 60% of patients experienced more than a 20% improvement in symptoms and had minimal associated side effects with a single IV injection of pamidronate. This reduction in symptoms lasted 12 weeks on average, and half of the patients who responded to the injection of pamidronate experienced continued relief of symptoms. Although it is unclear why some patients fail to respond, pamidronate represents an important therapy in patients with persistent or recurrent pain due to bone metastases. Because it inhibits osteoclast activity, pamidronate therapy represents a targeted approach that effectively treats hypercalcemia and promotes bone healing. The specific application of bisphosphonates as a high- vs. low-dose IV agent and the frequency of adminstration still need to be defined on the basis of clinical presentation. However, bisphosphonates are an effective means of treating patients who have failed other therapies, and they provide important understanding in the mechanism of pain due to bone metastases.—N.A. Janjan, M.D.

Intravenous Pamidronate Disodium Treatment of Bone Metastases in Patients with Breast Cancer: A Dose-Seeking Study

Glover D, Lipton A, Keller A, Miller AA, Browning S, Fram RJ, George S, Zelenakas K, Macerata RS, Seaman JJ (Presbyterian Univ, Philadelphia; Milton S Hershey Med Ctr, Hershey, Pa; Hematology Oncology Associates, Tulsa, Okla; et al)

Cancer 74:2949–2955, 1994 131-95-3-36

Background.—Nearly 70% of patients with breast cancer have metastases in bone that significantly decrease the quality of life. Symptomatic treatments include narcotics, radiation chemotherapy, or hormonal therapy. Bisphosphonates, which inhibit the osteoclast destruction of bone, are widely used to treat the hypercalcemia of malignancy. In a multicenter trial, the efficacy of 4 IV regimens of pamidronate was assessed in the palliative treatment of bone metastases.

Methods.—Sixty-one patients with breast cancer aged 18 years or older with a life expectancy of a least 3 months participated in the trial. Metastatic cancer to the bone was confirmed by a bone scan or a bone survey. The patients were randomized to 1 of 4 IV treatment regimens for 12 weeks: 30 mg every 2 weeks; 60 mg every 4 weeks; 60 mg every 2 weeks; or 90 mg every 4 weeks. The treatment was evaluated by the changes in pain scores (bone pain multiplied by the frequency of pain) over time. Other efficacy variables included narcotic scores, bone lesion response (International Union Against Cancer guidelines), and selected markers of osteoclast activity.

Results.—The patient characteristics on enrollment in the study were similar. After 3 months, only the smallest dose (30 mg every 2 weeks) failed to show a reduction in bone pain. The use of narcotics did not show any consistent changes. The biochemical variables were reduced, consistent with pain reduction. Healing lesions were seen in 25% of evaluable patients, and an additional 47% had stable disease. Transient (15–24 hours) side effects of fever (11.5 of patients), increased bone pain (10%), and myalgia (7%) were considered to be mild and not dose dependent.

Conclusions.—At the 3 highest doses tested, IV pamidronate was well tolerated and resulted in a significant reduction in bone pain. The decrease in biochemical markers was consistent with a reduction in osteoclast activity. Because the higher dose of pamidronate was most effective in patients with hypercalcemia, a multicenter, placebo-controlled trial is under way.

▶ Multiple centers have reported relatively consistent experience with palmidronate in the treatment of bony metastases. The relief of pain, however, is influenced by the dose administered. Therefore, further study is needed to account for potential variables in dose, frequency, and overall number of doses administered. These dose-response data will prove critical to subsequent studies that evaluate palmidronate used as a single agent and as an adjuvant to other therapies.—N.A. Janjan, M.D.

Pamidronate for Pain Control in Patients With Malignant Osteolytic Bone Disease: A Prospective Dose-Effect Study

Thürlimann B, Morant R, Jungi WF, Radziwill A (Kantonsspital, St Gallen, Switzerland)

Support Care Cancer 2:61–65, 1994 131-95-3–37

Introduction.—Osteolytic bone disease resulting from skeletal metastases affects approximately 70% of patients who die of cancer and causes significant long-term morbidity. Bisphosphonates, which inhibit osteoclast activity and therefore reduce bone resorption, are generally used to treat osteolytic bone disease and associated hypercalcemia. Recently, IV pamidronate, a second-generation bisphosphonate, has demonstrated an analgesic effect in these patients as well, but the optimal dose for palliative effect is not known. The safety of high doses of pamidronate and the dose-response relationship were investigated.

Methods.—Eighty patients with osteolytic bone metastases were treated with IV pamidronate given first at a dose of 30 mg every 4 weeks, then every 3 weeks, and every 2 weeks. Doses of 45 mg, 60 mg, and 90 mg were given on the same schedule. Palliative efficacy was evaluated by combining the pain and analgesic scores, using World Health Organization criteria, with the score documenting improvement of performance status, using Scandinavian European Oncology Study Group/Eastern Cooperative Oncology Group (SAKK/ECOG) criteria.

Results.—Although single doses of 30 mg usually brought measurable pain relief, infrequently administered low doses had little palliative effect. The most beneficial effect was achieved with 90 mg of pamidronate given every 2 or 3 weeks. Dose intensity and palliative effect correlated closely. Less than 10 mg/wk had no significant benefit, whereas 20–45 mg/wk produced significant palliative benefit. Two patients with myeloma who had elevated serum creatinine before treatment had further increases in serum creatinine. There were no other relevant toxic effects.

Discussion.—The palliative effect of IV pamidronate was dose dependent in patients with osteolytic bone metastases, with patients experiencing profound benefits only with a dose intensity of 20–45 mg/wk. The greatest pain relief was achieved at the highest doses without sacrificing safety. Therefore, pamidronate should be administered at a level of at least 20 mg/wk. Prospective, randomized trials should be performed to determine the optimal dose and schedule for palliative treatment.

► Pamidronate expands the armamentarium in the treatment of painful bony metastases. However, the indications and optimal dose and frequency of administration have yet to be defined. The mechanism of action may complement other therapies, allowing pamidronate to successfully treat bone metastases that fail to respond to other forms of treatment, e.g., chemotherapy, hormonal therapy, radiotherapy, and radiopharmaceuticals. Also, pamidronate may prove to be a significant adjuvant and may potentiate the response to these other types of treatment. Dose-response data are important to the design of subsequent clinical trials that stratify the type of prior therapy, the extent and location of bony metastases, and the primary histology. These factors should be incorporated into further trials that evaluate pamidronate, used either alone or as an adjuvant therapeutic agent.—N.A. Janjan, M.D.

Detection of Vertebral Metastases: Comparison Between MR Imaging and Bone Scintigraphy

Algra PR, Bloem JL, Tissing H, Falke THM, Arndt J-W, Verboom LJ (Free Univ, Amsterdam)

RadioGraphics 11:219–232, 1991 131-95-3–38

Introduction.—Bone scintigraphy is the method most often used to detect skeletal metastases. However, it can produce both false positive and false negative findings. Magnetic resonance imaging is highly effective for evaluating bone marrow and may be a more sensitive method of detecting bone metastases. The sensitivity of MRI vs. planar bone scintigraphy was compared by prospectively detecting vertebral metastases in patients with malignancy and known skeletal metastases.

Methods.—During a 2-year period, 71 patients with a primary tumor, biopsy specimen-proven skeletal metastases, and clinically or radiographically suspected vertebral metastases were evaluated with both MRI and bone scintigraphy. Two blinded observers interpreted the bone scintigrams, and 2 additional blinded observers interpreted the MR images. Proof of vertebral lesions was determined by the results of all other imaging studies and clinical follow-up, including vertebral biopsy in 12 patients.

Results.—Bone scintigraphy detected 499 vertebral lesions; MRI detected 818 vertebral lesions. Four distinct types of metastases, with characteristic signal intensity patterns, were recognized by MRI: focal lytic, focal sclerotic, diffuse inhomogenous, and diffuse homogenous metastases. Vertebral biopsy in 12 patients confirmed the metastases identified by MRI but not by scintigraphy. The use of MRI also allowed evaluation of soft tissue extension and compressive myelopathy, which scintigraphy could not do.

Discussion.—Magnetic resonance imaging detected vertebral metastases more sensitively than bone scintigraphy. It may also be useful for guiding needle biopsy or localizing lesions for surgical or radiation therapy. However, unlike with bone scintigraphy, long acquisition times and repeated examinations for imaging the entire skeleton are required.

▶ Detection of metastases in the vertebral body was more effective when MRI was performed. Magnetic resonance imaging primarily has been used to evaluate soft tissue extension and spinal cord compression, whereas bone scans have been regarded as the most sensitive assessment of bony metastases. This study, however, demonstrates that MRI more accurately identifies and characterizes metastatic involvement of the vertebral body. Another advantage of MRI is the evaluation of possible epidural disease, undetected by bone scans, that can result in progressive symptoms and compromise neurologic integrity.

It is unclear whether this additional information provided by MRI will significantly influence therapeutic decisions or outcomes. Palliative irradiation, for example, is only administered to symptomatic sites; knowledge of more extensive disease may or may not influence radiation fields.

The advantages of bone scans include a lower cost when compared with MRI and a more efficient means of evaluating the entire skeleton. Prospective trials should be considered to determine the cost-effectiveness relative to neurologic function. A subgroup of patients might be identified in whom bone scans do not provide adequate diagnostic information, and in whom MRI would significantly impact on therapy and clinical outcome. Further study will be required to define specific indications for MRI in assessing vertebral body metastases.—N.A. Janjan, M.D.

The Management of Cancer Metastatic to Bone
Aaron AD (Georgetown Univ, Washington, DC)
JAMA 272:1206–1209, 1994 131-95-3-39

Introduction.—As many as 85% of patients who die of breast, prostate, or lung cancer have bone involvement at the time of autopsy. Patients with bone metastasis generally describe constant, dull pain that becomes gradually more intense. Ultimately, the pain is not relieved by rest. Needle biopsy is preferable to an open procedure when diagnostic confirmation is necessary.

TABLE 1.—Indications for Prophylactic Fixation of Impending Long-Bone Fractures

1. Cortical bone destruction of 50% or more
2. Lesion of 2.5 cm or more in the proximal femur
3. Pathological avulsion fracture of the lesser trochanter
4. Persisting stress pain despite irradiation

(From Aaron AD: *JAMA* 272:1206–1209, 1994. Courtesy of Harrington KD: *Orthopedic Management of Metastatic Bone Disease*. St Louis, Mo, CV Mosby, 1988, p 7.)

Management.—Radiation is a very effective means of relieving pain that results from a progressive tumor. It is usually the initial treatment modality, particularly when a solitary metastasis is present. Hormonal and chemotherapeutic measures also may provide excellent pain relief, particularly in patients with primary disease in the breast or prostate. Diphosphonates are used to relieve hypercalcemia and the pain that results from bone metastases. Radionuclides also have been used to treat metastatic bone pain.

Pathologic Fracture.—Indications for prophylactic fixation in patients with impending pathologic fracture remain imprecisely defined (Table 1). A system of classifying the risk of such fracture (Table 2) might prove helpful. Once a fracture develops, aggressive surgical tretment generally is indicated.

▶ This is an excellent review article about the management of bone metastases. Therapeutic options include localized approaches, such as surgery, external-beam irradiation, and systemic therapy with diffuse involvement. Recent advances in the systemic options, including bisphosphonates and radionuclide therapy, are presented. Optimization of therapeutic and analgesic management should provide symptomatic relief for the majority of patients.—N.A. Janjan, M.D.

TABLE 2.—A Scoring System to Quantitate the Risk of Pathologic Fractures

	Score		
Variable	1	2	3
Site	Upper limb	Lower limb	Peritrochanter
Pain	Mild	Moderate	Functional
Lesion	Blastic	Mixed	Lytic
Size*	< 1/3	1/3-2/3	> 2/3

*Fraction of cross-sectional bone diameter apparent on roentgenograms.
(From Aaron AD: *JAMA* 272:1206–1209, 1994. Courtesy of Mirels H: *Clin Orthop* 249:256–264, 1989.)

Radiotherapy

Dosimetry and Toxicity of Samarium-153-EDTMP Administered for Bone Pain Due to Skeletal Metastases

Bayouth JE, Macey DJ, Kasi LP, Fossella FV (Univ of Texas MD Anderson Cancer Ctr, Houston)

J Nucl Med 35:63–69, 1994 131-95-3-40

Introduction.—The bone-seeking phosphonate ethylenediaminetetramethylenephosphonic acid (EDTMP), chelated with the β-emitter samarium-153 (^{153}Sm), is being tested at cancer centers for relief of bone pain caused by metastatic cancer. This phase I/II clinical trial was intended to define the pharmacokinetics of repeated injections of ^{153}Sm-EDTMP, define its skeletal uptake, and determine radiation doses to various organs.

Methods.—Nineteen patients received as many as 4 injections of ^{153}Sm-EDTMP in a dose of either .5 or 1 mCi/kg of body weight. The radiopharmaceutical was injected intravenously for 1 minute in a volume that did not exceed 1 mL. Skeletal retention of radioactivity was estimated from urinary excretion.

Findings.—The mean biological half-life of skeletal activity was 520 hours, or infinite for purposes of dosimetry because the biological half-life of the nuclide is 10-fold greater than its physical half-life. Blood activity declined rapidly in the first 30 minutes to about 20% of the injected dose, and then more slowly. Skeletal uptake varied widely but averaged 50% of the injected dose. Bone marrow toxicity, as reflected by changes in platelet counts, was dose related. Thirteen of the 19 patients (68%) reported significant relief of bone pain.

Conclusion.—Bone pain from metastatic cancer may be relieved by injecting ^{153}Sm-EDTMP, which results in a limited dose to the red marrow and has no toxic effects on other organs.

▶ A variety of radiopharmaceutical agents are currently being investigated. The advantages of these agents include the ability to treat diffuse disease, efficiency of therapy with a single injection, lack of systemic effects, and minimal hematologic toxicity. Response rates of 80% are reported with the use of strontium-89 to achieve palliation of bone metastases from prostate and breast cancers. Samarium-153 represents another radiopharmaceutical that has been shown to effectively palliate bony metastases. This bone-seeking radiopharmaceutical has limited hematologic toxicity, and no uptake has been documented in other organs. Repeated injections, resulting in limited bone marrow toxicity, can be performed in patients who experience a partial response. Larger clinical trials will be needed to determine overall rates of response and evaluate dose-response issues. Samarium-153 may expand the therapeutic options available in radiopharmaceutical therapy. Further experience is necessary to determine whether its efficacy is influenced by primary histology, characteristics of the metastatic involvement in the bones, and administered dose.—N.A. Janjan, M.D.

Results of a Randomized Phase-III Trial to Evaluate the Efficacy of Strontium-89 Adjuvant to Local Field External Beam Irradiation in the Management of Endocrine Resistant Metastatic Prostate Cancer

Porter AT, McEwan AJB, Powe JE, Reid R, McGowan DG, Lukka H, Sathyanarayana JR, Yakemchuk VN, Thomas GM, Erlich LE, Crook J, Gulenchyn KY, Hong KE, Wesolowski C, Yardley J (Wayne State Univ, Detroit; London Regional Cancer Inst, Ont, Canada; Cross Cancer Ctr, Edmonton, Alta, Canada)

Int J Radiat Oncol Biol Phys 25:805–813, 1993 131-95-3–41

Background.—Radiotherapy in patients with metastatic prostate adenocarcinoma is often associated with relief of pain from osseous disease and an improved quality of life. Radiotherapy may also effectively decrease the propensity for adjuvantly treated disease to become symptomatic. Strontium-89 is a systemic radionuclide that can relieve pain from bony metastases. The efficacy of strontium-89 adjuvant to local-field, external beam irradiation in the treatment of endocrine-resistant metastatic prostate cancer was studied.

Methods.—Eight Canadian centers participated in the phase III, randomized, placebo-controlled trial. One hundred twenty-six patients were enrolled and received local-field radiotherapy and either strontium-89 as one 10.8-mCi injection or placebo.

Findings.—There were no significant differences in survival or pain relief at the index site. Patients treated with strontium-89 had a significant reduction in analgesic intake and significantly fewer symptomatic sites that needed subsequent radiotherapy. These patients also had reduced tumor markers. Strontium-89 also resulted in a superior quality of life compared with placebo; because pain relief improved, physical activity increased significantly. However, patients receiving strontium-89 had increased hematologic toxicity.

Conclusion.—Strontium-89 is an effective adjuvant to local-field radiotherapy. It reduces disease progression and the need for analgesia and improves patients' quality of life.

▶ Many new agents are available for the treatment of diffuse bone metastases. Strontium-89, a radiopharmaceutical, administers relatively high radiation doses to the site of the metastases, yet has little overall effect on normal bone marrow. The half-life of strontium-89 in normal bone marrow is about 14 days compared with about 100 days at the metastatic sites. Although strontium-89 is reported to be 80% effective in patients with diffuse symptomatic bone metastases or in patients who have persistent localized pain after external-beam irradiation, its role as an adjuvant has yet to be determined. If analgesic effect is improved, and the subsequent need for radiotherapy is reduced, adjuvant strontium-89 may prove cost-effective.—N.A. Janjan, M.D.

Effect of High-Dose Dexamethasone in Carcinomatous Metastatic Spinal Cord Compression Treated With Radiotherapy: A Randomised Trial

Sørensen PS, Helweg-Larsen S, Mouridsen H, Hansen HH (Natl Univ, Copenhagen)

Eur J Cancer 30A:22–27, 1994 131-95-3–42

Objective.—The value of high-dose dexamethasone as an adjunct to radiotherapy was examined in a randomized study of 57 patients who had spinal cord compression with metastatic solid tumors.

Study Design.—A single-blind, randomized design was used. After myelography or MRI, the patients were randomly assigned to receive either no treatment or an IV bolus of 96 mg of dexamethasone; the same dose of dexamethasone was administered for 3 days, and was subsequently given orally in 4 divided portions when feasible. Treatment then was tapered for a total of 10 days. A total dose of 28 Gy delivered with 6-MV photon beams was given in 1 week.

Results.—The 27 dexamethasone-treated and 30 control patients were well matched clinically and demographically. About half the patients in each group had a complete spinal cord block on myelograph. A successful outcome was defined as preservation of gait or its restoration within 3 months of therapy. Functional preservation was achieved in 81% of steroid-treated patients and 63% of control patients. Thirty percent of the steroid-treated group and 20% of control patients remained alive and ambulatory 1 year after treatment.

Conclusion.—High-dose glucocorticoid treatment appears to be a useful adjunct to radiotherapy in patients who have spinal cord compression from a metastatic epidural tumor.

► This prospective, randomized study is an extremely important experience that justifies the administration of steroids to patients with spinal cord compression to maximize functional outcome. Increased rates of paraplegia represented the grave consequence of less aggressive therapy in this experience. Although not systematically evaluated in this study, steroids also are a well-recognized adjuvant analgesic, and they often serve to effectively treat the severe pain that prompts the diagnosis of spinal cord compression. Because of the significant impact on functional outcome and symptoms and the successful management of potential side effects, the emergent administration of steroids and radiotherapy should be considered standard of care in the treatment of spinal cord compression. However, the dose and route of steroid administration require further refinement. The specific indications for surgical decompression should also be prospectively considered. Functional outcome after the diagnosis of spinal cord compression remains the most important index for success of therapy. Ineffective therapy that results in a loss of neurologic integrity will result in higher health care costs because of the need for long-term supportive care.—N.A. Janjan, M.D.

Retreatment With Radiotherapy for Painful Bone Metastases

Mithal NP, Needham PR, Hoskin PJ (Royal London Hosp, Whitechapel, England; Mount Vernon Centre for Cancer Treatment, Northwood, Middlesex, England)

Int J Radiat Oncol Biol Phys 29:1011–1014, 1994 131-95-3–43

Introduction.—Irradiation has been established as the treatment of choice for painful bone metastatic disease. Although practice varies, the site is often re-irradiated if symptoms relapse after the initial treatment. A retrospective review of patient data was undertaken to determine the value of re-treatment of painful bone metastases with external-beam irradiation.

Methods.—Patient records for 97 of 105 patients who received local irradiation for metastatic bone pain from January 1991 to June 1991 were reviewed. The type of treatment (single-dose or a fractionated radiation regimen) and the number of sites requiring re-treatment were evaluated. The treatment response, defined as complete (no pain), partial (improvement with need for analgesics), no response, or unknown response, was recorded.

TABLE 1.—Percentage Response (Complete Response + Partial Response) With Dose/Fractionation

Dose/ fractionation	Retreatment 1	Retreatment 2
Single fractions		
8 Gy/1	11/14 (78%)	2/2 (100%)
10 Gy/1	3/3 (100%)	2/2 (100%)
Other	3/6 (50%)	0/1 (0%)
Multiple fractions		
26 Gy/6	12/12 (100%)	1/1 (100%)
28 Gy/7	3/3 (100%)	
30 Gy/10	11/11 (100%)	1/1 (100%)
Other	5/8 (57%)	1/1 (100%)
Total	48/57 (84%)	7/8 (87.5%)

(Courtesy of Mithal NP, Needham PR, Hoskin PJ: *Int J Radiat Oncol Biol Phys* 29:1011–1014, 1994.)

TABLE 2.—Retreatment Response and Initial Response

	First retreatment response				
Initial response	CR	PR	NR	NK	D
CR (12)	4 (33%)	6 (50%)	0	2	0
PR (37)	4 (11%)	28 (76%)	2	1	2
NR (8)	0	6 (75%)	1	0	1
Total = 57	8	40	3	3	3

Abbreviations: CR, complete response; PR, partial response, NR, no response; NK, not known.

(Courtesy of Mithal NP, Needham PR, Hoskin PJ: *Int J Radiat Oncol Biol Phys* 29:1011–1014, 1994.)

Results.—Pain relapse occurred in 69 of the 229 evaluable sites of response (30%). Re-treatment was done on 57 of these sites; either a complete or partial response was achieved in 48 cases. Relapse occurred in 12 of the 48 sites, and 8 received a second re-treatment (Table 1). No significant differences in response rates were noted based on the radiation dose or number of fractions. Of the 57 sites that relapsed, 12 had a complete response after initial treatment, 37 had a partial response, and 8 had no response (Table 2). The duration of response was shown to be shorter in patients with a partial response as compared with those achieving a complete response (Table 3).

Conclusion.—Re-treatment of bony metastases with localized irradiation is often effective in relieving pain. Single-dose irradiation appeared to be as effective as fractional dose treatment in the re-treatment of bone pain. Additionally, patient age, sex, or primary tumor type or site had no effect on response to treatment.

TABLE 3.—Response and Relapse

	Response	Number relapsed	Av Time to relapse (range/months)
First retreatment	CR 8	3 (38%)	9.7 (6–16)
	PR 40	9 (23%)	5 (2–14)
Second retreatment	CR 2	1 (50%)	37
	PR 5	None	—

Abbreviations: CR, complete response; PR, partial response.

(Courtesy of Mithal NP, Needham PR, Hoskin PJ: *Int J Radiat Oncol Biol Phys* 29:1011–1014, 1994.)

▶ Two important observations are reported in this study. First, symptomatic bone metastases can often be re-irradiated, and palliation of pain can be achieved without significant morbidity. Second, although a variety of fractionation schedules have been used for re-irradiation, often a single fraction of 8 Gy or 10 Gy is an efficient means of treating symptoms that have relapsed in a previously irradiated site. These findings provide more latitude in the radiotherapeutic options for patients with symptomatic bone metastases.—N.A. Janjan, M.D.

Radiotherapy for Bone Pain

Needham PR, Mithal NP, Hoskin PJ (Royal London Hosp; Mount Vernon Hosp, Northwood, Middlesex, England)

J R Soc Med 87:503–505, 1994 131-95-3–44

Introduction.—Patients with cancer often have painful bone metastases. Most of these patients are treated with external-beam irradiation. The choice of a single-fraction vs. a more fractionated regimen is controversial. A retrospective review of patients receiving various regimens of radiotherapy for the treatment of painful bone metastases was completed.

Methods.—The records of 97 patients were reviewed to collect data on the rates of response relative to the regimens used. The importance of the site of the primary tumor, the site treated, and the influence of other treatments on pain relief were also evaluated. Patients who achieved a complete response were pain-free and taking no analgesics within 1 month after radiotherapy. Patients who achieved a partial response were either pain-free with analgesics or had reduced pain.

Results.—The location of primary tumors in the 97 patients with painful bone metastases follows: 47% were in the breast; 21%, the prostate; 8%, the lung; 3%, the kidney; 11%, other sites; 5%, unknown; and 4%, myeloma (Table 1). There were 280 sites irradiated; 59% were treated

TABLE 1.—Number of Patients With Primary Tumor and Sites Irradiated

	No. *of patients*	*(%)*	No. *of sites*	*(%)*
Breast	46	(47)	166	(59)
Prostate	20	(21)	50	(18)
Lung	8	(8)	8	(3)
Unknown	5	(5)	6	(2)
Myeloma	4	(4)	14	(5)
Renal	3	(3)	5	(2)
Other	11	(11)	31	(11)
Total	97		280	

(Courtesy of Needham PR, Mithal NP, Hoskin PJ: *J R Soc Med* 87:503–505, 1994.)

TABLE 2.—Fractionation Related to Site Treated

Site*	No. of fractions 1	2–5	>5	Total
Spine	20 (18%)	3 (3%)	86 (79%)	109
Pelvis/hip(s)	14 (28%)	3 (6%)	33 (66%)	50
Ribs	37 (95%)		2 (5%)	39
Long bones	22 (54%)	3 (7%)	16 (39%)	41
Other	16 (42%)	2 (5%)	20 (53%)	38

* Seven sites are included in 2 categories.
(Courtesy of Needham PR, Mithal NP, Hoskin PJ: *J R Soc Med* 87:503–505, 1994.)

with fractionated radiotherapy, and 41% with a single radiation dose. The number of fractions was not related to primary tumor. It was, however, significantly influenced by the site of irradiation, with the spine and pelvis more commonly treated with multiple fractions, whereas ribs and long bones were more commonly treated with single fractions (Table 2). Younger patients were more likely to receive multiple fractions than patients older than age 70 years, but the association was not significant. There was an overall response rate of 82%, with complete response being achieved by 20% of the patients. Response was not related to age, sex, fractionation, total dose, primary tumor type, or treatment site. In all but 8 patients, response was achieved either at all or none of the sites.

Discussion.—These findings confirm that the majority of patients still are treated with fractionated radiotherapy regimens, even though current evidence has shown benefits with single fractions (Table 3). Both regimens were equally effective. Prospective, long-term studies are needed to assess the occurrence of relapse, retreatment, and late toxicity after single-fraction treatments.

▶ This study adds to the growing body of literature that reviews practice patterns and outcomes of patients who receive external-beam radiotherapy for bone metastases. As in earlier studies, administration of a single fraction of radiotherapy resulted in rates of pain relief that were comparable to those from treatment regimens that included more radiation fractions. Radiotherapists, however, were reluctant to treat the spine with a single large fraction because of concerns about response to therapy and normal tissue toxicity. Although detailed pain and analgesic diaries kept by patients are not included in this retrospective review, a complete response was defined as the absence of pain without the use of analgesics. Overall response rates were comparable to those from other published series. Prospective, randomized studies, however, will be necessary to establish appropriate criteria for the treatment of bone metastases with external-beam irradiation.—N.A. Janjan, M.D.

TABLE 3.—Response Rates From the Published Prospective, Randomized Trials

Reference	No. of *treatments*	*Total dose*	No. of *fractions*	*Overall response (complete response)*
Tong *et al.*	759	15–40.5	5–15	90 (54)
Blitzer reanalysis of RTOG trial	759	30 & 40.5	10 & 15	48
		15–25	5	35
Madsen *et al.*	57	24	6	47
		20	2	48
Price *et al.*	288	8	1	82 (45)
		30	10	71 (28)
Okawa *et al.*	92	30	15	76
		22.5	5	75
		20	10 (×2 per day)	78
Cole *et al.*	29	24	6	100
		8	1	100
Hoskin *et al.*	270	4	1	44 (36)
		8	1	69 (39)

(Courtesy of Needham PR, Mithal NP, Hoskin PJ: *J R Soc Med* 87:503–505, 1994.)

4 Basic Science

Introduction

The basic science reports summarized in this chapter illustrate the continuing interest in nitric oxide and the N-methyl-D-aspartate (NMDA) receptor in spinal cord plasticity and pain mechanisms. The involvement of the NMDA receptor and opioid tolerance is being clarified, and manipulations of the ions (Mg and Ca) associated with the NMDA receptor cation channel suggest potentially useful approaches to achieving control of pain. The presence of NMDA receptors on the terminals of primary afferent neurons in the spinal dorsal horn suggests that they may also function as "autoreceptors." Does glutamate regulate its own release? Or the release of peptides, such as substance P, from primary afferent terminals?

The central and noncyclooxygenase-mediated effects of nonsteroidal analgesic drugs were the focus of a number of studies. Some evidence suggests that drugs like acetaminophen have central antihyperalgesic actions that interfere with the nitric oxide cascade. More is likely to come regarding this topic. As knowledge about the different isoforms of cyclooxygenase (COX I and COX II) expands, it is likely that nonsteroidal anti-inflammatory and analgesic drugs with selectivity for the inducible COX II will be developed. Check this space next year.

Investigators who used the microneurographic approach made a number of important contributions this year. Muscle afferents subserving deep sensation in humans were studied for the first time, and insensitive *branches* of mechanosensitive C-fibers were found to become sensitized by chemical irritation of the mechanosensitive area of the C-fiber. Although inherently injurious to the nerve, microneurography was shown not to be associated with serious symptomatology in healthy humans.

Are there any new players this year? We have found two: nerve growth factor (NGF) and the peptide NPY. Neither is actually "new," but an appreciation of their potential importance to pain definitely is. The role of neurotrophins (e.g., NGF) in plasticity (e.g., hyperalgesia) is becoming more clear. Nerve growth factor and its receptor, TrkA, are rapidly affected when tissue is injured, and antagonists at the TrkA receptor may present a novel target through which the development of hyperalgesia associated with tissue injury may be minimized or prevented. The peptide NPY (and its receptor) also shows rapid changes after tissue injury. Because NPY is often localized with the inhibitory amino acid GABA, it may act presynaptically to inhibit spinal nociceptive transmission.

Finally, Thunberg's 1896 thermal grill illusion has been solved, but you should read about that interesting development on your own! (See Abstract 131-95-1-1.)

G.F. Gebhart, Ph.D.

The Thermal Grill Illusion: Unmasking the Burn of Cold Pain

Craig AD, Bushnell MC (Barrow Neurological Inst, Phoenix, Ariz; Université de Montréal)

Science 265:252–255, 1994 131-95-4-1

Purpose.—The parallel ascending sensory channels governing pain and temperature sensations are regarded as physiologically separate, but an interaction between the 2 can be demonstrated. In the Thunberg grill illusion, the simultaneous application of harmless warm and cool stimuli to the skin by means of interlocking spiral tubes elicits a sensation of strong heat. This sensation has been likened to the burning feeling that accompanies cold pain. Neurophysiologic and psychophysical techniques were used to study the causes of this illusion.

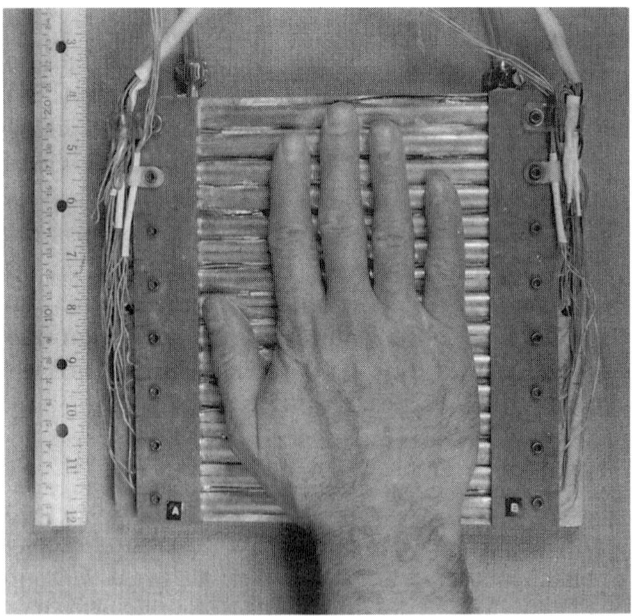

Fig 4–1.—The thermode used with human participants. The stimulus surface (20 by 14 cm) was made of fifteen l-cm-wide sterling silver bars, set approximately 3 mm apart. Underneath each bar were 3 longitudinally spaced thermoelectric (Peltier) elements (1 cm^2), and a thermocouple was located on top of each bar. Alternate (even- and odd-numbered) bars could be controlled independently. (Courtesy of Craig AD, Bushnell MC: *Science* 265:252–255, 1994.)

Methods.—A thermode was used to present thermal stimuli to the palmar surface of the hand in 11 normal human subjects (Fig 4–1). Three different 50-second stimuli were presented 3 times each in pseudorandom order: "warm," in which the temperature of the entire thermode surface was increased to 40°C; "cool," in which the interface temperature was decreased to 20°C; and "grill," in which alternating bars were warmed and cooled.

The same stimuli were applied to cats to assess the physiologic stimuli in the ascending thermosensory channels via recording from spinal cord neurons projecting to the brain in the spinothalamic tract (STT). The cells of the STT in lamina I of the dorsal horn were used because this lamina is the nearly exclusive termination site of cold-sensitive C polymodal primary afferent fibers and probably of cold-specific Aδ fibers as well. In addition, lamina I contains a unique concentration of thermoreceptive-specific neurons, and the lamina I STT axons ascend in a critical location for temperature and pain sensation. The experiment addressed the 3 major types of cat lamina I STT neurons: nociceptive-specific cells, thermoreceptive-specific (COLD) cells, and multimodal cells that respond to heat, pinch, and cold. The study hypothesis was that the sensation of heat evoked by the grill condition represented central unmasking of the cold-activated C polymodal nociceptive channel because of reduction in specific cold activity.

Results.—The human subjects described the warm and cold stimuli as moderate but not painful. Ten of 11 rated the grill stimulus as painful. They rated the grill condition as hotter than "warm" and less cold than "cool." Thus, adding interlaced warm bars to the cool stimulus not only decreased the sensation of cold but also resulted in a sensation of painful heat.

In the cat study, the warm stimulus did not activate the nociceptive-specific, COLD, or heat, pinch, and cold (HPC) cells, although it did partly inhibit the baseline ongoing discharge of COLD cells. The nociceptive-specific cells were unaffected by any of the 3 conditions, but both the COLD and HPC cells strongly responded to the cool stimulus. There was a strong reduction in the response of COLD cells to the grill condition, whereas the responses of the HPC cells to the grill and cool conditions were nearly the same. Thus, adding interlaced warm bars to the cool stimulus reduced activity in the cold-specific channel and shifted the relative pattern of activity toward the HPC or C polymodal channel.

Conclusions.—The Thunberg thermal grill illusion reflects the central integration of ascending pain and sensory channels. These findings add to recent evidence indicating that harmless cold inhibits central pain processing. This model may explain the burning pain and cold allodynia of classic thalamic pain syndrome.

▶ It's cool; it's warm. Both stimuli are accurately perceived without difficulty. About 100 years ago, however, Thunberg (1) showed that these sensations interact to produce an illusion. Innocuous cool and warm sensations applied *simultaneously* to the skin were found to elicit the sensation of strong heat, which was compared with the burning sensation that often accompanies cold pain. This study solves Thunberg's illusion.

In psychophysical studies in healthy subjects and electrophysiologic studies in rat spinal cord lamina I, Craig and Bushnell propose an integrative model. They conclude that the thermal grill illusion results from the central integration of ascending pain and temperature sensory channels. In practical application, the model explains how innocuous cold inhibits central pain processing. Put an ice bag on it.—G.F. Gebhart, Ph.D.

Reference

1. Thunberg T: *Uppsala Läkfören. Föhh.* 2:489, 1896.

A Thalamic Nucleus Specific for Pain and Temperature Sensation

Craig AD, Bushnell MC, Zhang E-T, Blomqvist A (Barrow Neurological Inst, Phoenix, Ariz; Université de Montréal; Univ of Linköping, Sweden)
Nature 372:770–773, 1994 131-95-4–2

Background.—A more complete understanding of the neural mechanisms of pain and temperature sensations requires identification of the thalamic terminations of the nociceptive and thermoreceptive components of the spinothalamic tract (STT). Half the STT originates in lamina I of the dorsal horn. This portion warrants particular attention because it receives input from small-diameter afferents from all body tissues, contains a specific concentration of nociceptive and thermoreceptive STT neurons, and projects ascending STT axons in the middle of the contralateral lateral funiculus. The STT terminations in the thalamus and their physiologic characteristics were studied in macaque monkeys.

Methods and Results.—Restricted injections of high-resolution anterograde tracers were made into lamina I. A dense, compact lamina I STT termination site was identified in the posterior part of the ventral medial nucleus. Recordings were made from single somatosensory neurons located histologically in the posterior part of the ventral medial nucleus. Ninety-seven percent of the characterized neurons responded specifically to noxious or thermal stimuli. The cells' small receptive fields were topographically organized anteroposteriorly. Discharge rates graded with stimulus intensity above threshold.

Conclusions.—The posterior part of the ventral medial nucleus appears to act as a specific thalamic relay nucleus for nociception and ther-

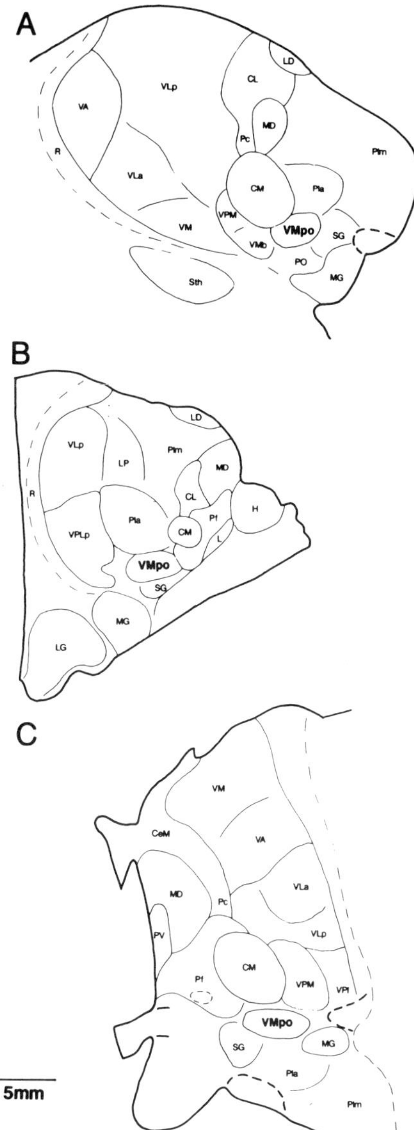

Fig 4–2.—Drawings of the cytoarchitectonic location of the human VMpo in the 3 standard stereotaxic planes: **A,** sagittal L + 14 mm; **B,** frontal, A + .5 mm; and **C,** horizontal, H 0.0. *Other Abbreviatons: CeM,* central medial n.; *CL,* central lateral n.; *H,* habenula; *L,* n. limitans; *LD,* lateral dorsal n.; *LG,* lateral geniculate n.; *LP,* lateral posterior n.; *MD,* medial dorsal n.; *Pc,* paracentral n.; *Plm,* medial pulvinar n.; *PO,* posterior complex; *PV,* paraventricular (thalamic) n.; *R,* reticular n.; *SG,* suprageniculate n.; *Sth,* subthalamic n.; *VA,* ventral anterior n.; *VLa,* anterior part of the ventral lateral n.; *VLp,* posterior part of the ventral lateral n.; *VM,* ventral medial n.; *VMpo,* posterior part of the ventral medial n.; *VP1,* ventral posterior inferior n.; *VPLp,* posterior part of the ventral posterior lateral n.; *VPM,* ventral posterior medial n. (Courtesy of Craig AD, Bushnell MC, Zhang E-T, et al: *Nature* 372:770–773, 1994.)

moreception. Its location in macaques corresponds to the general region in humans in which infarcts that produce analgesia and thermoanesthesia can occur (Fig 4–2). Stimulation of the same area can evoke thermal or painful sensations, and a few nociceptive neurons have been recorded there. The posterior part of the ventral medial nucleus is thus identified as a thalamic nucleus, homologous in humans and macaques, that relays specific pain and temperature activity.

▶ In this combined neuroanatomical and neurophysiologic study in the monkey, the authors identify the posterior part of the thalamic ventral medial nucleus (VMpo) as a specific relay for pain and temperature. Electrical stimulation in this area in humans evokes pain or cold sensations. Lesions in this area are associated with thalamic pain syndrome, and the area is strongly activated in studies of human pain sensibility as assessed by positron emission tomography. Accordingly, it is suggested that VMpo is homologous in macaque monkeys and humans, relaying specific pain and temperature information from lamina I nociceptive and temperature inputs to the insula of the cerebral cortex. Although VMpo is an important means of pain and temperature relay, it is probably not the only thalamic nucleus important to these sensations. How the VMpo relates to other thalamic (and nonthalamic) nuclei that have been shown to contain neurons that also respond to noxious or thermal input arriving via the spinothalamic tract awaits further investigation.—G.F. Gebhart, Ph.D.

Histopathology After Repeated Intrathecal Injections of Preservative-Free Ketamine in the Rabbit: A Light and Electron Microscopic Examination

Borgbjerg FM, Svensson BA, Frigast C, Gordh T Jr (Univ of Copenhagen, Herlev, Denmark; Univ Hosp, Uppsala, Sweden; The Royal Danish Veterinarian Univ, Frederiksberg, Denmark)

Anesth Analg 79:105–111, 1994 131-95-4–3

Background.—Ketamine, when used both intrathecally and epidurally in humans, produces analgesia in patients after surgery and in those with cancer, without motor blocking effects, in the dose range used. Single-dose studies suggest that preservative-free ketamine lacks neurotoxic effects. The effects of repeated intrathecal injections of preservative-free ketamine were assessed.

Methods.—In a randomized study, 14 New Zealand albino rabbits received intrathecal, preservative-free ketamine, .5 mL of 1% solution, or .5 mL of saline once a day for 14 consecutive days. On day 15, the animals were anesthetized and received transcardial perfusion of Tyrode's solution followed by a mixture of 2% glutaraldehyde and 1% formaldehyde in a .1-mol/L phosphate buffer. Five cm of the spinal cord caudal and rostral to the tip of the catheter were removed and studied under light and electron microscopy, combined with quantitative morphometric investigations.

Results.—Intrathecal ketamine produced motor impairment for 15 minutes, whereas intrathecal saline did not. Light and electron microscopy showed no significant morphologic differences between the saline controls and ketamine-injected animals. Furthermore, the total number of cells in laminae I–III of the dorsal horn, the ratio of neuronal cells bodies, and the mean cell volume did not differ significantly between saline- and ketamine-treated animals.

Conclusion.—Intrathecal or epidural preservative-free ketamine is devoid of neurotoxic effects both after single and repeated administration in animals. Preservative-free ketamine is safe for intrathecal administration in humans.

▶ Too often, drugs are given to humans epidurally or intrathecally without sufficient knowledge of the potential toxicologic effects unrelated to the effect for which the drug is given. This study documents that in the rabbit spinal cord, repeated intrathecal administration of ketamine, an *N*-methyl-D-aspartate receptor channel blocker, does not produce neurotoxic effects. For more, see Abstract 131-95-4–4.—G.F. Gebhart, Ph.D.

Spinal Delivery of Sufentanil, Alfentanil, and Morphine in Dogs: Physiologic and Toxicologic Investigations

Sabbe MB, Grafe MR, Mjanger E, Tiseo PJ, Hill HF, Yaksh TL (Univ of Leuven, Belgium; Univ of California, San Diego, La Jolla; Med College of Wisconsin, Milwaukee; et al)

Anesthesiology 81:899–920, 1994 131-95-4–4

Introduction.—Studies in several animal models have shown that intrathecal or epidural administration of μ-opioid agonists results in potent, dose-dependent antinociception. Spinal administration of the anilinopiperidines (e.g., as sufentanil and alfentanil) has received special attention. This is because the anilinopiperidines typically have higher lipid partition coefficients and a greater intrinsic activity than morphine, i.e., greater effects for a given fractional receptor occupancy. A study was conducted in dogs to determine the behavioral effects and possible neurotoxicity of sufentanil, alfentanil, and morphine after chronic epidural and intrathecal administration.

Methods.—Beagle dogs underwent implantation of a chronic lumbar intrathecal or epidural catheter. They then received daily injections of saline or 1 of 3 μ-agonists: sufentanil, alfentanil, or morphine. The sufentanil dose was 5, 25, or 50 μg/.5 mL intrathecally, or 10, 50, or 100 μg/2 mL epidurally. The alfentanil dose was 40 or 400 μg/.5 mL intrathecally, or 80 or 800 μg/2 mL epidurally. The morphine dose was .5 or 5 mg/.5 mL intrathecally, or 1 or 10 mg/2 mL epidurally. Epidural injections continued for 15 days; intrathecal injections continued for 28 days. Antinociception was assessed in terms of skin twitch; neurobehavioral changes were assessed as well. After the dogs were killed, their cisternal CSF and spinal cord tissue were analyzed.

Results.—All 3 μ-agonists by both routes produced dose-dependent antinociception, bradycardia, initial tachypnea followed by decreased respiratory rate, hypothermia, and somnolence. On all measures, sufentanil was the most potent, followed by alfentanil, followed by morphine. Loss of response, or tolerance, was observed on all measures during the prolonged period of drug delivery. Comparison of the various drug and dose groups showed no abnormal morphologic or histologic effects. All dogs had an inflammatory reaction to the catheter. Intrathecal catheters caused significant increases in CSF protein and cell counts in dogs receiving placebo, although epidural catheters did not. These values were not significantly different in drug-treated animals vs. their respective vehicle controls. All 3 drugs demonstrated rapid systemic redistribution, with no differences in pharmacokinetics measured at day 1 vs. the day of killing for either route.

Conclusions.—The expected pharmacologic potency and tolerance development of spinal sufentanil, alfentanil, and morphine in dogs were illustrated. The 3 μ-agonists show no evidence of neurotoxicity throughout a wide range of doses when given intrathecally or epidurally. The canine model used in this study appears to be appropriate for testing the safety of these drugs in concentrations greater than those used for daily intermittent epidural and intrathecal administration in humans.

▶ The antinociceptive and potential neurotoxic effects of 3 opioids were studied in dogs. The order of antinociceptive potency of the 3 opioids when given epidurally or intrathecally was confirmed in this dog model. Daily injections of the opioids were found to be unassociated with neurotoxicity over the dose range studied. It is important to emphasize that, in this study, the safety of opioids (and, in Abstract 131-95-4–3, the safety of ketamine) does not necessarily extend to the dosages and durations of treatment that exceed those studied. These 2 studies (and the one described in Abstract 131-95-4–5) attest to the growing awareness of the need for such information.—G.F. Gebhart, Ph.D.

Laser-Doppler Evaluation of Spinal Cord Blood Flow After Intrathecal Administration of an *N*-Methyl-D-Aspartate Antagonist in Rats

Kristensen JD, Karlsten R, Gordh T (Univ Hosp, Uppsala, Sweden)

Anesth Analg 78:925–931, 1994 131-95-4–5

Introduction.—Drugs administered directly to the spinal cord may be neurotoxic. The N-methyl-D-aspartate (NMDA) receptor system is involved in the transmission and modulation of nociceptive information. Suppression of the NMDA receptor produces antinociception in experi-

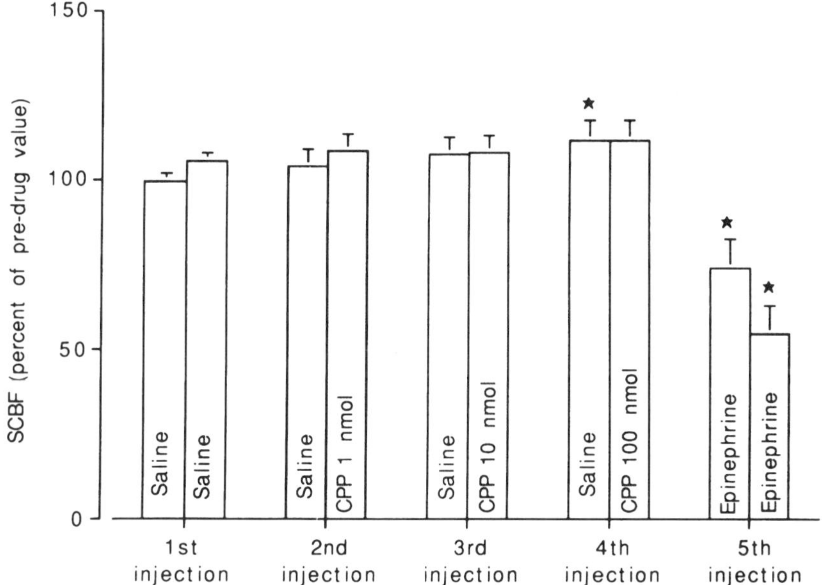

Fig 4–3.—Spinal cord blood flow after intrathecal injection of saline or 3-(2-carboxypiperazin-4-y1) propyl-1-phosphonic acid (CPP) in increasing doses. The values are determined 20 minutes after each injection. No differences were evident between the saline- and CPP-injected animals. Spinal cord blood flow increased by about 10% in both groups during the study, but the increase was statistically significant only in the saline groups. *Stars* indicate a significant difference from baseline (paired *t*-test). Values are means ± standard error of the mean from 8 animals. (Courtesy of Kristensen JD, Karlsten R, Gordh T: *Anesth Analg* 78:925–931, 1994.)

mental animals, and 1 of the most potent antagonists of the NMDA receptor is 3-(2-carboxypiperazin-4-yl)propyl-1-phosphonic acid (CPP). The effect of NMDA antagonists on spinal cord blood flow (SCBF) has to be established before it can be safely used for spinal application in humans.

Methods.—Spontaneously breathing rats anesthetized with inhaled nitrous oxide and enflurane received repeated intrathecal administration of saline or CPP in increasing doses of 1–100 mmol (i.e., from doses within the pharmacologic range to approximately 400-fold the lowest antinociception dose). Laser-Doppler flowmetry was used to measure SCBF. Because of the acidic properties of the CPP solution, saline at pH 6.0, 5.0, 4.0, 3.0, and 2.0 was injected intrathecally to analyze the effect of pH on SCBF.

Results.—There were no significant differences in SCBF between the saline- and CPP-injected animals (Fig 4–3). Although the animals were anesthetized for 2.5 hours, mean arterial pressure and arterial blood gas values remained stable and did not differ significantly between the 2 groups before or after the 80-minute observation period. In saline-treated animals, SCBF increased smoothly, by about 10% during the 80-minute period, and each injection resulted in a minor reduction in SCBF

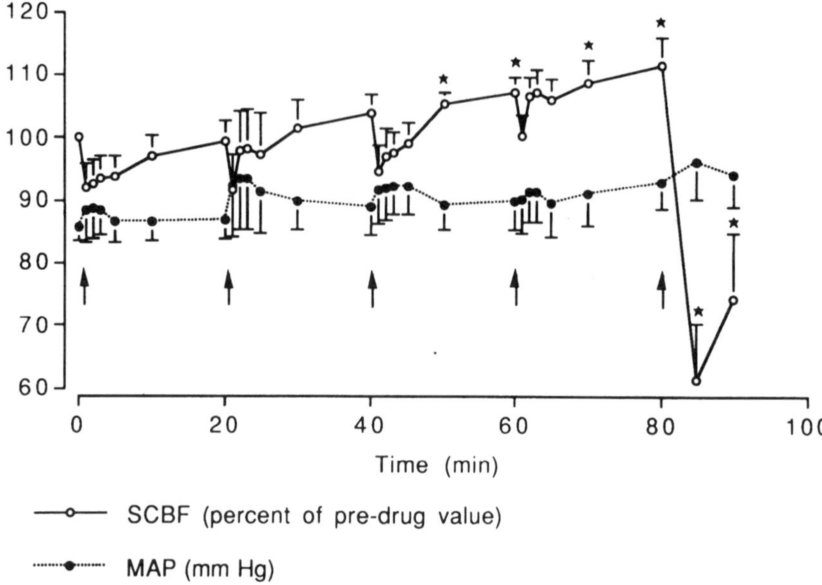

Fig 4–4.—Spinal cord blood flow (*SCBF*) and mean arterial blood pressure (*MAP*) after intrathecal injections of saline. Four consecutive injections of saline were given at 20-minute intervals. After each injection, a transient disturbance in SCBF, lasting 5–10 minutes, was evident. During the 80 minutes of observation, SCBF increased by approximately 10%. Epinephrine injected at the end of the study reduced SCBF by approximately 40%. *Arrows* indicate saline injection. *Stars* indicate a significant difference from baseline (paired *t*-test). Values are means ± standard error of the mean from 8 animals. (Courtesy of Kristensen JD, Karlsten R, Gordh T: *Anesth Analg* 78:925–931, 1994.)

of 6% to 9% that lasted less than 10 minutes (Fig 4–4). When acidic solutions were injected, the SCBF increased in inverse proportion to the pH of intrathecally administered saline.

Discussion.—Intrathecal administration of CPP does not affect SCBF, even in doses 400-fold higher than the smallest dose that induced antinociception. This finding suggests that antinociception and neurotoxicity are likely to occur as a result of vasoconstriction of spinal cord microcirculation, and it does not contraindicate the use of CPP in clinical pain treatment. A gradually developing increase in SCBF (about 10%) should be expected during the observation period; the pH of the injected substance also affects SCBF. Laser-Doppler flowmetry measures only a small part of SCBF; hence, other methods, such as quantitative autoradiographic analysis, should be used before making conclusions regarding the drug's effect on SCBF.

▶ This is another study examining the potential neurotoxic effects of a drug, CPP, that has been given intrathecally in humans (1). When given intrathecally, epinephrine (a "positive" control in these experiments), but neither saline nor CPP, significantly reduced spinal cord blood flow (Fig 4–3) and mean arterial blood pressure (Fig 4–4). This study and those immediately preceeding it establish the safety of drugs that already are, or are likely in the future, to be used with greater frequency in humans. Neurotoxicologic studies are necessary before new drugs are "tested" in humans.—G.F. Gebhart, Ph.D.

Reference

1. Kristensen JD, Svensson B, Gordh T Jr: *Pain* 51:249–253, 1993.

The Consequences of Microneurography Electrode-Induced Injury of Peripheral Nerves Observed in the Rat and Man

Rice ASC, Andreev NY, McMahon SB (St Thomas' Hosp, London)

Pain 59:385–393, 1994 131-95-4-6

Background.—Microneurography has proved to be a helpful tool for investigating neural function since it was introduced in the 1960s, but little is known regarding its tissue effects and safety.

Methods.—The sequelae of microneurography were examined in both a rat sciatic nerve model and human volunteers. Both tungsten and coaxial electrodes were used. Expression of the injury-associated protein GAP-43 was examined by immunofluorescence in the rat sciatic nerve and dorsal root ganglia at 3 and 28 days after the nerve was injured by microneurography electrodes. The ability of unmyelinated afferent nerve fibers to induce neurogenic edema was determined by estimating the extravasation of Evans' Blue dye. In addition, the hind limb withdrawal response to noxious stimulation was monitored.

Animal Observations.—No increase in GAP-43 was noted 3 days after nerve injury, but increased expression was seen 28 days after the application of a coaxial electrode. Both electrodes led to increased expression of GAP-43 in the dorsal root ganglia 28 days after injury. The tungsten electrode decreased dye extravasation at 28 days, but the coaxial electrode had a more transient effect. Both electrodes altered the hind limb withdrawal time but only in the short term.

Human Studies.—Two of 32 volunteer subjects described mild paresthesias after application of the coaxial electrode; the condition resolved within 24 hours. A few volunteers had dull aching at the recording site, which most often disappeared within 24 hours.

▶ Microneurography allows direct electrophysiologic recording from identified primary afferent fibers and has been instrumental in documenting the existence of tissue receptors that respond to specific energies (i.e., stimuli) applied to their receptive endings. Human psychophysical studies using the microneurographic technique to record from afferent nerve fibers innervating the skin have analyzed the elementary sensations of applied stimuli, confirming the validity of the "specificity theory" of pain. Although it is a powerful approach, the technique has been criticized as potentially injurious to nerves when they are penetrated transcutaneously by recording electrodes.

In this study, the inevitable neural injury is shown to be unassociated with serious symptomatology in healthy human volunteers.—G.F. Gebhart, Ph.D.

Identification of Muscle Afferents Subserving Sensation of Deep Pain in Humans

Simone DA, Marchettini P, Caputi G, Ochoa JL (Univ of Minnesota, Minneapolis; Istituto Scientifico H San Raffaele, Milan, Italy; Oregon Health Sciences Univ, Portland)

J Neurophysiol 72:883–889, 1994 131-95-4–7

Background.—Muscle pain and deep tenderness are prominent features of crippling pain syndromes (e.g., "fibromyalgia," trigger point pains, muscle ischemia, some types of low back pain, various athletic injuries, and peripheral neuropathy). However, there are few data on the neural mechanisms that encode and transmit muscle pain under normal

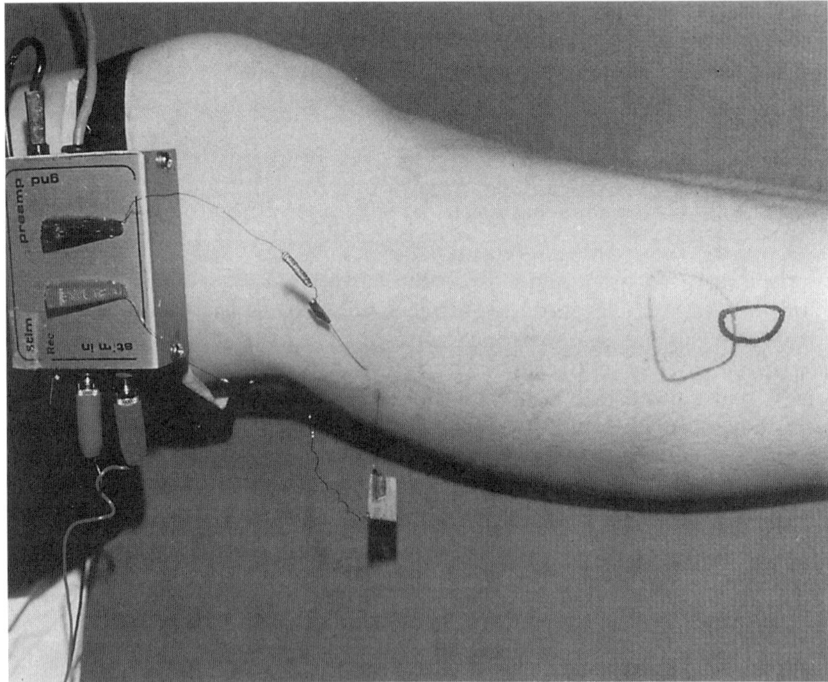

Fig 4–5.—General setup to search for and identify muscle nociceptors. The preamplifier is attached behind the knee. A microelectrode (distal) was inserted into the common peroneal nerve, and a reference electrode (proximal) was inserted into subcutaneous tissue nearby. The outlined area to the left represents the projection of deep pain to the underlying muscle during intraneural microstimulation (INMS) at threshold for pain sensation. The outlined area to the right represents the mechanosensitive receptive field of a group IV nociceptor with conduction velocity of 1.9 m/s. (Courtesy of Simone DA, Marchettini P, Caputi G, et al: *J Neurophysiol* 72:883–889, 1994.)

conditions. A combination of intraneural microstimulation (INMS) and microneurography was used to identify nociceptors in human skeletal muscle and to describe the elementary sensations evoked by their activation.

Methods.—Eleven healthy adult volunteers were studied. Intraneural microstimulation and microneurography were used to stimulate and record from muscle nociceptor primary afferent fibers of the subjects' common peroneal nerves (Fig 4–5). When INMS-evoked pain was projected to muscle, innocuous and noxious pressure was applied to the projected painful area to evoke afferent activity.

Results.—The pain projected to muscle during INMS trains of 5–10 seconds' duration at threshold intensity was well localized and described as cramping in nature. Within or near the painful projected field (PF), slowly adapting mechanoreceptors were identified with receptive fields in muscle and with moderate-to-high receptor thresholds. Overlap was usually noted between the receptive field areas of all units and PFs of sensation evoked during INMS. The areas of PFs evoked by INMS were no different in size from receptive fields.

Conclusions.—Group III and IV nociceptors appear to subserve muscle pain in humans. When these nociceptors are activated, the primary sensation evoked is cramp-like pain. The same quality of sensation is evoked by myelinated and small unmyelinated nociceptive muscle afferents; this is in contrast to the situation with cutaneous nociceptors. The finding that the subjective quality of muscle pain and tendon pain are clearly distinguishable supports the results of classic psychophysical studies.

▶ In this important report, muscle afferent fibers were studied by using the microneurography recording electrode to electrically stimulate the afferent fiber. The major findings: pain projected to muscle by stimulation of afferent fibers was generally well localized and overlapped with the mechanosensitive receptive field of the fiber (Fig 4–5); cramp-like pain was the only sensation evoked from muscle; and activation of both group III (thinly myelinated) and group IV (unmyelinated) muscle afferents evoked the same quality of pain. As previously documented for cutaneous nociceptors, low-frequency stimulation of muscle afferent fibers produced no sensation; a minimum frequency of stimulation of 5–6 Hz was required to evoke pain referred to muscle.—G.F. Gebhart, Ph.D.

Sensitization of Insensitive Branches of C Nociceptors in Human Skin

Schmelz M, Schmidt R, Ringkamp M, Handwerker HO, Torebjörk HE (Univ Hosp, Uppsala, Sweden; Univ of Erlangen/Nürnberg, Germany)

J Physiol 480.2:389–394, 1994 131-95-4–8

Background.—Primary hyperalgesia has been ascribed to a single peripheral neural mechanism, an inflammation-induced reduction in the threshold of nociceptive afferent nerve fibers. Apart from central mechanisms that may account for secondary hyperalgesia in the setting of trauma, another peripheral mechanism may be involved: "awakening" of additional nociceptors that are insensitive in the absence of tissue inflammation. Recruitment of such units would be expected to result in spatial—rather than temporal—summation at central synapses.

Methods.—Recordings were made from 18 cutaneous mechanosensitive C nociceptors in the peroneal nerves of healthy humans. The identity of these fibers was monitored by intracutaneous electrical stimulation, and their activation (by mechanical or transcutaneous electrical stimulation) was monitored by slowing conduction velocity during the relative refractory period. Mechanoreceptive fields (mRFs) were mapped with suprathreshold von Frey hair stimuli.

Results.—The successive topical application of mustard oil and capsaicin expanded the mRFs (initially covering an area of 99 mm^2) by 57 mm^2 in 8 of 15 units. In only 2 of 12 units subjected to electrical stimulation were the borders of the electroreceptive fields and the mRFs identical. In the remaining units, an additional mechano-insensitive area averaging 55 mm^2 was found from which electrical stimulation activated the unit. The application of mustard oil and capsaicin to the mechano-insensitive area sensitized 5 of 8 units to mechanical stimulation. The mRF, after sensitization, corresponded exactly to the electroreceptive field.

Conclusion.—Insensitive nerve branches are present in mechanosensitive cutaneous C nociceptors that, in the presence of inflammation, may be activated and may contribute to hyperalgesia.

▶ How does one explain the lowered pain thresholds in humans and exaggerated nociceptive behaviors in nonhuman animals after tissue inflammation in the absence of sensitization of peripheral nociceptors? Central changes play a role, as does the awakening of so-called "sleeping nociceptors." In this microneurographic study, another mechanism is uncovered, i.e., insensitive branches of mechanosensitive C fibers become sensitive after the application of mustard oil or capsaicin to the mechanosensitive area of the C fiber. Unlike the conventional sensitization of nociceptors, this study found that silent branches of a nociceptive axon acquired mechanical sensitivity.—G.F. Gebhart, Ph.D.

Different Patterns of Hyperalgesia Induced by Experimental Inflammation in Human Skin

Kilo S, Schmelz M, Koltzenburg M, Handwerker HO (Univ of Erlangen-Nürnberg, Germany; Univ of Würzburg, Germany)

Brain 117:385–396, 1994 131-95-4–9

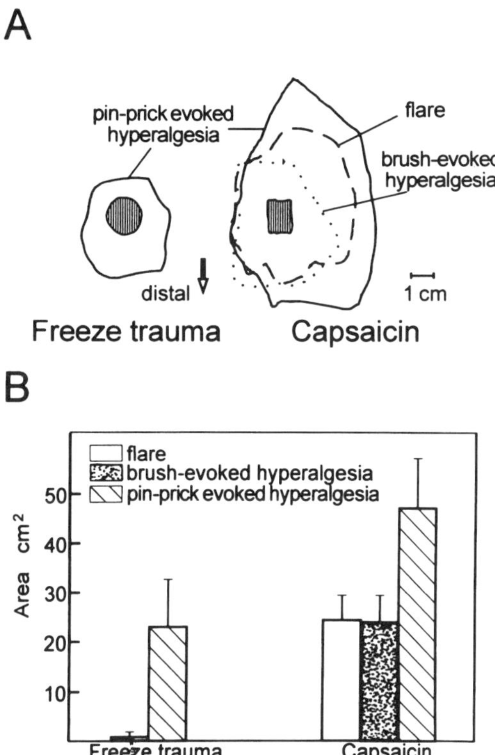

Fig 4–6.—**A,** specimen records of the areas treated with capsaicin or by freezing (*hatched*), the extension of the flare after capsaicin (*broken line*), and the hyperalgesia to punctate stimuli (*solid line*) and brush-evoked (*dotted line*) pain. Applications at the volar site of the forearm. **B,** mean areas of flare and 2 types of hyperalgesia after freeze trauma and after capsaicin. All *error bars* represent SEM. (Courtesy of Kilo S, Schmelz M, Koltzenburg M, et al: *Brain* 117:385–396, 1994.)

Introduction.—Patients with skin injuries and partial lesions of the peripheral nerves commonly have hyperalgesia to mechanical and thermal stimuli. Topographic and stimulus quality considerations are able to distinguish several types of hyperalgesia. Previous studies have characterized 2 zones of abnormal pain sensitivity after focal experimental skin injuries: a primary zone that is directly affected by the injury stimulus and a secondary zone of apparently undamaged tissue around the focus of injury. Differing types of mechanical hyperalgesia appear to arise from different neural mechanisms and may coexist after experimental skin injury. Two models of experimentally induced skin inflammation were used to study different types of hyperalgesia.

Methods.—Inflammation was induced in small skin areas of healthy volunteers by 1 of 2 methods: topical application of 1% capsaicin solution in 70% ethanol or brief freezing of a similar-sized area to −28°C. Sensory tests were conducted 30 minutes after application of capsaicin and 22 hours after freezing, including assessment of the responses to 4 different types of mechanical stimulation.

Results.—Both experimental treatments led to lowered heat pain thresholds, probably because of nociceptor sensitization. In both models, punctate stimuli resulted in hyperalgesia at the skin site directly affected by the injury stimulus and in the surrounding skin. The area of secondary hyperalgesia to punctate stimuli was smaller after freezing than after capsaicin. In the capsaicin model, there was prominent hyperalgesia to gentle brushing of the skin in both the primary and secondary zones; this response was nearly absent after freezing (Fig 4–6). Differential nerve block testing showed that brush-evoked pain was mediated by low-threshold mechanosensitive Aβ fibers, whereas hyperalgesia to punctate stimuli was elicited when only C fibers were conducting. Hyperalgesia to brushing required continuous background discharges in nociceptor units.

On tonic stimulation with a blunt probe, pressure hyperalgesia was noted in the primary zone in both models, probably because of recruitment of sensitized nociceptor units. When small bullets were shot against the skin at predetermined velocities, impact hyperalgesia was noted in the primary zone after freezing but not after capsaicin application. Impact hyperalgesia appeared to be mediated by sensitized C fibers.

Conclusion.—Different types of experimentally induced inflammation in human skin may result in characteristically different patterns of hyperalgesia. Central nervous plasticity changes, rather than nociceptor sensitization, appear to be responsible for hyperalgesia to punctate stimuli and pain evoked by gentle brushing. Rather than a generalized increase in excitability, the neural basis for pain and hyperalgesia appears to be a combination of distinct pathophysiologic events.

▶ Cutaneous inflammation can lead to qualitatively different patterns of hyperalgesia, including a unique type of mechanical hyperalgesia found in this study in 1 of 2 models tested in human volunteers. Freeze trauma and topical capsaicin both produced tissue inflammation and hyperalgesia (Fig 4–6) but differed significantly. Capsaicin produced background pain and hyperalgesia to mechanical brush, punctate, and pressure stimuli but not to mechanical impact stimulation. The freeze lesion produced no background pain and no hyperalgesia to mechanical brush stimulation. Hyperalgesia to mechanical punctate, pressure, *and* impact stimulation characterized and distinguished the freeze lesion from capsaicin-induced hyperalgesia. Impact hyperalgesia is the new type of mechanical hyperalgesia described here, believed by the authors to arise from peripheral sensitization of the unmyelinated nociceptors.—G.F. Gebhart, Ph.D.

Modality-Dependent Modulation of Conduction by Impulse Activity in Functionally Characterized Single Cutaneous Afferents in the Rat

Thalhammer JG, Raymond SA, Popitz-Bergez FA, Strichartz GR (Harvard Med School, Boston; Brigham and Women's Hosp, Boston)

Somatosens Mot Res 11:243–257, 1994 131-95-4–10

Background.—The peripheral axon generally is viewed as a "labeled line" that carries signals from receptors to spinal synapses. The process of impulse conduction in axons is not a static one, but it depends on the history of preceding activity. All axons initially are subexcitable for a few milliseconds. In many axons, the membrane subsequently becomes hyperexcitable for a "supernormal" period lasting tens of milliseconds.

Methods.—Changes in axonal excitability consequent to neuronal firing were related to the functional type of axon in studies of 39 cold fibers and 51 nociceptors of rats. The latency of the conducted impulse was taken as a measure of altered axonal excitability induced by electrical stimulation.

Observations.—Latency increased after natural stimulation of the receptive fields and also after electrical stimulation. The increase in latency correlated with the number of impulses and with the frequency of the preceding discharge. Increased latency after either natural or electrical stimulation was associated with decreased responsiveness to natural stimulation. In nociceptors, latency continued to increase during a train of stimuli, but in cold fibers it increased only for a few seconds and then plateaued even when firing continued. Impulse failure occurred more often during repetitive stimulation in both Aδ and C nociceptors than in velocity-matched cold fibers.

Conclusions.—The pattern of latency change during neural activity is modality-specific in a given type of fiber. Activity-dependent axonal processes have a role in adaptation and encoding in cutaneous sensory afferent nerves.

▶ Here is evidence of the importance of modality, as opposed to axon diameter, in conduction in the cutaneous afferent fibers. These authors document that the slowing of conduction and the rate of recovery after repetitive stimulation correlate better with axon function than axon diameter, suggesting that activity-dependent shifts in the latency changes in the discharge pattern and changes in latency during recovery from trains of stimulation provide better physiologic characterization than do the conventional means of characterization based solely on conduction velocity. Therefore, the axon may do more than just ax.—G.F. Gebhart, Ph.D.

Properties of Afferent Nerve Fibres Supplying the Saphenous Vein in the Cat

Michaelis M, Göder R, Häbler H-J, Jänig W (Christian-Albrechts-Universität zu Kiel, Germany)

J Physiol 474.2:233–243, 1994 131-95-4–11

Introduction.—The human peripheral veins do not normally act as a source of conscious sensations, although pain may result from venous puncture and IV infusion of drugs with unphysiologic osmolarity or pH. In addition, tenderness and persistent pain frequently result from inflammation of superficial veins. Psychophysical studies have shown that various noxious stimuli applied to the inside of the hand vein segment can induce pain. The reported quality of these sensations was the same regardless of whether the stimulus was mechanical, osmotic, thermal, or electric, suggesting that polymodal nociceptive afferents were stimulated. The responses of small-diameter venous afferents to mechanical and chemical stimuli were analyzed in cats.

Methods.—Mechanical and chemical stimuli were applied to a vascularly isolated saphenous vein segment in anesthetized cats to assess the responses of the primary afferent neurons supplying this segment. Centrally cut axons of afferent nerve fibers were isolated from the saphenous nerve near its junction with the femoral nerve, and activity was recorded from these axons.

Results.—Of 30 units responding to 1 of the stimuli, 23 were activated by local mechanical stimulation of the venous wall. The receptive fields were mainly circular spots (Fig 4–7). Of 15 venous segments tested for a response to distention, 8 were activated. Discharges were induced at a mean intravasal threshold pressure of 120 mm Hg. Of 27 units tested for mechanosensitivity and chemosensitivity, 13 were classified as A fibers and 14 as C fibers. Conduction velocities were 5–30 m s^{-1} and less than 2.5 m s^{-1}, respectively. Twelve of the A fibers and 8 of the C fibers were mechanosensitive. Two thirds of the mechanosensitive A fibers and all of

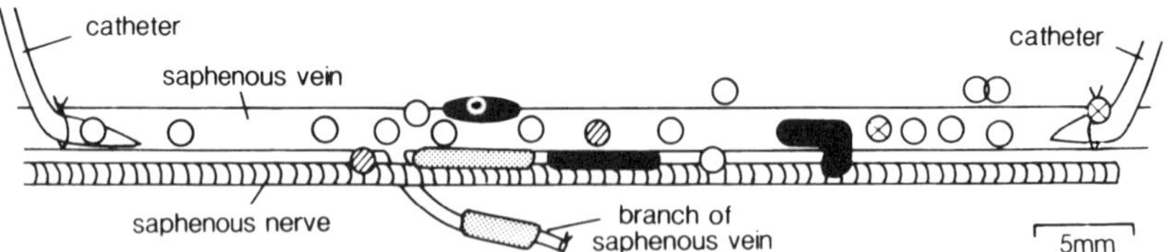

Fig 4–7.—Receptive fields and conduction velocity of mechanosensitive afferent units. Located on the medial or lateral surface of the vein, the receptive fields were usually spotlike (*open circle*, if the unit was excited by probing the receptive field but not by stroking; *circle with diagonal lines*, if the unit additionally responded to stroking). A few receptive fields were elongated (*dotted area*, if units were activated by probing, but not stroking; *filled areas*, if units also responded to stroking). One unit had 2 receptive sites (*circle with* X). (Courtesy of Michaelis M, Göder R, Häbler H-J, et al: *J Physiol* 474.2:233–243, 1994.)

the mechanosensitive C fibers also responded to 1 or more chemical stimuli, including hypertonic saline, bradykinin (BK), or capsaicin.

All 7 remaining units were activated by venous injection of BK but not by mechanical stimuli. Six of these units were identified during experiments using BK as a search stimulus. When BK was injected into the isolated venous segment, an increase in systemic blood pressure resulted. In further systematic experiments, only about 1% of unmyelinated fibers in the saphenous nerve responded to mechanical stimulation of the venous segment.

Conclusions.—A small percentage of saphenous nerve afferent fibers respond to noxious mechanical and/or chemical stimuli applied to the saphenous vein. Acting with chemospecific venous afferents, these fibers may be able to encode nociceptive information from the vein, particularly under disease conditions.

▶ For some time, it has been appreciated that veins can be a source of pain, but experimental investigation of venous afferent fibers has been limited. In this quantitative study, the authors overcame the problems of controlled stimulus application (Fig 4–7) to investigate the receptive fields and sensitivity of small-diameter venous afferent fibers. They document that the majority of small-diameter myelinated and unmyelinated sensory fibers studied were sensitive to mechanical and/or chemical stimuli. Mechanosensitive fibers did not encode changes well in venous pressure in the physiologic range; many were polymodal in character in that they also responded to chemical stimulation. The receptive endings of the fibers studied are considered to be in the venous wall, where they may play a role in tenderness and pain in pathologic conditions.—G.F. Gebhart, Ph.D.

Sympathetic Activation of Cat Spinal Neurons Responsive to Noxious Stimulation of Deep Tissues in the Low Back

Gillette RG, Kramis RC, Roberts WJ (Good Samaritan Hospital and Med Ctr, Portland, Ore; Western States Chiropractic Coll, Portland, Ore)

Pain 56:31–42, 1994 131-95-4–12

Background.—Axons located in the lumbar sympathetic chains contribute to the activation of spinal pain pathways and to low back pain, as shown by studies that use sympathetic blocks in patients, electrical stimulation of the chain in conscious humans, and neuroanatomical mapping of afferent fiber projections. Two mechanisms may explain the activation of spinal "pain pathways" (Fig 4–8). One mechanism involves primary afferent fibers that ascend through the sympathetic trunk and project directly or polysynaptically onto somatosensory neurons. The other involves sympathetic efferent fibers exciting primary afferent fibers in somatic and/or visceral tissues via sympathetic-sensory interactions.

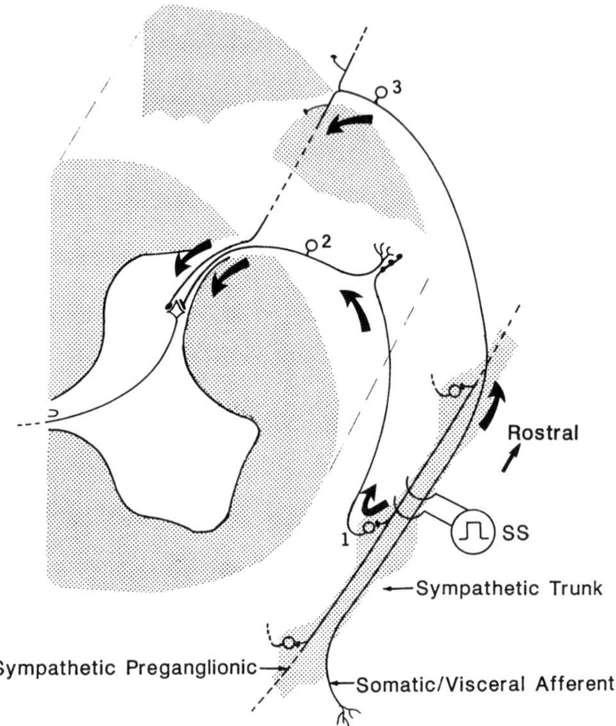

Fig 4–8.—Schematic diagram of neuronal pathways proposed to mediate responses to sympathetic trunk stimulation in spinal neurons. Sympathetic stimulation activates descending preganglionic axons that excite postganglionic neurons (*1*), which excite primary afferents (2) via sympathetic-sensory interactions to produce ***nonentrained*** responses in dorsal horn neurons. Sympathetic stimulation (*SS*) can also activate ascending somatic/visceral afferents (3) that act directly (or via interneurons) to produce *entrained* responses. (Courtesy of Gillette RG, Kramis RC, Roberts WJ: *Pain* 56:31–42, 1994.)

Method.—In anesthetized cats, dorsal horn neurons receiving nociceptor input from lumbar paraspinal tissues were tested for activation by electrical stimulation of the lumbar sympathetic chain.

Results.—Of the 83 spinal neurons tested, 70% were responsive to sympathetic trunk stimulation. The excitatory responses were of 2 distinct types. Nonentrained excitatory responses were elicited in 48% of neurons and resulted from sympathetic efferent activation of primary efferents in the units' receptive fields. Intravenous administration of the α-adrenergic antagonist, phentolamine, reversibly blocked the nonentrained excitatory responses. Entrained responses to sympathetic stimulation were observed in 29% of neurons and resulted from the electrical stimulation of somatic and/or visceral afferent fibers ascending through the sympathetic trunk into the dorsal horn. Entrained responses were not affected by phentolamine. Furthermore, a higher percentage of neurons gave entrained responses in preparations in which the sympathetic trunk was not crushed rostral to the stimulating electrode, suggesting that conduction along axons that ascend in the trunk from the sympathetic electrode significantly contributed to entrained responding. Nonentrained responses were absent in nociceptive-specific neurons but common in multireceptive/wide-dynamic-range neurons, suggesting that nonentrained responses were mediated by non-nociceptive sensory input.

Conclusion.—Low back pain may be exacerbated by activity in both afferent and efferent fibers located in the lumbar sympathetic chain. Nonentrained responses are elicited via noradrenergically mediated, sympathetic efferent interactions with primary afferents in somatic or visceral tissues, whereas entrained responses result from direct electrical activation of primary afferents that ascend through the sympathetic trunk to the spinal cord.

▶ Low back pain, which often exists in the absence of clear pathology, remains largely unexplained. This laboratory has been examining contributions of the sympathetic nervous system to low back pain. Spinal cord neurons receiving input from paraspinal tissues are shown to receive convergent input from the lumbar sympathetic chain. The authors suggest that non-somatic/non-nociceptive input from the sympathetic chain can affect spinal neurons that are responsive to paraspinal inputs, possibly contributing to low back pain.—G.F. Gebhart, Ph.D.

Magnesium Suppresses Neuropathic Pain Responses in Rats Via a Spinal Site of Action

Xiao W-H, Bennett GJ (Natl Inst of Dental Research, Bethesda, Md)

Brain Res 666:168–172, 1994 131-95-4–13

Objective.—In pharmacologic doses, magnesium has anticonvulsive action, as well as neuroprotective effects in models of cerebral ischemia, trauma, and excitatory amino acid-evoked neurotoxicity. In rats subjected to peripheral nerve transection, magnesium pretreatment can slow the onset and reduce the severity of self-mutilation. A voltage-dependent Mg^{2+} ion blockade modulates the N-methyl-D-aspartate receptor-gated ion channel, and previous reports have suggested that the effects of Mg^{2+} therapy may be at least partly mediated via augmentation of this channel-blocking mechanism. The ability of Mg^{2+} therapy to block the pain responses in rats with an experimental peripheral neuropathy was examined.

Methods.—Chromic gut ligation of the sciatic nerve was performed in rats to create a painful peripheral neuropathy. Magnesium was administered by varying routes and dosages to determine whether it blocked the heat-hyperalgesia, mechano-allodynia, and mechano-hyperalgesia seen in this model.

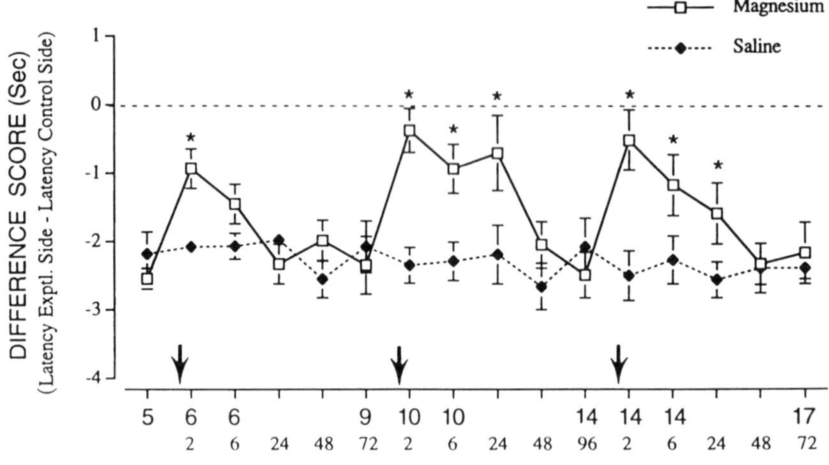

Fig 4–9.—Effects of subcutaneous injections of saline ($n = 5$) or 600 mg of $MgSO_4$ per kg ($n = 6$) on neuropathic heat-hyperalgesia. The test was repeated 3 times. Difference scores (mean ± SEM) are the latency of the nocifensive withdrawal reflex on the control (sham-operated) side subtracted from the latency on the nerve-injured side. Negative difference scores thus indicate hyperalgesia; the difference score of normal rats is 0 (*dashed line*). Injections of Mg^{2+} (*arrows*) produced statistically significant reductions in the severity of heat-hypralgesia for 2–24 hour post injection ($P < .05$ compared with immediately preceding no-injection trials; one-tailed paired *t*-tests). Injections of Mg^{2+} had no statistically significant effect on the withdrawal latencies on the control, sham-operated side. Saline injections (*arrows*) had no effect on the responses from either side. Note abscissa: upper row = days postoperative; lower row = hours after last injection. (Courtesy of Xiao W-H, Bennett GJ: *Brain Res* 666:168–172, 1994.)

Results.—Subcutaneous magnesium sulfate in a dose of 600 mg/kg produced significant reductions in heat-hyperalgesia and mechano-allodynia for 2–24 hours after injection (Fig 4–9). Mechano-hyperalgesia was unaffected. Given intrathecally at doses of 185–750 μg at the level of the lumbar spinal cord, Mg^{2+} significantly reduced heat-hyperalgesia. However, perineural application of Mg^{2+} to the site of nerve injury, at doses of 750–7,000 μg, had no such effect. Magnesium did not affect responses from the sham-operated side, whether given subcutaneously or intrathecally.

Conclusions.—In a rat model of peripheral neuropathy, Mg^{2+} administration suppresses heat-hyperalgesia and mechano-allodynia via a spinal site of action. It does not affect the mechano-hyperalgesia seen in this model. Magnesium therapy may have only a limited role in the treatment of painful peripheral neuropathies in humans.

▶ The spinal *N*-methyl-D-aspartate (NMDA) receptor has been shown to mediate much of the hypersensitivity exhibited by rats after loose ligation of the sciatic nerve, a model developed in this laboratory. The NMDA receptor is voltage-dependent and is normally blocked by Mg^{2+}. Accordingly, one would expect that Mg^{2+} would suppress hypersensitive responses in sciatic nerve–ligated rats, an effect that the authors of this study document. Although it appears that the effect of Mg^{2+} is at a spinal site, it may not necessarily be at the NMDA receptor. Regardless of the mechanism, Mg^{2+} may prove useful, after further study, for relief of neuropathic pain in humans.—G.F. Gebhart, Ph.D.

Voltage-Sensitive Calcium Channels in Spinal Nociceptive Processing: Blockade of N- and P-Type Channels Inhibits Formalin-Induced Nociception

Malmberg AB, Yaksh TL (Univ of California, San Diego, La Jolla)

J Neurosci 14:4882–4890, 1994 131-95-4–14

Background.—Regulation of synaptic transmission is thought to involve calcium influx through voltage-sensitive calcium channels (VSCC). This type of calcium influx also plays an essential role in such cellular functions as neurotransmitter release, enzyme activity, and membrane excitability. The pharmacologic and electrophysiologic evidence suggests

Mean Effective Dose Values and 95% confidence Interval (CI) for Intrathecal Conopeptides on Phase I (0–9 Minutes) and Phase 2 (10–60 Minutes) of the Formalin Test

Drug	n*	ED_{50} (nmol. IT) = 95% CI Phase 1 (0–9 min)	Phase 2 (10–60 min)
N-type channel antagonists			
SNX-111	13	0.003 (0.001–0.006)	0.003 (0.002–0.004)
SNX-159	12	> 0.26	0.12 (0.01–1.3)
SNX-183	16	0.010 (0.007–0.014)	0.009 (0.007–0.013)
SNX-199	12	> 0.30	0.23 (0.03–1.7)
SNX-239	12	0.54 (0.09–2.2)†	0.052 (0.02–0.23)
L-type channel antagonists			
Nifedipine	6	> 29	> 29
Nimodipine	6	> 24	> 24
Verapamil	6	> 200	> 200
Diltiazem	6	> 220	> 220
P-type channel antagonists			
Agatoxin IVA	12	> 0.006†	0.001 (0.0008–0.002)
Non-N/non-L-type channel antagonists			
SNX-231	10	> 0.24	> 0.24
Trivalent cations			
Lanthanum	13	> 0.3‡	0.11 (0.06–0.19)
Neodymium	13	> 0.3‡	0.06 (0.02–0.14)

**Abbreviation:* n, number of animals in the dose-response curve for calculation of mean effective dose (ED_{50}).
†The highest dose produced about a 60% inhibition of the first-phase control.
‡Highest dose produced a 40% to 50% reduction of the first-phase response.
(Courtesy of Malmberg AB, Yaksh TL: *J Neurosci* 14:4882–4890, 1994.)

that there are at least 3 types of neuronal, high-voltage-activated calcium channels: the L, N, and P types.

Methods.—Antagonists of the L, N, and P types, as well as nonselective VSCC antagonists, were intrathecally injected in rats to assess their potential behavioral effects and modulation of formalin-induced nociceptive behaviors. The ability of selected agents to suppress the escape response to high-threshold thermal stimulus was also examined.

Findings.—Use of the trivalent cations, neodymium and lanthanum, for VSCC blockade resulted in dose-dependent suppression of both phases of the response to formalin. Selective blockade of N-type VSCC with Ω-conopeptides also yielded dose-dependent inhibition of both the initial behavior and the facilitated-response phases of the formalin test. Also, SNX-231—, which selectively blocks a non-L/non-N site, and the L-type VSCC blockers nifedipine, nimodipine, verapamil, and diltiazem had few effects on either phase of the formalin test, even at the highest doses. Ω-Agatoxin IVA, a P-type channel blocker, yielded a 40% inhibition of phase 1 at the highest dose. Phase 2 was suppressed in dose-dependent fashion (table).

Neodymium and SNX-111 yielded a moderate increase in the response latency to a high-threshold thermal stimulus, i.e., the hot plate test. Verapamil and Ω-agatoxin IVA produced no such change. At high doses, the N-type VSCC produced characteristic shaking behavior, as well as serpentine tail movements and impaired coordination. Antinociceptive doses of these blockers produced no significant motor effects, although 3 of the N-type antagonists produced some tail movements.

Conclusions.—The N-type VSCC may play a role in inducing facilitated states of large and small afferent processing in the spinal cord. The L-type VSCC appears to have no such role. The link between N-type calcium channels and small primary afferent neurotransmitter release may help to explain the selective effect on spinal nociceptive transmission. However, the functional characteristics of these agents suggest a more complicated organization.

► Calcium is an ion important to synaptic transmission and neuron excitability. Despite their potential importance to sensory transmission, particularly nociception, the role of calcium channels has not been studied behaviorally. Not surprisingly, antagonists of VSCC were antinociceptive in formalin test in rats. As with the *N*-methyl-D-aspartate receptor, which also gates calcium, these author conclude that the N-type VSCC may be important to facilitated nociceptive transmission in the spinal cord.—G.F. Gebhart, Ph.D.

Antinociceptive Actions of R(−)-Flurbiprofen, A Non-Cyclooxygenase Inhibiting 2-Arylpropionic Acid, in Rats

Geisslinger G, Ferreira SH, Menzel S, Schlott D, Brune K (Univ of Erlangen-

Nürnberg, Germany; Univ of Sao Paulo, Brazil)
Life Sci 54:173–177, 1994 131-95-4–15

Background.—Recent studies have suggested that nonsteroidal anti-inflammatory drugs (NSAIDs) possess antinociceptive effects independent of their anti-inflammatory actions, but these studies have mainly focused on their peripheral mode of action. It has become increasingly evident that NSAIDs have a central antinociceptive action. Whether systemic administration of enantiomers of flurbiprofen was antinociceptive in the formalin-induced hyperalgesia model in the rat was studied.

Methods.—In male rats, R(−)-flurbiprofen and S(+)-flurbiprofen were administered intraperitoneally before injection of formalin on the right paw. Flinches were counted at 2-minute intervals for 60 minutes. A modification of the Randall Sellito rat paw pressure test was also used, in which hyperalgesia was induced by intraplantar injection of prostaglandin E_2 (PGE_2).

Results.—In the rat paw formalin test, intraperitoneal administration of R(−)-flurbiprofen and S(+)-flurbiprofen resulted in a dose-dependent antinociceptive behavior, with S (+)-flurbiprofen being 3 times more potent than R(−)-flurbiprofen (Fig 4–10). Because the cerebrospinal levels of metabolically formed S(+)-flurbiprofen after R(−)-administration remained low and constant despite increasing doses of R(−)-flurbiprofen, it was unlikely that the antinociceptive action of R(−)-flur-

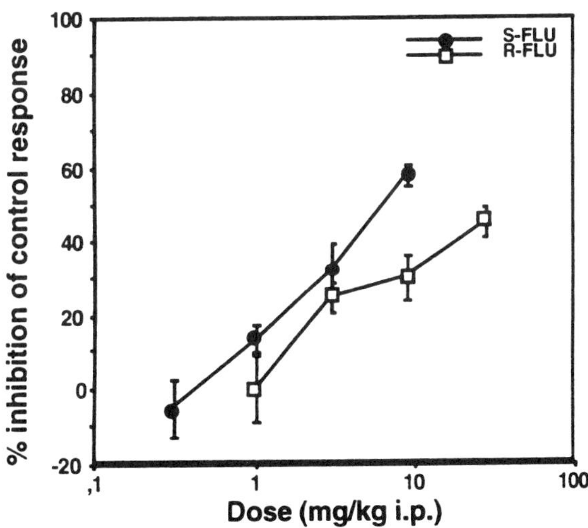

Fig 4–10.—Dose response curve for intraperitoneally administered R(−)- and S(+)-flurbiprofen presented as % inhibition of control response during phase 2a vs. dose (mg/kg) in the formalin-induced hyperalgesia model of the rat. Each data point represents the mean ± standard error of the mean of 8 rats. The statistical calculations for dose response relationships were as follows (analysis of variance): S(+)-flurbiprofen, $F = 76.5$, $P < .001$; R(−)-flurbiprofen, $F = 32.6$ $P < .001$. (Courtesy of Geisslinger G, Ferreira SH, Menzel S, et al: *Life Sci* 54:173–177, 1994.)

biprofen was via chiral inversion to the S-enantiomer. In a modified Randall Sellito assay, both enantiomers caused significant antinociception when administered systemically (subcutaneous). When administered locally (intraplantar), only S(+)-flurbiprofen significantly reduced the intensity of hyperalgesia. In contrast, R(−)-flurbiprofen did not block PGE_2-induced hyperalgesia when given locally.

Implication.—These findings suggest the involvement of alternative mechanisms apart from inhibition of prostaglandin production at the spinal cord level. Because R(−)-flurbiprofen is unable to block PGE_2-induced hyperalgesia when given locally, it may be that its antinociceptive effects after systemic administration involve a central site of action either at the spinal cord or supraspinal levels.

▶ In recent years, it has become accepted that NSAIDs have central as well as peripheral actions that contribute to their antinociceptive effect. Whether cyclooxygenase inhibition is important to the central antinociceptive action of these drugs is unclear. This study provides indirect evidence for a central antinociceptive action of a noncyclooxygenase-inhibiting enantiomer of flurbiprofen. By what other mechanism might these effects occur? See Abstract 131-95-4–16.—G.F Gebhart, Ph.D.

Acetaminophen Blocks Spinal Hyperalgesia Induced by NMDA and Substance P

Björkman R, Hallman KM, Hedner J, Hedner T, Henning M (Univ of Gothenburg, Sweden; Sahlgren's Hosp, Gothenburg, Sweden)

Pain 57:259–264, 1994 131-95-4–16

Background.—Acetaminophen is widely used, and yet its therapeutic mechanism of action remains unclear. It has been reported that acetaminophen inhibits spinally substance P (SP)–mediated hyperalgesia and that postsynaptic structures in the CNS produce nitric oxide (NO) from L-arginine by an enzymatic process in response to activation of SP and excitatory amino acid receptors. Inhibition of the L-arginine-NO pathway may represent a potential central mechanism of action for acetaminophen.

Study Design.—In Sprague-Dawley rats, acetaminophen (1.3 mmol/kg) or saline was given intraperitoneally 15 minutes before intrathecal injection of N-methyl-D-aspartic acid (NMDA), α-amino-3-hydroxy-5-methyl-4-isoxazolepropionate (AMPA), or SP. The number of caudally directed "bites, scratches, and licking" was counted at 1-minute intervals for 10 minutes and compared between treatment groups. In addition, the natural substrate for NO synthetase, L-arginine, and its isomer, D-arginine, were given intraperitoneally at 5 and 20 minutes before injection of NMDA, AMPA, or SP.

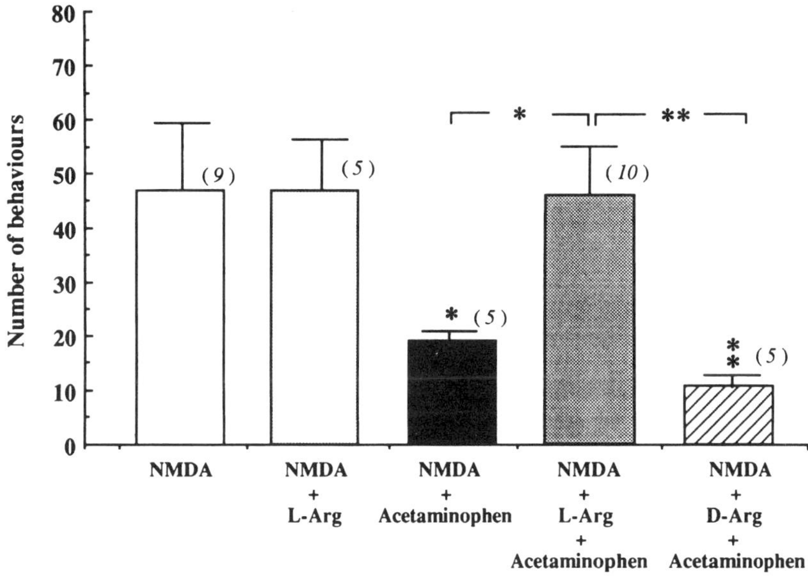

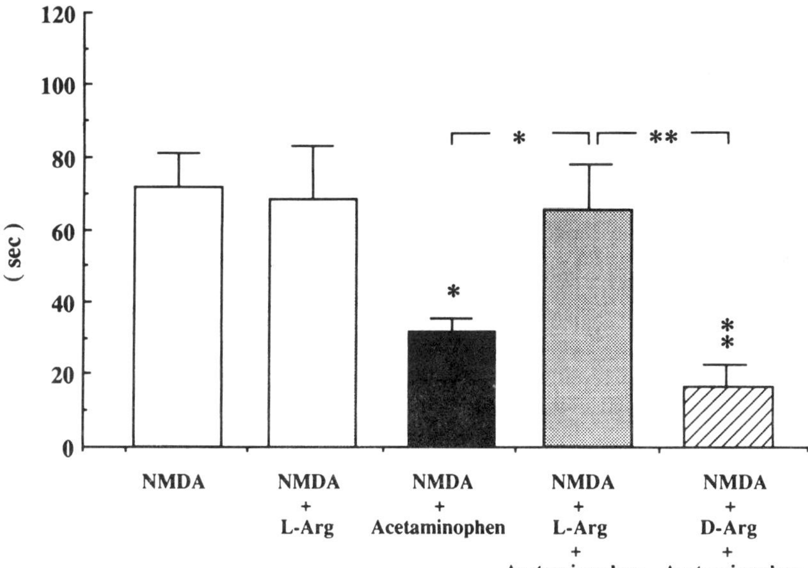

Fig 4–11.—Effects of acetaminophen on the N-methyl-D-aspartic acid (NMDA)-induced biting, scratching, and licking (BSL) response in rats. The effect of pretreatment with L-arginine or D-arginine at 20 and 5 minutes before NMDA is also shown. Shown are means ± standard error of the mean of the number of behaviors of BSL responses (**upper panel**) and the total duration in seconds of the behavioral response (**lower panel**). The number of animals in each group is show within brackets. $^{*}P < .05$, $^{**}P < .01$. (Courtesy of Björkman R, Hallman KM, Hedner J, et al: *Pain* 57:259–264, 1994.)

Results.—The animals exhibited a characteristic biting, scratching, and licking response after spinal administration of NMDA, AMPA, or SP. Pretreatment with acetaminophen reduced the number of behaviors in response to NMDA and SP, but not AMPA. The effect of acetaminophen on NMDA-induced hyperalgesia was dose-dependent and competitive. Pretreatment with L-arginine, but not D-arginine, reversed the acetaminophen-induced inhibition of behaviors after administration of NMDA and SP, but not AMPA (Fig 4–11).

Discussion.—Acetaminophen inhibits spinal hyperalgesia induced by both NMDA and SP, but not by AMPA. The effect of acetaminophen is readily and selectively reversed by L-arginine, but not by D-arginine, suggesting that the analgesic effect of acetaminophen is related to inhibition of NO generation, with NMDA and SP receptors modulating nociceptive activity at the spinal level. It appears that a significant portion of the analgesic effect of acetaminophen, when used clinically, may be related to an interaction with neuronal L-arginine-NO pathway.

▶ In this study, a weakly effective nonsteroidal anti-inflammatory drug, acetaminophen, was shown to attenuate the effects of NMDA given intrathecally. Because NMDA and SP, which was also used, produce hyperalgesic effects in the spinal cord via the arginine-NO-cyclic guanosine monophosphate cascade, acetaminophen is thought to interfere with this cascade. Acetaminophen was given systemically in this study, as was the NO precursor L-arginine; therefore, the site of the interaction is uncertain. Regardless, acetaminophen appears to have a supraspinal and/or spinal site of action that is unrelated to an involvement with cyclooxygenase but contributes to its antinociceptive effect.—G.F. Gebhart, Ph.D.

Intraarticular Morphine for Postoperative Analgesia Following Knee Arthroscopy

Björnsson A, Gupta A, Vegfors M, Lennmarken C, Sjöberg F (Univ Hosp, Linköping, Sweden)

Reg Anesth 19;104–108, 1994 131-95-4–17

Background.—The effectiveness of local anesthetics directly injected into the articular space is not clear. One study indicated that 1 mg of intra-articular morphine provides significant analgesia for up to 6 hours after the operation. This effect can be reversed by the injection of naloxone, confirming specific action to local opioid receptors. The analgesic effects of low- and high-dose morphine or bupivacaine injected intra-articularly after arthroscopic procedures were assessed.

Study Design.—A total of 149 healthy young patients undergoing arthroscopic knee surgery participated in a 2-stage, prospective, double-blind, randomized, and controlled study. All patients received standard general anesthesia. In the first study, at the end of surgery, 78 patients were injected intra-articularly with either 1 mg of morphine diluted in 19 mL of .9% saline, 20 mL of .9% saline (placebo), 20 mL of .25% bupivacaine (50 mg), or 1 mg of morphine plus 19 mL of .25% bupivacaine. In the second part of the study, at the end of the operation, 71 patients were treated with either 5 mg of morphine mixed with 35 mL of .9% saline given intra-articularly, 40 mL of .9% saline given intra-articularly, or 40 mL of .9% saline given intra-articularly plus 5 mg of morphine given intramuscularly. Using a linear visual analogue scale, postoperative analgesia was assessed at 30, 60, 90, and 120 minutes and repeated at home at 8, 24, and 48 hours.

Outcome.—There were no significant differences in visual analogue scores between the different groups in both parts of the study. Furthermore, the postoperative analgesic requirement was similar in all groups.

Conclusion.—This study fails to confirm the beneficial analgesic effects of 1 mg or 5 mg of morphine, or 50 mg of bupivacaine when given intra-articularly in patients undergoing minor diagnostic arthroscopic surgery. In contrast, Stein et al. have shown a beneficial effect of morphine between 3–6 hours after the operation, and Khoury et al. showed a lasting effect of morphine from 4 hours up to 48 hours. The differences may be a result of the earlier assessment and use of regular alfentanil during the operation in the present study.

▶ Morphine has been reported in some, but not all, studies to have a potent, peripheral analgesic effect. Several different experimental approaches support the peripheral action of morphine: morphine reduces the release of peptide neurotransmitters from peripheral nerve terminals, and opioid receptors have been reported to be present in peripheral tissues. This report, however, did not find a peripheral analgesic action for morphine when injected intra-articularly. The authors acknowledge that the intraoperative use of another opioid may have confounded the outcome, but other factors that may be important in such experiments also need to be considered because this approach is potentially very useful. What are the pharmacokinetics of morphine given intra-articularly? Would a more or less hydrophilic opioid be a better choice? What role is played by general anesthesia or by local post-surgical inflammation?—G.F. Gebhart, Ph.D.

Influence of Morphine on the Activity of Low-Threshold Visceral Mechanoreceptors in Cats With Acute Pericarditis

Balkowiec A, Kukula K, Szulczyk P (Warsaw Med School, Poland)

Pain 59:251–259, 1994 131-95-4–18

Introduction.—Opioid receptors, because of their location on peripheral sensory terminals, are thought to be involved in the activity relayed along sensory fibers. Some experiments have suggested that peripherally acting opioid agonists inhibit pain perception, possibly more effectively for pain caused by inflammation, through suppression of excitation of pain-encoding afferent fibers. However, other data indicate that opioids may stimulate vagal afferents. To determine the reaction of afferent fibers to opioids, morphine was topically applied to sensory fibers of the thoracic viscera of cats with induced pericarditis.

Methods.—The thoracic visceral sympathetic and vagal afferent fibers from 23 anesthetized cats were dissected and identified by electrical stimulation. Pericarditis was induced with injection of 1 mL of 4% kaolin suspension in .9% saline. Four concentrations of morphine (0.001, 0.01, 0.1, and 1.0 mg/mL) were sequentially applied to the afferent fibers for 5 minutes. Electrocardiogram limb leads I, II, and III were then recorded before and after induction of pericarditis, and then every 2 hours during the experiment. In an experiment to block the afferent fiber's reaction to morphine, naloxone, 1 mg/mL, was applied topically prior to the application of morphine.

Results.—A dose-dependent increase in activity occurred when morphine was applied to the receptive field of the afferent sympathetic fibers in 12 of 12 fibers tested. Morphine failed to evoke excitation in the fibers tested when applied immediately after the application of naloxone. Similarly, 7 of 9 afferent vagal fibers showed dose-dependent activity after the application of morphine. Application of naloxone also inhibited vagal fiber excitation to morphine application. Although not significant, the mean increase in activity observed was larger for the vagal afferent fibers as compared with the sympathetic afferent fibers.

Conclusion.—Vagal and sympathetic group III and IV afferent fibers were activated in a dose-dependent manner after application of morphine to the receptive fields of these fibers. The location of the receptive field, either in inflamed or noninflamed tissue, did not affect the reaction of the fibers to morphine. Considering the peripheral location of opioid receptors, the effect of morphine observed in this study may be the result of its direct influence on the activity of peripheral endings. Alternatively, morphine may exert its action indirectly on sensory fibers and act on opioid receptors in non-neuronal tissues.

▶ The location of opioid receptors on peripheral nerve terminals suggests an opportunity for modulation by opioids of afferent fibers. The expectation is that morphine would attenuate activity of afferent fibers innervating inflamed tissue. Not so, according to this study. After experimental induction of pericarditis, the activity of 19 of 21 low-threshold mechanoreceptors innervating thoracic viscera was increased by morphine in a dose-dependent, receptor-selective manner. One could interpret this outcome to mean that morphine can make visceral pain worse. More likely, morphine activates vagal afferent fibers that contribute to pain modulation through a brain stem circuit.—G.F. Gebhart, Ph.D.

Subarachnoid Morphine Reduces Stimulation-Induced But Not Basal Expression of Preproenkephalin in Rat Spinal Cord

Crosby G, Marota JJA, Goto T, Uhl GR (Harvard Med School, Boston; Massa-

chusetts Gen Hosp, Boston; Johns Hopkins School of Medicine, Baltimore, Md)
Anesthesiology 81:1270–1276, 1994 131-95-4–19

Background.—Tissue damage in the periphery causes many changes in central neural function that affect the subsequent pain experience. The central release of excitatory neurotransmitters facilitates or sustains pain, whereas the release of neurochemical mediators with inhibitory functions may modulate nociceptive transmission. The possibility that the potent exogenous opioid analgesic morphine may change the neuronal expression of opioid peptide genes was explored.

Methods.—The effect of subarachnoid morphine on basal and noxious stimulation-induced expression of preproenkephalin in spinal cord neurons was studied using male Sprague-Dawley rats. Twenty rats were prepared 48 hours in advance with lumbar subarachnoid catheters. Initially, basal expression was assessed in rats receiving morphine 10 μg or saline intrathecally. The experiment was then repeated, except that 10 minutes after administration of morphine or saline, rats were given a hindpaw footpad injection of 50 μL of 5% formalin. Two hours later, the rats were killed during pentobarbital anesthesia. Messenger RNA transcribed from preproenkephalin was measured in the lumbar spinal cord with quantitative in situ hybridization with a complementary sulfur 35-labeled oligonucleotide probe and emulsion autoradiography.

Findings.—In unstimulated rats, 20% of the neurons in laminae I–II and 10% of those in laminae III–IV expressed preproenkephalin. Injection of formalin increased the fraction of positive neurons in laminae I–II and V–VI by 34% and 20%, respectively, but it did not affect expression in laminae III–IV. Subarachnoid morphine administration did not change the basal expression of preproenkephalin, but it substantially attenuated the noxious stimulation-induced increase in laminae I–II and V–VI by preventing the stimulation-evoked recruitment of preproenkephalin-expressing neurons that would have occurred with it.

Conclusions.—Morphine acts indirectly to decrease stimulation-evoked expression of preproenkephalin by blocking noxious excitatory inputs into opioid neurons. This mechanism is consistent with reports that the ability of morphine and other μ opioid receptor agonists inhibit stimulation-evoked release of primary afferent neurotransmitters through a presynaptic action on the central terminals of primary afferent fibers. In addition, it does not preclude the possibility that morphine decreases the sensitivity of second-order neurons to noxious inputs.

► Among the many things morphine does, in this study it was shown to significantly attenuate the inflammation-induced increase in spinal neuron preproenkephalin expression. Because morphine did not alter basal expression of preproenkephalin in spinal neurons, the effect of morphine is indirect (e.g., on the release of excitatory amino acids or peptides from primary afferent nerve terminals in the dorsal horn). The more interesting speculation is that morphine interferes with c-*fos*–mediated regulation of the preproenkephalin gene.—G.F. Gebhart, Ph.D.

Prolonged Analgesia and Decreased Toxicity With Liposomal Morphine in a Mouse Model

Grant GJ, Vermeulen K, Zakowski MI, Stenner M, Turndorf H, Langerman L (New York Univ, NY)

Anesth Analg 79:706–709, 1994 131-95-4–20

Background.—Patients undergoing surgery often do not receive sufficient postoperative analgesia. As-needed pain treatment with IM narcotics is not optimal. A reliable method of long-lasting postoperative analgesia in a single dose would be very useful.

Methods.—A liposomal morphine formulation was synthesized and compared with free morphine in a mouse model. Analgesia was tested by tail-flick after intraperitoneal injection. The duration of analgesia and systemic toxicity were compared, and the release rate of morphine from liposomes was assessed in vitro.

Findings.—The lethal free morphine dose in 50% of the mice was 400 mg/kg. The maximum safe dose was 130 mg/kg. The highest dose of liposomal morphine administered—1,650 mg/kg—did not kill any mice. The duration of analgesia associated with the highest dose of liposomal morphine was 21.5 hours, which was significantly longer than the 3.7 hours associated with the maximum safe dose of free morphine. A slow release rate of morphine from the liposome depot was noted in the in vitro experiments (Fig 4–12).

Conclusions.—The significant prolonged analgesia with liposomal morphine in this mouse model may be useful in the treatment of postoperative pain in humans. Slow liposomal release of morphine should re-

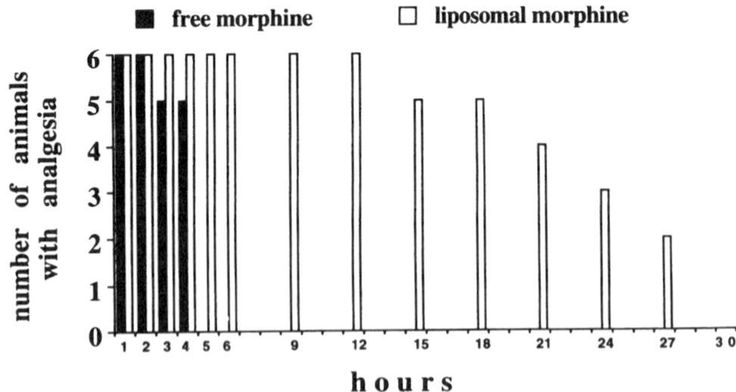

Fig 4–12.—Duration of analgesia in mice after intraperitoneal injection of free or liposomal morphine. Number of animals with analgesia ($n = 6$ per group) is plotted against time. There was a significant difference in the mean duration of analgesia between the groups ($P < .01$). (Courtesy of Grant GJ, Vermeulen K, Zakowski MI, et al: *Anesth Analg* 79:706–709, 1994.)

sult in a sustained treatment effect with a single dose and minimize the likelihood of systemic morphine toxicity.

▶ Is this a means for improving postoperative pain control? Liposomes are biocompatible vesicles synthesized from phosphocholine and cholesterol and are thus nontoxic. Drugs can be encapsulated in liposomes for slow release in vivo. In this study, a more than fivefold increase in duration of action with no significant toxicity was realized. If safe in humans, a liposomal morphine formulation could be good news for pain control.—G.F. Gebhart, Ph.D.

Modulation of Morphine Tolerance by the Competitive *N*-Methyl-D-Aspartate Receptor Antagonist LY274614: Assessment of Opioid Receptor Changes

Tiseo PJ, Cheng J, Pasternak GW, Inturrisi CE (Cornell Univ Med College, New York; The Cotzias Lab of Neuro-Oncology, New York; Mem Sloan-Kettering Cancer Ctr, New York)

J Pharmacol Exp Ther 268:195–201, 1994 131-95-4–21

Background.—The development of tolerance to the analgesic effects of morphine reduces its effectiveness and complicates the treatment of patients with persistent pain. Laboratory animals can also develop tolerance to opioid effects such as analgesia. The competitive N-methyl-D-aspartate (NMDA) antagonist, LY274614 ([±]-6-phosphonomethyl-decahydroisoquinolin-3-carboxylic acid), can reverse morphine tolerance and restore morphine sensitivity in tolerant animals that continue to receive morphine. The influence of LY274614 on morphine tolerance and the affinity and density of CNS opioid receptors were studied in rats.

Methods.—Adult male Sprague-Dawley rats were investigated using 75 mg of morphine or placebo pellets implanted subcutaneously. The rats received continuous subcutaneous infusions of LY274614 (24 mg/kg of body weight per 24 hours) or saline. Each animal's analgesic response was assessed at 1 hour after the administration of a challenge dose of morphine with a 52.5°C HP.

Results.—Co-administration of morphine and LY274614 significantly attenuated the development of tolerance to morphine. Rats that were made tolerant to morphine and were then infused with LY274614 regained their analgesic sensitivity to morphine faster than did control rats infused with saline. Some nontolerant animals were infused with LY274614 for 1 week. One week after the infusion was stopped, they received a morphine challenge. There was no difference in the expression of morphine analgesia or in the development of morphine tolerance between the rats infused with LY274614 and the rats infused with saline. The density or affinity of *mu, delta, kappa*-1 or *kappa*-3 opioid receptors in rat brain homogenates was not increased by a 1-week infusion of LY274614. The IC_{50} values for LY274614 in *mu*-1, *mu*-2, *delta, kappa*-1, or *kappa*-3 ligand binding assays were greater than 10 μM.

Conclusions.—The competitive NMDA receptor antagonist LY274614 can both attenuate and reverse the development of morphine tolerance in rats. This modulation of tolerance is not caused by a change in the affinity or number of opioid receptors. After LY274614 administration is ended, its ability to moderate tolerance expires in less than 1 week. The NMDA receptor system seems important in the development of tolerance to morphine.

▶ From this study we learn what is *not* the means by which NMDA receptor antagonists can attenuate or reverse tolerance to the antinociceptive effects of morphine. Neither the number nor the affinity of any of the 3 principal opioid receptor subtypes (μ, δ, or κ) is affected by administration of LY274614. What is unchanged by this study is our lack of understanding about this potentially important interaction with NMDA receptors (see, however, Abstract 131-95-4–22). Interestingly, in the absence of tolerance, NMDA receptor antagonists appear to potentiate the antinociceptive effects of morphine, which is another reason why development of a safe and effective NMDA receptor antagonist for use in humans is a high priority—G.F. Gebhart, Ph.D.

The NMDA Receptor Antagonists, LY274614 and MK-801, and the Nitric Oxide Synthase Inhibitor, NG-Nitro-L-Arginine, Attenuate Analgesic Tolerance to the Mu-Opioid Morphine But Not to Kappa Opioids

Elliott K, Minami N, Kolesnikov YA, Pasternak GW, Inturrisi CE (Cornell Univ, New York; Mem Sloan-Kettering Cancer Ctr, New York)

Pain 56:69–75, 1994 131-95-4–22

Introduction.—The development of tolerance to the analgesic effects of opioids is poorly understood. Previous reports have indicated that LY274614 (LY), a competitive, and MK-801, a noncompetitive, N-methyl-D-aspartate (NMDA) receptor antagonist can attenuate the development of morphine tolerance in rats, in part through inhibition of the formation of nitric oxide (NO). The latter is supported by the observation that the NO synthase (NOS) inhibitor, NG-nitro-L-arginine (NorArg) attenuates the development of analgesic tolerance to morphine in the mouse.

Study Design.—The effects of LY, MK-801, and NorArg in models of μ and κ tolerance were studied in the CD-1 adult mouse. Tolerance to the μ-opioid agonist, morphine sulfate; the κ_1-opioid agonist, U50488H; and the κ_3-opioid agonist, naloxone benzoylhydrazone (NalBzoh), was produced by once-daily injection of opioid for 5 days. A standardized tail-flick apparatus was used to assess the antinociceptive (analgesic) response.

Results.—Once-daily administration of the opioid agonists resulted in a two- to threefold shift to the right of the respective analgesic dose-response curves, indicating the development of tolerance. Concurrent administration of LY in an infusion of 24 mg/kg/day or 6 mg/kg given intraperitoneally (IP) once daily, with morphine, attenuated the development of tolerance on day 5 compared with the use of saline plus morhphine. Similarly, administration of MK-801 at .3 mg/kg IP once daily or NorArg at 1 mg/kg IP twice daily attenuated the development of morphine tolerance. None of these drugs modified the tail-flick response or altered the ED_{50} for morphine. In contrast, co-administration of LY, MK-801, or NorArg in doses that attenuated morphine tolerance failed to attenuate the development of tolerance to the analgesic effect of U50488H or to NalBzoh.

Conclusion.—The μ-opioid tolerance, but not κ_1- or κ_3-opioid tolerance, involves the mediation of NMDA receptors and the NO system. The NMDA antagonist and NOS inhibitors may provide a means of attenuating opioid analgesic tolerance in patients with chronic pain.

► Some refinement in our understanding comes courtesy of the same laboratory. The NMDA receptor antagonists (and inhibition of NOS) attenuate tolerance only to the μ-opioid receptor agonist morphine; tolerance produced by repeated administration of κ-opioid receptor agonists was unaffected. If NMDA receptors are co-localized with μ-opioid receptors, we know from this study that manipulation of the NMDA receptor that blocks tolerance does not upregulate or downregulate the μ-opioid receptor. We are still looking for the link. An important conclusion to take from this study is that the mechanisms of analgesia and tolerance differ between μ- and κ-opioids.—G.F. Gebhart, Ph.D.

The NMDA Antagonist 3-(2-Carboxypiperazin-4-yl)Propyl-1-Phosphonic Acid (CPP) has Antinociceptive Effect After Intrathecal Injection in the Rat

Kristensen JD, Karlsten R, Gordh T, Berge O-G (Univ Hosp, Uppsala, Sweden; Astra Pain Control AB, Södertälje, Sweden)

Pain 56:59–67, 1994 131-95-4–23

Background.—The N-methyl-D-aspartate (NMDA) receptor may be involved in the transmission and modulation of nociceptive information in the spinal cord. Studies in mice using the competitive NMDA antagonist D-2-amino-5-phosphonopentanoate (and noncompetitive or nonspecific antagonists) show that antinociception in phasic tests requires doses that impaired motor function. Although 3-(2-carboxypiperazin-4-yl)propyl-1-phosphonic acid (CPP) is a potent NMDA receptor antagonist, it lacks agonistic properties and does not affect a broad spectrum of non-NMDA receptor systems in the CNS. Three different antinociceptive tests were used to analyze the pharmacologic effects of intrathecally administered CPP in rats, to assess its antinociceptive effects, and to learn the relation between its antinociceptive effects and motor function.

Methods.—Each male Sprague-Dawley rat was anesthetized, and a polyethylene catheter was inserted into its subarachnoid space through the cisterna magna. After a 5-day recovery period, the 8 animals in each of the 5 groups received an intrathecal injection of either saline or CPP (.5, 1, 5, or 10 nmol). After drug injection, each animal was tested frequently for as long as 4 hours, starting with the tail-flick test and followed immediately by the hot-plate test and motor function evaluation. For the formalin test, a separate set of rats was divided into 4 groups of 8 to 9 animals each, that were injected intrathecally with either saline or with CPP (.25, .5, or 1 nmol, respectively).

Results.—No motor dysfunction was seen at doses less than 1 nmol; 1 nmol produced slight ataxia in 2 of 8 rats. After injections of 5 nmol and 10 nmol, dose-related apparent sedation and motor dysfunction were observed. The thermal tests showed dose-related antinociception after doses that caused little or no motor dysfunction. The antinociceptive effect was attenuated at higher doses in the tail-flick test, resulting in a bell-shaped dose-response curve. The formalin test showed dose-related antinociception after doses from .25 to 1 nmol.

Conclusions.—In rats, the competitive NMDA antagonist CPP has an antinociceptive effect at low doses that do not affect motor function. Both phasic and tonic nociceptive tests show antinociception. The dose-response relation in the tail-flick test is bell-shaped, which suggests that NMDA is involved in functionally divergent nociceptive systems.

▶ In previous studies, NMDA receptor antagonists were reported to have effects on phasic pain tests only at dosages that also impaired motor function, thus confounding interpretation of outcomes. The novel finding in this study is that CPP is antinociceptive in both phasic and tonic pain tests without affecting motor function. Maybe NMDA receptor antagonists should not be considered as antihyperalgesic only.—G.F. Gebhart, Ph.D.

Injury-Induced Plasticity of Spinal Reflex Activity: NK1 Neurokinin Receptor Activation and Enhanced A- and C-Fiber Mediated Responses in the Rat Spinal Cord In Vitro

Thompson SWN, Dray A, Urban L (Sandoz Inst, London)

J Neurosci 14:3672–3687, 1994 131-95-4–24

Background.—The prolonged hypersensitivity caused by peripheral tissue injury results from increased sensitivity of the nociceptors innervating the area of peripheral damage, as well as from changes in the excitability of spinal cord neurons. Induction of this central sensitization depends on activation of nociceptive afferent fiber inputs. The primary afferent fibers responsible for inducing central sensitization have the unique ability to evoke prolonged postsynaptic potentials in spinal cord neurons. Studies of in vitro spinal cord preparations have found that such long-duration prolonged postsynaptic potentials can be recorded extracellularly as a prolonged ventral root potential (VRP). The A- and C-fiber evoked VRP responses were studied in isolated spinal cord preparations from young rats with and without experimentally induced behavioral hyperalgesias.

Methods.—Thermal and mechanical hyperalgesias were produced by ultraviolet irradiation of 1 hindpaw. The evoked VRPs in isolated spinal cord preparations from these animals were compared with those in preparations from untreated rats.

Results.—The treated animals had significantly longer A- and C-fiber–evoked VRPs. The prolonged VRP evoked by single-shock C-fiber stimulation in untreated rats was antagonized by the NMDA receptor antagonist D-AP5 and by the NK2 receptor antagonist MEN,10376, but not by the NK1 receptor antagonists CP-96,345 or RP,67580. Only D-AP5 antagonized the summated VRPs evoked by repeated C-fiber stimulation in untreated animals. In the rats with behavioral hyperalgesias, NK1, NK2, and NMDA antagonists significantly reduced the prolonged VRPs evoked by C-fiber stimulation, as well as the summated VRP. In both groups, only D-AP5 antagonized the single-shock–evoked A-fiber ventral root response. In the rats that were hyperalgesic, NMDA, NK1, and NK2 receptor antagonists reduced the summated VRP evoked by repeated A-fiber stimulation.

Conclusions.—Spinal cord preparations from rats with behavioral hyperalgesias induced by peripheral injury show enhanced A- and C-fiber–evoked responses in vitro. In this model, repetitive stimulation of A-fiber primary afferents enhances spinal excitability to an extent similar to that evoked by C-fibers in untreated animals. The C-fiber–evoked response induced by peripheral injury shows an NK1 receptor component. The phenomenon of central sensitization may be influenced by the enhanced ventral root responses and the changes in receptor sensitivity. These factors may be directly related to behavioral hyperalgesia.

▶ Here is more information on peripheral injury, central hyperexcitability, and hyperalgesia. It has been documented by several workers that C-fiber–evoked responses from inflamed tissue can be attenuated by *N*-methyl-D-aspartate (NMDA) or NK1 receptor antagonists; there is typically no effect of these agents on C-fiber–evoked responses from noninflamed tissue or on A-fiber–evoked responses. The important findings of this study are the effects of NMDA, NK1, and NK2 receptor antagonists on A-fiber–evoked ventral root responses recorded in vitro after induction of a peripheral injury. Thus, the effects of repetitive A-fiber stimulation are similar to those evoked by C-fiber stimulation in this model, suggesting that inputs from both nociceptive and non-nociceptive afferent fibers can contribute to behavioral hyperalgesia.—G.F. Gebhart, Ph.D.

The Correlation Between the Distribution of the NK_1 Receptor and the Actions of Tachykinin Agonists in the Dorsal Horn of the Rat Indicates That Substance P Does Not Have a Functional Role on Substantia Gelatinosa (Lamina II) Neurons

Bleazard L, Hill RG, Morris R (Univ of Liverpool, England; Neuroscience Research Centre, Essex, England)

J Neurosci 14:7655–7664, 1994 131-95-4–25

Introduction.—Substance P and neurokinin A are tachykinins that are localized within small-diameter primary afferents. These afferents terminate mainly in the substantia gelatinosa (SG) of the spinal cord and trigeminal nucleus caudalis. Release of substance P in the SG results from noxious peripheral stimuli. The cloning and sequencing of tachykinin receptor subtypes have been reported, and selective agonists for these receptors are available. The direct actions of selective tachykinin receptor agonists on the membrane potentials and primary afferent evoked synaptic responses of SG neurons were investigated in neonatal rats. In addition, an antibody to the C-terminal sequence of the rat NK_1 receptor was used to locate this receptor in rats of the same age.

Findings.—Just 10.5% of neurons in lamina II of a neonatal spinal cord splice showed any response to the application of a selective NK_1 receptor agonist. In contrast, 48.3% of neurons in deeper dorsal horn laminae responded to the same agonist. Selective NK_2 and NK_3 agonists produced no response in lamina II neurons. Similarly, synaptic potentials in lamina II neurons evoked by periphral nerve stimulation were unaffected by the NK_1 agonist. Very few lamina II neurons were found to express NK_1 receptors in immunocytochemical studies using an antibody directed against the C-terminal of the NK_1 receptor.

Conclusions.—Neurons in the deep laminae have functional NK_1 receptors, but those in the SG do not. Although incomplete, these findings suggest that current models of the operation of the small-diameter primary afferent system in acute pain must be reconsidered.

▶ This transmitter-receptor mismatch raises interesting questions. Substance P, an NK1 receptor agonist, is contained in small-diameter primary afferent terminals that terminate in the superficial dorsal horn, including the SG. Noxious stimuli release substance P in the SG, and one would expect NK1 receptors to also be located in the SG. This intracellular electrophysiologic and immunocytochemical study found that neurons in the superficial dorsal horn, however, were generally insensitive to NK1, NK2, and NK3 receptor agonists; neurons in the deep dorsal horn were responsive to a NK1 receptor agonist. In support of this finding, there were few immunocytochemically labeled NK1 receptors in the superficial dorsal horn. These results suggest that the role of the SG in spinal nociceptive processing requires reevaluation.—G.F. Gebhart, Ph.D.

Evidence for Presynaptic *N*-Methyl-D-Aspartate Autoreceptors in the Spinal Cord Dorsal Horn

Liu H, Wang H, Sheng M, Jan LY, Jan YN, Basbaum AI (Univ of California, San Francisco)

Proc Natl Acad Sci U S A 91:8383–8387, 1994 131-95-4–26

Objective.—Previous research has suggested that the N-methyl-D-aspartate (NMDA)-type glutamate receptor is involved in neuronal excitoxicity, degenerative disorders, and various neuropathic pain conditions after nerve injury. Changes in neurotransmitter release play a role in NMDA-regulated synaptic plasticity. However, the general assumption is that NMDA receptor-mediated increases in intracellular Ca^{2+} in the postsynaptic neuron are responsible for initiating presynaptic mechanisms of potentiation. The distribution of the NMDA receptor in the spinal cord and the CA1 region of the hippocampus—2 regions in which NMDA-mediated long-term plasticity has been found—was studied in rats.

Methods and Results.—Electron microscopic immunocytochemistry was used, as was an antibody directed against an alternatively spliced exon near the C terminus of NMDAR1, the NMDA receptor's essential functional subunit. In the CA1 hippocampal region, the NMDA receptor was expressed only on postsynaptic structures. In approximately one third of labeled synapses in the spinal cord, the receptor was located in the presynaptic terminal, immediately adjacent to the vesicle release site at the active zone. Combined postembedding immunocytochemical studies showed that more than 70% of the NMDA receptor immunoreactive terminals were positive for glutamate, suggesting that the presynaptic NMDA receptor was an autoreceptor. On nerve ligation studies, this receptor was found to be transported by dorsal roots to the spinal cord and by the sciatic nerve to the periphery.

Conclusions.—Expression of presynaptic NMDA receptors is demonstrated in glutamatergic terminals in the spinal cord dorsal horn. The NMDA autoreceptor is found in terminals of primary afferent fibers. In this location, it may facilitate the transmission of input to the spinal cord by increasing the release of neurotransmitters from the primary afferent terminal.

▶ It has generally been assumed that the NMDA receptors that are important to increased excitability of neurons in the spinal cord are located in the spinal cord postsynaptic to primary afferent input. The important finding of this report is that, in addition to their localization postsynaptically, NMDA receptors in the spinal cord are also localized to terminals of primary afferent fibers that contain glutamate as a neurotransmitter. If these receptors function as "autoreceptors," then glutamate released from an afferent terminal in the spinal cord could act to modulate the release of additional glutamate from the same afferent terminal. In cases of persistent peripheral input (e.g., inflammation), positive feedback control at the NMDA autoreceptor could be associated with enhanced release of glutamate, as well as substance P and calcitonin gene-related peptide (both of which are co-contained with glutamate in some nerve terminals) and other putative mediators of nociception.—G.F. Gebhart, Ph.D.

The Role of Nitric Oxide in Spinal Nociceptive Reflexes in Rats With Neurogenic and Non-Neurogenic Peripheral Inflammation

Semos ML, Headley PM (Univ Walk, Bristol, England)

Neuropharmacol 33:1487–1497, 1994 131-95-4–27

Background.—Tissue injury results in hypersensitivity and hyperalgesia. Among the mechanisms that probably underlie hyperalgesia is activation of N-methyl-D-aspartate (NMDA) receptors, which can release nitric oxide (NO) in the CNS. Apart from serving as a second messenger in NMDA receptor–mediated synaptic transmission, NO may modulate inflammation through peripheral mechanisms. Nitric oxide is released by agents such as substance P that mediate peripheral inflammation.

Methods.—An in vivo electrophysiologic study was planned to examine the role played by NO in mechanical and thermal spinal nociceptive reflexes in rats anesthetized with α-chloralose. The effects of N^G-nitro-L-arginine methyl ester (L-NAME), a NO synthase inhibitor, on these reflexes were compared in normal rats and those having peripheral inflammation that was induced neurogenically, with mustard oil, or non-neurogenically with carrageenan. Methoxamine was administered to mimic the marked hypertensive response to L-NAME.

Results.—Thermal nociceptive reflexes were comparably reduced by methoxamine and L-NAME in both normal rats and those with inflammation. In contrast, mechanical reflexes were significantly inhibited by L-NAME (but not D-NAME) in a dose-dependent manner in rats with either type of inflammation. The effect was more pronounced than that of methoxamine. Mechanical reflexes were not influenced by L-NAME in rats without inflammation or in spinalized rats with inflammation. The suppressive effect of L-NAME on mechanical reflexes in carrageenan-treated rats was prevented and reversed by either pretreatment or post-treatment with L-arginine (but not with D-arginine).

Conclusion.—Nitric oxide appears to mediate mechanical nociceptive reflexes through a supraspinal mechanism in rats with induced peripheral inflammation.

▶ Nitric oxide is generally considered to be pro-nociceptive in the spinal cord, where it is thought to be released upon activation of spinal NMDA receptors. Not new: In this study, NO is shown to be important to the hyperalgesia associated with tissue inflammation. New: The nitric oxidase inhibitor L-NAME was without effect in spinally transected rats. This result suggests a reevaluation in our thinking about the source of NO that mediates hyperalgesia after tissue inflammation. Supraspinal sites appear to be important. Does the NO that is synthesized and released locally in the spinal cord arise from the terminals of axons that descend from the brain stem, or does it arise from interneurons under control from such descending axons? Certainly, there is more to come on this issue.—G.F. Gebhart, Ph.D.

Peripheral and Central Mechanisms of NGF-Induced Hyperalgesia

Lewin GR, Rueff A, Mendell LM (State Univ of New York, Stony Brook; Max-Planck-Inst for Psychiatry, Planegg-Martinsried, Germany)

Eur J Neurosci 6:1903–1912, 1994 131-95-4–28

Background.—A single injection of nerve growth factor (NGF) produces marked, long-lasting hyperalgesia to heat and mechanical stimulation in the adult rat. In the setting of tissue damage, an increased tissue concentration of NGF may play a physiologic role in the development of hyperalgesia.

Objective.—The mechanisms by which NGF may normally produce hyperalgesia were studied by administering single systemic injections of the factor to adult rats.

Results.—A single dose of NGF produced hyperalgesia to radiant heat within minutes, and the effect lasted for days. The same response developed in animals pretreated with a mast cell degranulating agent or 1 of 2 specific 5-hydroxytryptamine (5-HT) receptor antagonists, but its onset was delayed by more than 3 hours. Initial hypoalgesia was noted in animals given a 5-HT receptor antagonist. The later phase of thermal hyperalgesia was selectively blocked by a noncompetitive N-methyl-D-aspartate (NMDA) receptor antagonist. Injection of NGF produced hyperalgesia to mechanical stimulation after a 7-hour latency period, and none of the agents that attenuated thermal hyperalgesia blocked this response. Hyperalgesia induced by NGF was not maintained by increased spontaneous activity in C-fibers. When inflammation was produced by injecting complete Freund adjuvant, thermal hyperalgesia was blocked by the concomitant administration of anti-NGF antiserum.

Conclusion.—The hyperalgesic responses to thermal and mechanical stimuli induced by NGF appear to be mediated by different mechanisms. The early component of thermal hyperalgesia is mediated by a peripheral mechanism entailing mast-cell degranulation, whereas the late component involves central NMDA receptors. Mechanical hyperalgesia is seemingly independent of both these mechanisms.

▶ The role of neurotrophins like NGF in plasticity in the nervous system has become an area of promising investigation. Nerve growth factor has been documented by this laboratory to produce thermal and mechanical hyperalgesia when administered systemically. In this report, NGF-produced thermal hyperalgesia was found to be composed of both peripheral (competent mast cells) and central (NMDA receptors) components. Nerve growth factor was also shown to be required for the generation of thermal hyperalgesia after tissue injury, suggesting that NGF and antagonists at the receptor at which it acts, TrkA, may be appropriate targets for development of novel strategies to modulate hyperalgesia associated with tissue injury.—G.F. Gebhart, Ph.D.

Inflammation-Induced Release of Excitatory Amino Acids Is Prevented by Spinal Administration of a $GABA_A$ But Not by a $GABA_B$ Receptor Antagonist in Rats

Sluka KA, Willis WD, Westlund KN (Marine Biomedical Inst, Galveston, Tex; Univ of Texas, Galveston)

J Pharmacol Exp Ther 271:76–82, 1994 131-95-4–29

Background.—Previous research suggests that primary afferent depolarization (PAD) and the accompanying dorsal root reflexes may contribute to joint inflammation. Primary afferent depolarization is known to be mediated through $GABA_A$ receptor activation on the central terminals of primary afferent fibers. Therefore, $GABA_A$-mediated dorsal root reflexes triggered by PAD of the central terminals of the primary articular afferent fibers may lead to the peripheral release of inflammatory neuropeptides into the joint. It was hypothesized that the late phase of excitatory amino acid release after the induction of arthritis would not occur in animals pretreated with a $GABA_A$ antagonist, which would decrease joint inflammation.

Methods and Findings.—Injection of kaolin and carrageenan into the knee joint of rats reduced paw withdrawal latency (PWL) to radiant heat ipsilaterally, indicating hyperalgesia. This reduction was blocked by the

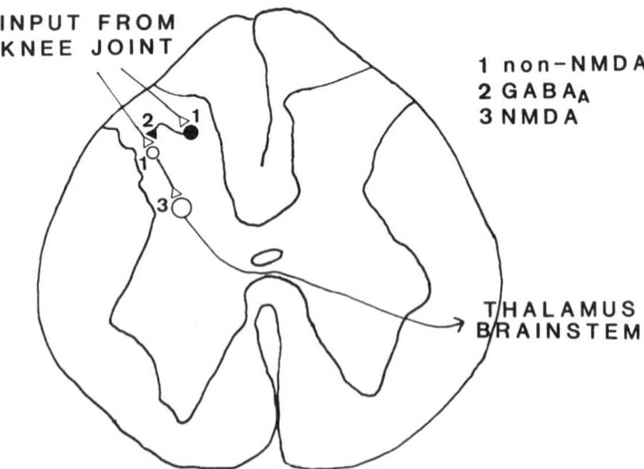

Fig 4–13.—Diagram representing a proposed model for the spinal cord control of peripheral inflammation and nociceptive transmission. (Courtesy of Sluka KA, Willis WD, Westlund KN: *J Pharmacol Exp Ther* 271:76–82, 1994.)

pretreatment of the spinal cord dorsal horn with the $GABA_A$ receptor antagonist bicuculline, but not with the $GABA_B$ receptor antagonist CGP35348 given by microdialysis. The inflammation-induced release of amino acids from the spinal dorsal horn occurred in 2 phases, 1 at the time of injection and 1 at 3.5–8 hours. In the late phase, aspartate (ASP), glutamate (GLU), and glutamine were released. The inhibitory amino acids serine and glycine were also released during the PWL test after arthritis induction. The elevated release of excitatory amino acids at injection was not affected by bicuculline or CGP35348 pretreatment. Amino acid release during the late phase and PWL test was blocked by pretreatment with bicuculline but not CGP35348. The increased joint circumference that usually occurs with this model did not occur with bicuculline pretreatment. Joint circumference change and the last-phase release of ASP and GLU were correlated positively (Fig 4–13).

Conclusions.—Concentrations of ASP and GLU did not increase above baseline in bicuculline-treated arthritic rats with minimal joint inflammation. The $GABA_A$-mediated spinal events appear to be important factors in the spinal cord release of ASP and GLU as well as in the peripheral neurogenic edema leading to increased joint circumference in this model of arthritis.

▶ Bicuculline, the $GABA_A$ receptor antagonist, when given to the spinal cord via a microdialysis fiber inserted through the dorsal horn, reduced peripheral joint inflammation and the spinal release of putative amino acid transmitters in the spinal dorsal horn. A $GABA_B$ receptor antagonist was without effect. This is strong support for an important spinal interaction between GABA and excitatory amino acids. The role of the CNS in peripheral inflammation is gaining attention. It has been known for decades that peripheral inflammation is altered in spinal-transected animals.—G.F. Gebhart, Ph.D.

Some Inhibitory Neurons in the Spinal Cord Develop c-*fos*-Immunoreactivity After Noxious Stimulation

Todd AJ, Spike RC, Brodbelt AR, Price RF, Shehab SAS (Univ of Glasgow, Scotland)

Neuroscience 63:805–816, 1994 131-95-4–30

Background.—Because c-*fos* is one of a number of immediate early genes that are induced in neurons after appropriate stimulation, immunocytochemical detection of its protein product has been used as a marker for neuronal activation in the CNS. Neurons immunoreactive for c-*fos* are found throughout the spinal gray matter after noxious peripheral stimulation. Some of these cells are known to be projection neurons, but most of them probably are interneurons.

Objective and Methods.—An attempt was made to learn which neurochemical types of spinal neurons produce c-*fos* in response to noxious stimulation (subcutaneous injection of formalin into a rat hindpaw). The c-*fos* protein was sought immunocytochemically in nonembedded sections of rat lumbar spinal cord 2 hours after noxious stimulation. Immunoreactivity for GABA and glycine was sought in embedded semithin sections cut through c-*fos*-immunoreactive neurons.

Results.—From 72% to 81% of neurons throughout the spinal cord that were immunoreactive for c-*fos* lacked GABA- and glycine-like immunoreactivity. As many as 20% of c-*fos*-reactive neurons in the superficial dorsal horn and dorsal white matter were immunoreactive for GABA, and some were also glycine-immunoreactive. In other parts of the cord, up to 35% of c-*fos*-reactive cells also were immunoreactive to GABA, glycine, or both.

Conclusion.—Noxious stimulation appears to lead to the expression of c-*fos* protein in several types of spinal neurons, including projection cells and both excitatory and inhibitory interneurons.

▶ The immediate early gene c-*fos* has been widely used to provide information about the spatial characteristics of noxious input to the spinal cord. Neither the functions of c-*fos* nor the types of spinal neuron that produce c-*fos* in response to noxious input are fully understood. In this report, a small but significant proportion of spinal neurons that were c-*fos* immunoreactive were found also to be immunoreactive for the inhibitory amino acid neurotransmitter GABA. Whereas c-*fos* has generally been taken as a marker of neuronal activation, those neurons that are activated (as reported in this study) include neurons (most likely interneurons) that have an inhibitory function in the spinal cord.—G.F. Gebhart, Ph.D.

Identification of a Human Delta Opioid Receptor: Cloning and Expression

Knapp RJ, Malatynska E, Fang L, Li X, Babin E, Nguyen M, Santoro G, Varga EV, Hruby VJ, Roeske WR, Yamamura HI (Univ of Arizona, Tucson)

Life Sci 54:PL463–469, 1994 131-95-4–31

Introduction.—There is increasing evidence that selective δ-receptor agonists may have superior therapeutic properties relative to currently used μ-receptor selective opioid drugs. Identification of δ-opioid receptor clones from human cDNA libraries and the preparation of a human δ-receptor cDNA in the pcDNA3 expression vector for transfection studies are reported.

Results.—The cDNA encodes a 372 amino acid protein that has 93% amino acid identity to both mouse and rat δ-receptors. Membranes from COS-7 cells transfected with pcDNA3 show high specific binding for δ-receptor-selective radioligands compared with cells transfected with nonrecombinant pcDNA3. The highly selective δ-receptor ligands, including naltrindole benzofuran (NTB), 7-benzylidenenaltrexone (BNTX), [4'-C1-Phe^4]DPDPE, and [D-Ala^2, Glu^4]deltorphin have Ki values under 10 nM, whereas the affinities of the μ- and κ-opioid receptor ligands CTAP and U-69593, respectively, are over 4.0 μM. The agonists show binding to multiple affinity states of the receptor consistent with the presence of G-protein coupled and uncoupled forms of the expressed receptor. Furthermore, the eightfold higher affinity of NTB relative to BNTX suggests that this receptor is a δ_2-receptor subtype.

Conclusion.—The amino acid sequence of a human δ-opioid receptor that is likely to be of the δ_2-subtype was reported. The cDNA clone produced can be transfected into COS-7 cells to express a functional receptor protein with the expected high binding affinity for δ-receptor ligands. The precise characterization of the ligand requirements for this receptor may lead to the development of safer and more effective analgesic drugs.

▶ The opioid receptors resisted attempts to be cloned, and other receptors seemed to be cloned with relative ease. Now that the opioid receptors have been cloned, the characterization of ligand requirements will lead to the development of better opioid analgesics. This is the first report of the human δ-receptor, which the authors report is like the δ_2-subtype better characterized in nonhuman animals.—G.F. Gebhart, Ph.D.

Effect of Fedotozine on the Cardiovascular Pain Reflex Induced by Distension of the Irritated Colon in the Anesthetized Rat

Langlois A, Diop L, Rivière PJM, Pascaud X, Junien J-L (Institut de Recherche Jouveinal, Fresnes France)

Eur J Pharmacol 271:245–251, 1994 131-95-4-32

Background.—A number of studies have indicated that the antinociceptive actions of opioid receptor agonists are increased during inflammatory states. Several animal models of colitis have been developed to simulate the changes seen in clinical disease states.

Objective.—The antinociceptive effects of reference agonists of the κ- and μ-types were assessed in rats in which colonic irritation was induced by instilling .6% acetic acid.

Results.—Intracolonic instillation of acetic acid solution significantly increased the hypotensive reflex response to colonic distention. In control rats having saline infused intracolonically, fedotozine had no antinociceptive effect when given intravenously in a dose of .6 mg/kg or 1 mg/kg at a noxious pain pressure level of 75 mm Hg. In contrast, fedotozine, .6 mg/kg, was 38% antinociceptive in acetic acid–treated animals, and 1 mg/kg produced 54% antinociception. Comparable results were achieved using PD-117,302, a κ-opioid receptor agonist. The antinociceptive actions of morphine and U-50,488H, also a κ-opioid receptor agonist, were identical in saline- and acetic acid–treated animals. The selective κ-opioid receptor antagonist nor-binaltorphimine reversed the antinociceptive actions of both fedotozine and PD-117,302.

Conclusion.—Some, but not all, κ-opioid receptor ligands effectively lessen colonic hypersensitivity to painful mechanical stimulation in rats given acetic acid intracolonically.

▶ In an effort to model the altered sensitivity of the gastrointestinal tract that characterizes the functional bowel disorders, acetic acid was instilled into the colon in these experiments, producing an exaggerated response to balloon distension of the colon. In this study, the interesting finding is the effect of κ-opioid receptor agonists on the responses to balloon distension. Fedotozine, U-50,488H and PD-117,302 all act at κ-opioid receptors and were found to attenuate responses to colonic distension in a dose-dependent, receptor-selective manner. As has been reported for morphine when tested in the presence of hindpaw inflammation, fedotozine and PD-117,302 were more potent in the presence of colonic irritation.—G.F. Gebhart, Ph.D.

Central Effects of Baroreceptor Activation in Humans: Attenuation of Skeletal Reflexes and Pain Perception

Dworkin BR, Elbert T, Rau H, Birbaumer N, Pauli P, Droste C, Brunia CHM (Pennsylvania State Univ, Hershey; Univ of Münster, Germany; Eberhard-Karls Universität Tübingen, Germany; et al)

Proc Natl Acad Sci U S A 91:6329–6333, 1994 131-95-4–33

Background.—Mechanoreceptors in the carotid sinus and aortic arch comprise the afferent limb of the reflexes regulating blood pressure. Reflex effects of baroreceptor activation are known to help buffer rapid changes in arterial pressure. Baroreceptor stimulation produces clearly documented, but less well understood, general inhibition of central nervous processes. In animal models, activating the arterial baroreceptors blunts pain sensation and produces other types of CNS inhibition. Although these effects may be important to the regulation of blood pressure, they have not been rigorously verified in humans.

Methods and Findings.—A noninvasive, behaviorally unbiased method for stimulating baroreceptors was applied to the measurement of baroreceptor-mediated attenuation of pain perception and of Achilles tendon reflex. In 3 experiments, the control and stimulation neck-chamber method was combined with brief stimuli positioned differentially in the cardiac cycle. Stimulation of the high-pressure baroreceptors was found to have general CNS inhibitory effects. Baroreceptor CNS inhibition was found to be a robust physiologic mechanism that probably has a unique regulatory function. When acute sensory or emotional excitation excessively increases blood pressure, CNS dampening may augment vagal and sympathoinhibitory negative feedback mechanisms to help restore safer levels.

Conclusions.—These findings are relevant to the basic mechanisms of blood pressure stabilization and cardiovascular reactivity. They may also have implications for noncompliance with antihypertensive medications as well as the pathophysiology of essential hypertension.

▶ This study provides further evidence that activation of high-pressure baroreceptors can significantly attenuate perception of pain in humans. Findings in different individuals at 3 institutions, who were subjected to the same procedures for baroreceptor stimulation, attest to the robust nature of the experimental outcomes. The significance of the results extend beyond the potential importance to pain mechanisms.—G.F. Gebhart, Ph.D.

5 Biobehavioral Advances in the Assessment, Treatment, and Consequences of Pain

Introduction

In last year's introduction to this chapter of the YEAR BOOK OF PAIN, I apologetically stated that this chapter appeared to contain a review of articles that did not fit nicely into the other chapters. The inherent complexity of the pain experience has not changed during the past year. Therefore, this chapter again contains a wide array of articles on psychosocial and biobehavioral topics.

The past year has, however, resulted in some important advances in our understanding of chronic pain conditions. The importance of sound measurement, an essential component in any scientific undertaking, and the unique difficulties inherent in measurement of pain have again resurfaced in the pain literature and are highlighted in several articles in this chapter. A second important theme that has appeared in several articles seen in the literature during the past year is the importance of predicting treatment outcomes. With the shrinking health care dollar, like it or not, pain practitioners are being asked to define those patient populations that their treatment programs are best designed to serve.

Establishing clinical practice guidelines, quality assurance procedures, clinical pathways and algorithms, and so forth, is becoming essential for the survival of pain management practice. Thus, I have included articles that address clinical practice issues. Closely aligned with practice issues is the importance of conducting more carefully designed clinical trials to establish the usefulness of many common, yet scientifically undocumented, clinical procedures used in treatment of pain. These types of studies have been included, particularly those with adequate follow-up data that address the essential question of maintenance of change. It is important to inform the reader up front that an increasing bias of mine with respect to studies of chronic pain outcome is the importance of including behavioral/functional measures of outcome. Therefore, studies that merely documented that patients "felt better" after treatment have not been included in this chapter.

All in all, this year has been a productive year from a biobehavioral perspective, as reflected in the diversity and quality of the literature reviewed in this chapter. I am grateful to pain investigators for providing me with a substantial literature from which to select.

Thomas E. Rudy, Ph.D.

Measurement Issues

Introduction

Sound measurement, an essential component of any scientific discipline, remains a particular problem in pain research. The measurement of pain intensity, for example—particularly in clinical settings—is a difficult and often subjective undertaking. This is of little surprise to clinicians and clinical investigators, because it is well recognized that pain intensity, like other sensations and perceptions, is a private experience that displays considerable variability both across patients and within a patient across time. Nonetheless, pain quantification and discerning factors that may affect its measurement are important for evaluation purposes and to determine the effectiveness of treatment interventions.

Thomas E. Rudy, Ph.D.

What Is the Maximum Number of Levels Needed in Pain Intensity Measurement?

Jensen MP, Turner JA, Romano JM (Univ of Washington, Seattle)
Pain 58:387–392, 1994 131-95-5–1

Purpose.—There is continuing disagreement as to the number of measurement levels needed to assess self-reported intensity of pain. Different measures include 4 to 101 levels, or even an "infinite" number of levels, as with the visual analogue scales. It is often argued that more levels allow for more accurate pain assessment. However, if too few levels could result in the underestimation of the effects of treatment, too many levels could result in an overestimation. An empiric evaluation of the number of response levels needed to assess pain intensity in chronic pain patients was presented.

Methods.—The subjects were 124 patients with chronic pain who took part in a multidisciplinary treatment program. Each used the 101-point Numerical Rating Scales (NRS) to provide pretreatment and post-treatment measures of least, most, current, and average pain. These responses were analyzed to determine the actual number of levels the patients used. The responses to the 101-point scale were recorded to form

Percentage of Patients Reporting Pain Intensity in Multiples of 5 and 10 Pretreatment and Post-Treatment on the 101-Point Numerical Rating Scales

Time of assessment	Multiples of Five (0, 5, 10, 15, etc.)	Ten (0, 10, 20, 30, etc.)
	Average Pain	
Pretreatment	98%	74%
Post-treatment	97%	74%
	Current Pain	
Pretreatment	91%	73%
Post-treatment	96%	74%
	Worst Pain	
Pretreatment	96%	78%
Post-treatment	95%	74%
	Least Pain	
Pretreatment	97%	81%
Post-treatment	95%	77%

(Courtesy of Jensen MP, Turner JA, Romano JM: *Pain* 58:387–392, 1994.)

2-, 3-, 4-, 6-, 11-, and 21-point scales, and the sensitivity of the re-coded scales was examined.

Results.—Little information was lost by using the 11- or 21-point scales rather than the 101-point scale. These 2 re-coded scales were strongly correlated with the original 101-point scale; the correlation coefficients were somewhat lower for the 6-point scale and much lower for the 2- and 4-point scales. The 11-, 21-, and 101-point scales had essentially identical means, standard deviations, and t and P values associated with the t tests of treatment changes in pain intensity. The 6-point scale yielded similar results for measures of average, current, and most pain; the variation was greater for the lower point scales. On the 101-point scale, nearly all the patients used multiples of 5 or 10 to rate their pain, essentially reducing it to a 21-point scale. Well over half of the patients used multiples of 10 only in rating pain (table).

Conclusion.—As demonstrated previously, most patients with chronic pain respond to numeric pain intensity measures as if they were 11- or 21-point scales. The sensitivity of these scales can vary as the number of pain levels decreases. When present, these changes in sensitivity do not occur until the number of levels falls below 11 points. Thus, pain intensity measures with 11 or more levels are probably sufficient to detect changes in pain intensity for patients with chronic pain. Because shorter scales are easier to use than visual analogue scales and 101-point NRS, they may be preferable for research and clinical purposes.

Increasing the Reliability and Validity of Pain Intensity Measurement in Chronic Pain Patients

Jensen MP, McFarland CA (Univ of Washington, Seattle)

Pain 55:195–203, 1993 131-95-5–2

Background.—It has been postulated, based on psychometric theory, that the reliability and validity of pain intensity measurement (as measures of average pain) can be improved by increasing the number of pain assessments. The effects of increasing the number of evaluations were investigated to verify this theory.

Patients and Methods.—A total of 200 patients with chronic pain (average age, 44 years) were included in a study. Over 2 weeks, all patients completed a series of hourly pain ratings. Afterward, a sequence of regression analyses was conducted. Specifically, test-retest stability, internal consistency, and validity coefficients were computed to ascertain whether reports of chronic pain are similar from 1 day to another, and whether a single pain intensity reading, when used as an indicant of average pain, is both reliable and valid. In addition, the number of assessments (data points) needed to obtain estimates of average pain intensity with adequate-to-excellent psychometric properties, and the importance of sampling pain from different days were also determined (table).

Results.—The study results were consistent with predications based on patients' self-reports of pain and on psychometric theory. Most patients did not report comparable levels of pain from 1 day to the next. Furthermore, average pain scores computed from ratings obtained from a single day were less stable than those computed from ratings obtained from multiple days. As expected, the results also revealed that a single pain intensity rating is not adequately reliable or valid as a measure of average pain. A composite pain intensity score computed from an average of 12 ratings over a 4-day period, however, yielded both adequate reliability and excellent validity as a measure of average pain in this population of patients with chronic pain.

Conclusion.—Based on study results, the importance of averaging multiple measures of pain intensity across time to maximize the reliability and validity of pain assessment, and to provide empirical guidelines for determining how many observations to make has been underscored.

Test-Retest Stability: Correlation Coefficients Between Pain Intensity Measures from Week 1 and Week 2 as a Function of Number of Ratings

Number of ratings/day	Number of days of ratings						
	One	Two	Three	Four	Five	Six	Seven
One (hour 2)	0.63 (1)	0.79 (2)	0.83 (3)	0.86 (4)	0.88 (5)	0.91 (6)	0.92 (7)
Two (hours 2 and 6)	0.77 (2)	0.80 (4)	0.85 (6)	0.89 (8)	0.91 (10)	0.92 (12)	0.93 (14)
Three (hours 2, 6, 10)	0.73 (3)	0.84 (6)	0.88 (9)	0.91 (12)	0.92 (15)	0.93 (18)	0.94 (21)
Four (hours 2, 6, 10, 14)	0.72 (4)	0.84 (8)	0.88 (12)	0.91 (16)	0.93 (20)	0.94 (24)	***0.95*** (28)

Note: Stability coefficients greater than .90 are underlined. The number of assessments used to calculate each pain intensity measure, from which each test-retest stability coefficient was calculated, is listed in parentheses under the coefficient.

(Courtesy of Jensen MP, McFarland CA: *Pain* 55:195–203, 1993.)

A Comparison of Pain Measurement Characteristics of Mechanical Visual Analogue and Simple Numerical Rating Scales

Price DD, Bush FM, Long S, Harkins SW (Med College of Virginia, Richmond)
Pain 56:217–226, 1994 131-95-5–3

Introduction.—It is important that a pain scale be validated as a ratio scale because only ratio scales provide accurate estimates of ratios of pain intensity and percentage changes in pain. A comparison was made between numerical rating scales and mechanical visual analogue scales (M-VAS) to determine their ability to provide ratio scale measures of pain.

Methods.—Both tools used scales of 0–10 and were anchored by identical verbal descriptors. Experiment 1 consisted of 23 patients with orofacial pain. Patients rated 7 intensities of thermal stimuli applied to the forearm by a contact thermode, then rated stimuli on numerical scales or M-VAS. Ratios of perceived pain sensation intensity were determined by temperature increases of .5°C/sec, starting at 45°C. Patients

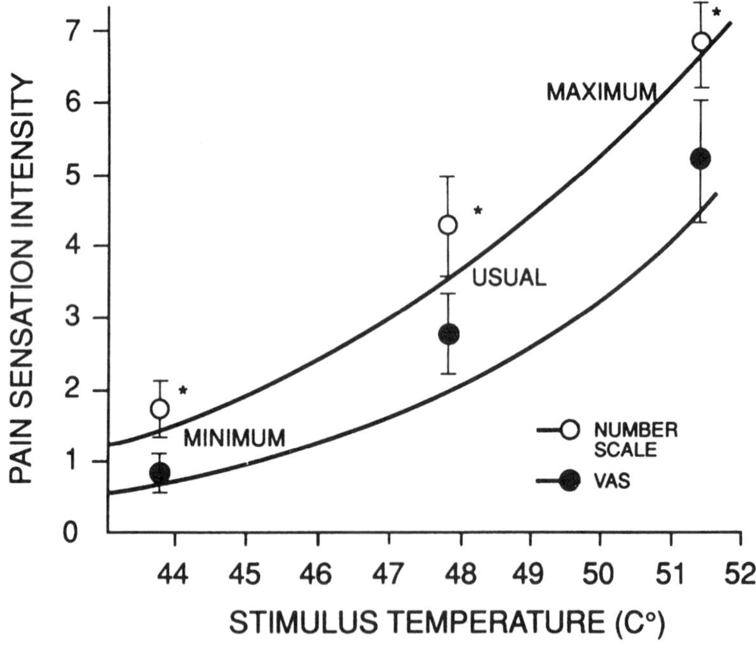

Fig 5–1.—Mean numerical ratings **(top)** and mean mechanical visual analogue scale (VAS) ratings **(bottom)** of clinical orofacial pain at minimum, usual, and maximum levels (along Y-axis) during the preceding week, shown in relation to mean temperature matches (along the X or temperature stimulus axis) and temperature stimulus-response regression lines. Because the intersection of the temperature matches and rating scale responses occur close to the corresponding regression lines, patients appear to use these rating scales in a consistent manner to rate both experimental and clinical pain. *Vertical bars* are standard deviations. (Courtesy of Price DD, Bush FM, Long S, et al: *Pain* 56:217–226, 1994.)

were asked to acknowledge the temperature they perceived as being twice as intense as the standard temperature. Experiment 2 consisted of 10 patients with chronic upper body myofascial pain. Patients in group 2 were tested as were patients in group 1, but they were asked to rate stimuli on the M-VAS or the pencil-and-paper VAS. Research assistants were employed to minimize bias, because the first author has a financial interest in M-VAS.

Results.—Numerical ratings were significantly higher than M-VAS ratings, a finding consistent with prior investigations. Both ratings increased with temperature sensation and pain unpleasantness ratings. Predicted temperature judgments were within the 95% confidence range for the M-VAS, but not the numerical scale. The systematic differences between numerical and M-VAS ratings of minimum, usual, and maximum orofascial pain were consistent with those observed for experimental pain (Fig 5–1). Both M-VAS and pencil-and-paper VAS gave similar ratings of clinical pain.

Conclusion.—Numerical and M-VAS ratings are consistent measures of experimental and clinical pain. However, only the M-VAS gives ratio scale measurements of pain sensation intensity.

▶ Abstracts 131-95-5–1 through 131-95-5–3 highlight the fact that pain measurement has been deeply influenced by 2 major research traditions that have guided measurement theorists during the 20th century. One tradition has its roots in the psychometric work of Charles Spearman, which is focused on the test score and is primarily concerned with measurement error and reliability and validity coefficients. This approach is commonly called test theory. The work of Jensen and colleagues (See Abstracts 131-95-5–1 and Abstract 131-95-5–2) is within this measurement tradition.

A second research tradition, which developed in a parallel fashion, has its roots in 19th-century work in psychophysics and has been called scaling theory. The focus of this research tradition is on the calibration of both individuals and items onto a latent variable scale, with particular emphasis placed on explicitly testing whether scores adequately fit well-defined and mathematically sound measurement models and whether the derived measures are invariant. The goal of invariant measurement has been succinctly stated by Stevens: "The scientist seeks measures that will stay put while his back is turned" (1). Aspects of this measurement approach are represented by the work of Price et al. (Abstract 131-95-5–3).

Both traditions have aspects that are important to consider in the field of pain measurement, and are not necessarily mutually exclusive. For example, the work of Jensen et al. (Abstract 131-95-5–1) can also be understood in terms of scaling theory, which suggests that it is important to distinguish observations from measurement. The rating scales provided to patients enable us to collect observations; in and of themselves, they are not measures. We give patients numbers to rate their pain intensity, primarily out of convenience to help them describe their pain experience, because most individuals have some notion of "measurement" from common, well-established physical measuring systems (e.g., larger numbers mean greater distance or more weight). However, like the pain experience they are used to represent, the numbers collected are indirect or abstract representations of this experience. How patients use these scales and whether the numeral observations collected can be used to derive meaningful, quantitatively sound measures are empirical questions that need to be tested explicitly.

Here, however, is where the measurement traditions described above part company. Proponents of the scaling tradition would argue that all pain severity ratings (patient observations), despite the number of categories or points on a scale, are ordinal because it cannot be assumed that distances between categories are equivalent across the range of the scale (2). Thus, whether the data fit certain mathematical models that permit observations to be transformed onto an interval (or ratio) measurement scale should be tested first before conducting linear statistics or concluding that one has a measurement system that can be generalized beyond the patient sample used to collect the observations. To summarize, because none of the 3 papers discussed demonstrated that fundamental measurement (invariance) was achieved, the conclusions reached have to be considered as *sample specific.* Thus, whether 7-, 11-, 21-, or 101-point scales lead to better, more treatment-sensitive measures of pain severity remains an unanswered question.—T.E. Rudy, Ph.D.

References

1. Stevens, SS: Mathematics, measurement, and psychophysics, in Stevens SS (eds): *Handbook of Experimental Psychology.* New York, Wiley, 1951, pp 1–49.
2. Wright BD, Linacre JM: Observations are always ordinal: Measurements, however, must be interval. *Arch Phys Med Rehabil* 70:857–860, 1989.

Sensory and Affective Predictors of Overall Pain and Emotions Associated With Affective Pain

Fernandez E, Milburn TW (Southern Methodist Univ, Dallas; Ohio State Univ, Columbus)

Clin J Pain 10:3–9, 1994 131-95-5-4

Background.—Pain is acknowledged to have both sensory qualities, such as throbbing or pinching, and affective qualities, such as vicious or frightful. It is also assumed that these components of pain can be measured separately. The relative contributions of the sensory and affective components of pain and the contribution of different emotions to the affective component were studied in 40 patients with chronic pain.

Methods.—The study participants were recruited from a pain management program. The mean age of the group was 44 years, and the average duration of pain was 63 months. Both the sites and etiology of chronic pain were varied. In a correlational design, participants used visual analogue scales to quantify overall pain, sensory pain, affective pain, and individual emotions. Ten emotions were listed: anger, fear, sadness, guilt, shame, disgust, contempt, surprise, interest, and joy. The data were examined by multiple regression techniques to express overall pain as a mathematical function of sensation and affect and to express the affective component of pain as a function of various emotions.

Results.—The overall pain could be expressed as a linear combination of sensory pain and affective pain by using a regression equation. There was a significant correlation between sensory and affective components. The sensory pain accounted for a sizeable portion of the variance in overall pain, whereas the variance in affective pain was best explained by anger, fear, and sadness.

Discussion.—Although pain has both sensory and affective components, the whole is more than a simple additive combination of these components. Overall, pain can be expressed in linear regression terms as a summation of the magnitude of physical sensation (multiplied by a coefficient of .58) and the degree of affective distress (multiplied by a coefficient of .18), plus a constant of 3.64. Both components exert reciprocal effects and should be assessed separately as features of the pain experience.

▶ There remains considerable debate in the pain literature as to whether affective components of the pain experience can be disentangled from sensory components, at least from a measurement standpoint. This paper provides additional insights into this controversy, particularly the role of anger in affective aspects of pain perception. However, the small sample size combined with the large unexplained variance in the authors' regression equations and the lack of adjusted for measurement error require that these findings be replicated.—T.E. Rudy, Ph.D.

Effects of Present Pain Level on Recall of Chronic Pain and Medication Use

Smith WB, Safer MA (The Catholic Univ of America, Washington, DC)

Pain 55:355–361, 1993 131-95-5–5

Introduction.—Patients with chronic pain that varies in intensity may have difficulty in recalling both the pain they experienced over a given period and their use of medication for the pain. With the use of an electronic diary, 30 patients with chronic pain recorded every change in their pain levels and each use of medication over the course of a week. Their recall of pain and medication use was then assessed.

Patients and Methods.—The study participants were 23 women and 8 men, ranging in age from 28 to 53 years, who had been receiving weekly outpatient physical therapy (PT) for chronic pain for at least 3 months. One patient did not complete the interview. The patients had been asked to volunteer for a study of a new type of pain diary, but they were not told they would be questioned about their recall of pain and medications. The data were collected with the Symtrack, a portable electronic diary, and pain was rated on a visual analogue scale. Also recorded were each use of medication, meals, and sleep and waking times. The recall of both pain and medication use was evaluated either before (15 patients, control group) or immediately after (15 patients, PT group) a PT session.

Results.—The patients had no difficulty in using the Symtrack, and the control and PT groups appeared to interpret the visual analogue scale similarly. The mean levels of pain obtained from the Symtrack records did not differ significantly for the 2 groups during the study week. As expected, patients who had completed a session of PT reported lower present pain than did controls, who had not yet had their PT session. However, in addition, the patients in the PT group recalled their pain during the previous day and week as being less severe than their diaries indicated. The control patients significantly overestimated their lowest and highest levels of pain for the previous day and their usual and lowest levels of pain for the previous week. Patients who had just completed a PT session also recalled taking significantly less medication than they had recorded in their diaries.

Conclusion.—According to their Symtrack diary, both the control and PT groups inaccurately recalled their pain and medication use. Present pain intensity was found to strongly influence the recall of past pain intensity. Thus, when assessing a patient's pain history, clinicians should take present pain status into account.

▶ A comprehensive history is essential in the evaluation of individuals experiencing persistent pain. This article, however, reminds us that the data we collect in these histories can be substantially biased by the patient's present condition, particularly pain severity. A logical extension of these findings is that treatment outcome studies that use respective recall of pretreatment pain levels and behaviors for evaluating treatment gains are probably on "thin ice."—T.E. Rudy, Ph.D.

Pain Assessment With Interactive Computer Animation

Swanston M, Abraham C, Macrae WA, Walker A, Rushmer R, Elder L, Methven H (Dundee Inst of Technology, Scotland; Univ of Dundee, Scotland; Dundee Royal Infirmary, Scotland)

Pain 53:347–351, 1993 131-95-5-6

Background.—Improved methods of evaluating pain should entail quantitative measures and, at the same time, be able to capture the various qualitative dimensions of pain. They also should not rely on liguistic competence, and should use measures that relate to the patient's experience. Most computer-based questionnaires have consisted of purely textual displays, but the advent of color graphics has made visual symbols a valid means of communicating with users. Interactive computer animation was compared with a conventional questionnaire-based assessment.

An Interactive Approach.—Interactive animation (IA) software was developed from spontaneous drawings made by adults to represent their experiences of pain. Five animation modules were developed, 4 representing categories of pain (pressure, burning, throbbing, piercing) and 1 being an interactive version of a visual analogue scale. The actual images are in color and simulate the qualities represented (e.g., a continuously changing symbol for throbbing).

Assessment.—Fifty patients attending a pain clinic were evaluated using IA software and the short-form McGill Pain Questionnaire. The patients were typical of clinic attendees with respect to age and gender. Nearly 40% of them had pain in more than one site. The back, shoulders, and neck were the most common sites of pain.

Results.—Correlations between the traditional and animated visual analogue scales indicated that animated measures are not less reliable than paper-based reports of pain. Animated measures reflecting the different qualities of pain correlated significantly with responses to the McGill Pain Questionnaire. Thirty-two of the 50 patients preferred the animated method, and 9 others had no preference. Patients who selected a single quality-of-pain animation appeared to differ from those choosing more than 1.

Discussion.—This unique approach, based on interactive computer-generated animations, appears to be a valid means of assessing pain. Preliminary observations suggest that IA may be used to assess well-being in elderly patients who undergo physical fitness training.

▶ This article suggests that computer-administered pain assessment can produce results comparable to those obtained by more traditional paper-and-pencil methods. Additionally, interactive computer graphics may give evaluators unique information that is not obtainable by traditional methods. However, I believe that in evaluation of pain, the real power and advantage of the computer can best be realized by what is called computer-adaptive testing. During the past 10 years, computer-adaptive testing methodology has advanced considerably in many areas of tests and measurements (e.g., national certification and licensing examinations). Derived from newer psychometric techniques, computer algorithms can be used to administer questionnaires that are adaptive, i.e., the inclusion and/or ordering of additional questions is based on responses to preceding questions. This type of computer interviewing may hold considerable promise for clinicians in that information not only can be collected in more time- and cost-efficient ways, but it can be dynamically tailored to individual patients or unique patient populations.—T.E. Rudy, Ph.D.

What Does the BDI Measure in Chronic Pain?

de C Williams AC, Richardson PH (St Thomas Hosp, London)

Pain 55:259–266, 1993 131-95-5-7

Introduction.—The Beck Depression Inventory (BDI), one of the most widely used measures of depressive symptomatology, has been questioned as an accurate measure of depression for medical patients. Because of the multiple somatic complaints affecting medical patients,

3-Factor Orthogonal Solution Excluding Irritability (*K*) and Crying (*J*)

F1	'Sadness about health'	F2	'Self-reproach'	F3	'Somatic disturbance'
T	Somatic preoccup. 70	–		–	
A	Mood 68	–		–	
L	Social withdrawal 68	–		–	
B	Pessimism 65	–		–	
D	Lack satisfaction 59	–		–	
M	Indecisiveness 56	–		–	
U	Loss of libido 50	–		–	
I	Self-punitive wishes 49	–		–	
–		C	Sense of failure 80	–	
–		E	Guilty feeling 71	–	
–		G	Self-hate 71	–	
–		H	Self-accusation 69	–	
–		F	Sense of punishment 63	–	
–		N	Body image 47	–	
–		–		R	Loss of appetite 65
–		–		S	Weight loss 59
–		–		P	Sleep disturbance 51
–		–		Q	Fatigability 41
–		–		O	Work inhibition 41

Note: Variance in factor space: F1 64.2%, F2 20%, F3 15.8%.
(Courtesy of de C Williams AC, Richardson PH: *Pain* 55:259–266, 1993.)

they resemble depressed psychiatric patients in their somatic item ratings on the BDI. However, they resemble normal controls in their cognitive and affective item ratings. Somatic complaints tend to increase with age. The older-age population is not represented by the BDI because the upper age limit was 44 when the tool was developed. Chronic pain is associated with somatic disturbances—such as sleep disturbances, fatigability, and irritability—that are similar to depressive symptomatology. An analysis was done to define the usefulness of the BDI in patients with chronic pain.

Methods.—A total of 207 patients with chronic pain completed the BDI, the Speilberger State Anxiety Inventory, and the Pain Self-Efficacy Questionnaire. Physical measures were 10 minutes of walking and 2 minutes of stair climbing. Pain was rated on a scale of 0 to 100.

Results.—The mean BDI score was 18.1, indicating mild depression for 71.7% of those tested. Sadness about health, self-reproach, and somatic disturbances were 3 meaningful labeled factors (table). Somatic factors were scored greater than zero in 65% to 94% of the population. By comparison, only 7 of 14 cognitive-affective items were rated as present by a majority of patients. Patients with chronic pain tended to report problems with work, sleep, and fatigue; health concerns; irritability; and dissatisfaction with daily life.

Conclusion.—Caution must be used in interpreting total BDI scores in patients with chronic pain. Somatic manifestations may create an exaggerated impression of cognitive and affective disturbances.

► All too frequently, pain investigators select measures from other disciplines and apply scale scores derived from these measures to patients with chronic pain. In this process, an appreciation of the fundamental role played by the items used to compute scale scores is lost. Item bias—more generally called differential item functioning (DIF)—has become an important topic in the field of tests and measurements, where developing tests free of gender and cultural biases is essential because of social, legal, and political consequences. Although these authors are to be congratulated for addressing these issues in assessment of depression in patients with chronic pain, and although their study provides some useful findings, unfortunately, widely accepted and more powerful DIF-type analyses were not performed. Therefore, definitive conclusions regarding item bias on the BDI when applied to patients with chronic pain are not possible.—T.E. Rudy, Ph.D.

Validity of Self-Reported Exposures to Work Postures and Manual Materials Handling

Wiktorin C, Karlqvist L, Winkel J, Stockholm MUSIC I Study Group (Karolinska Hosp and Institute, Stockholm; Natl Inst of Occupational Health, Solna, Sweden)

Scand J Work Environ Health 19:208–214, 1993 131-95-5–8

Relation Between the Self-Reports and Reference Measurements for the 12 Group 1 Variables, According to the Kappa Coefficients and the Percentage of Full Agreement (Full %) for All Subjects Participating in the Study

Variables	Kappa	Full %
Trunk bent forward >60° (time)	0.43	88
Trunk rotation >45° (time)		61
Hands above shoulder level (time)	0.17	57
Head rotation (time)	0.17	58
Kneeling or squatting (time)	0.76	88
Carrying, pushing or pulling		
1–5 kg (time)	0.26	63
6–15 kg (time)	0.50	79
16–45 kg (time)	0.64	90
>45 kg (time)		90
Lifting		
6–15 kg (frequency)	0.66	86
16–45 kg (frequency)	0.65	93
>45 kg (frequency)		90

Note: Number of participants equals 97.
(Courtesy of Wiktorin C, Karlqvist L, Winkel J, et al: *Scand J Work Environ Health* 19:208–214, 1993.)

Introduction.—Quantitative data on the validity of work postures and manual materials handling are gathered primarily by self-reports. A questionnaire was used to determine the accuracy of self-reports compared with actual reference measurements of exposure to work postures and manual materials handling.

Methods.—Of 72 research subjects, 27 were men and 45 were women. A questionnaire with 9 illustrated questions about varying work postures and 8 regarding manual materials handling was administered. Four questions were validated by comparison with reference measurements. Walking was measured by a pedometer, a posimeter registered the time spent standing and sitting, and an inclinometer measured trunk flexion. Other criteria were measured by direct computerized observation.

Results.—The dichotomous level of agreement between self-reports and reference measurements was satisfactory for 9 of 17 questions (table). Poor agreement was found in 5 questions, and 3 were discarded because exposure concerned less than 10% of the group. Agreement was poor in the 5 questions that could quantify the duration or frequency of exposure by using a 4- or 6-point scale. Agreement for group 1 was better because variables were of short duration and low frequency, compared with group 2 variables, which were of varied duration and frequency. Errors in self-reporting may have been attributable to the way questions were asked, the length of the recording period, or the fact that the report scales assessed several factors vs. a "yes" or "no" answer.

Conclusion.—Self-reporting for certain postures and the handling of loads greater than 5 kg were accurate and could be used in epidemiologic studies. When more detailed information is needed, self-reporting lacks accuracy. Further analysis is needed to determine whether musculoskeletal complaints influence self-reported exposure.

▶ The validity of self-reported information has always been of concern to pain investigators. The findings of this study should also be of interest to pain clinicians, because pain rehabilitation programs are increasingly focusing on work performance and assessment issues. From an economical perspective, using self-report instruments to evaluate patients' particular work environments would be advantageous compared with more expense and labor-intensive job site visits. These findings, however, question the utility and accuracy of these self-reports. The behaviors that were questioned were very concrete and specific, yet they were still inaccurate by self-report. What does that tell us about some of the more general self-report behavioral and activity inventories used in pain research and treatment?—T.E. Rudy, Ph.D.

Low Back Pain

Chronic Low Back Pain: The Relationship Between Patient Satisfaction and Pain, Impairment, and Disability Outcomes

Hazard RG, Haugh LD, Green PA, Jones PL (Univ of Vermont, Burlington)

Spine 19:881–887, 1994 131-95-5–9

Background.—The biopsychosocial complexity of low back pain and disability cannot be measured simply. Past discrepancies among biological, psychological, social, and economic variables have resulted in the use of employment as a general indicator of treatment effectiveness. Quality and outcome assessments also differ with method and observer. In this study, the relationship between long-term patient satisfaction and the more traditional outcomes in patients disabled by chronic low back pain was investigated.

Methods.—Ninety patients with chronic low back pain were studied. Initial pain was assessed using a 10-cm visual analogue scale of pain (VAS), impairment was determined by a physical impairment score (PIS), and disability was evaluated using the Oswestery pain questionnaire (OPQ).

Findings.—Correlations of initial VAS, PIS, and OPQ were all less than .5. Pain and disability levels were matched more closely at the 5-year follow-up. Among 65 patients in rehabilitation, 5-year patient satisfaction scores were not closely associated with VAS, PIS, or OPQ improvements during therapy. Five-year satisfaction was weakly associated with current pain and disability. Satisfaction levels were greater among workers than among the unemployed after 1 and 5 years.

Conclusion.—These findings are consistent with those of other studies showing weak correlations among pretreatment pain, impairment, and disability levels in patients with chronic back pain. Functional restoration program graduates' pain and disability scores on completing therapy did not differ significantly between eventual workers and nonworkers. At 1 year after study entry, graduates' self-assessments of disability were significantly higher for those remaining out of work. However, pain complaints were comparable for workers and nonworkers. The dissociation of pain, impairment, and disability before and after treatment must be considered in assessing clinical trials and in prescribing treatment.

▶ Clinicians are frequently called upon to make predictions about patients' rehabilitation potentials. To date, models predicting treatment success have been weak at best, particularly when pretreatment data are considered. This study adds to those findings, and it incorporates patient satisfaction ratings as part of their multidimensional outcome and prediction models. With the increased emphasis on including patient satisfaction within program evaluation plans, I find this study of interest because there are very weak correlations between satisfaction and changes in measures of pain, impairment, and disability (all < .15). Future research may need to define differential weightings for primary measures of outcome, those aspects that the patient considers to be most important, and those that are rated as more important by the treating clinicians.—T.E. Rudy, Ph.D.

Successful Treatment of Low Back Pain and Neck Pain After a Motor Vehicle Accident Despite Litigation

Schofferman J, Wasserman S (San Francisco Spine Inst, Daly City, Calif)

Spine 19:1007–1010, 1994 131-95-5–10

Background.—Low back pain or neck pain after a motor vehicle accident occurs in a significant number of patients. In a small number of these patients, the structural source of the pain is readily identifiable. In a larger group, however, imaging studies reveal no abnormalities or only mild structural changes. The medical and legal communities may consider such patients to have "accident neurosis." Patients with low back pain or neck pain resulting from a motor vehicle accident and who were involved in litigation were studied prospectively and longitudinally to assess their outcomes.

Methods.—Thirty-nine consecutive patients with low back pain or neck pain and litigation pending were studied. They completed a McGill Pain Questionnaire (MPQ) to quantify pain and an Oswestry Low Back Disability Questionnaire (OSW) to quantify function. The patients were also interviewed about medications being taken and work status at the initial and final visits.

Findings.—Thirty-three patients completed the MPQ at the first and last assessment. Pain decreased in 88% and increased in 12%. Of 38 patients completing the OSW at the initial and final visits, 34 had improved function, and 4 had worse function. Significant improvements were noted in pain, function, and medication use.

Conclusion.—In this study, patients with low back pain or neck pain sustained in a motor vehicle accident significantly improved with treatment, despite ongoing litigation. These findings are consistent with a large body of evidence indicating that such patients are not "cured by verdict."

▶ With continued debate related to the potential adverse effects of compensation on rehabilitation outcomes, better designed, prospective studies are needed to help resolve this controversy. This study moves in the right direction, although measures other than just self-reported changes on functional/behavioral factors would have strengthened the conclusions.—T.E. Rudy, Ph.D.

Use of Psychometric Measures and Nonorganic Signs Testing in Detecting Nomogenic Disorders in Low Back Pain Patients

Hayes B, Solyom CAE, Wing PC, Berkowitz J (Univ of British Columbia, Vancouver, Canada; Berkowitz and Assoc, Vancouver, BC, Canada)

Spine 18:1254–1262, 1993 131-95-5–11

Background.—Assessment of low back pain largely relies on patients' self-report, which is problematic, especially in patients involved in litigation and in those receiving or expecting disability benefits. The effect of financial compensation on responses to psychometric testing was studied in a large series of patients with chronic back pain.

Methods.—Two hundred thirty-one patients were studied. Ninety-seven patients were anticipating or receiving financial compensation, and 134 patients were not. Two tests were administered within 4 hours, and an item-by-item comparison of responses was done to produce inconsistency scores. These scores, in addition to scores on other psychometric measures and Waddell's nonorganic signs test, were compared between groups.

Findings.—Patients expecting or receiving compensation had significantly greater mean inconsistency scores than did patients who were not expecting or receiving compensation. The former group also had significantly higher mean scores on almost all psychometric tests and nonorganic signs. Eighty-three percent of the former group had a score of 2 or higher on nonorganic signs, whereas almost all of those in the latter group had a score of 0. The nonorganic signs score alone predicted group status, correctly classifying 90% of the subjects. Using the inconsistency scores, 78% were correctly classified. The 2 assessment measures together classified 93% of the subjects.

Conclusion.—Nonorganic and inconsistency scores can distinguish between patients with chronic back pain who are receiving compensation and those who are not. These findings suggest that the psychometric tests used yield unreliable results and are, therefore, not valid for patients receiving or anticipating compensation.

▶ This study "claims" to have demonstrated that patients expecting or receiving compensation have greater inconsistency scores than patients not receiving compensation when repeated testing is conducted on self-report assessment instruments. However, patients in the former group also had higher scores on these instruments than did noncompensation patients. Thus, the inconsistency scores are probably biased in that it is well recognized in the psychometric literature that higher scores also lead to higher variability among scores; therefore, the inconsistency measures created are most likely an artifact rather than a true effect. Similarly, without psychometric analysis related to differential item functioning between these 2 patient samples—including the real possibility that scale reliability coefficients are different between samples—the conclusions reached are unwarranted.—T.E. Rudy, Ph.D.

Objective Assessment for Exercise Treatment on the B-200 Isostation as Part of Work Tolerance Rehabilitation: A Random Prospective Blind Evaluation With Comparison Control Population

Sachs BL, Ahmad SS, LaCroix M, Olimpio D, Heath R, David J-A, Scala AD (Tufts Univ, Boston; Thomas Jefferson School of Medicine, Philadelphia; Parkland Med Ctr, Derry, NH; et al)

Spine 19:49–52, 1994 131-95-5–12

Objective.—The B-200 Isostation was evaluated as part of a rehabilitation program for patients with lumbar dysfunction syndrome. Patients who participated in a standard work tolerance program were compared for muscle strength and lumbar range of motion with patients who had exercised on the B-200 Isostation in addition to the standard program.

Methods.—All patients were referred for conservative treatment. Fourteen patients were randomized to B-200 exercise and 16 to non–B-200 exercise. Eighteen normal volunteers without spinal pathology also completed an exercise program using the B-200 machine. A standard work tolerance program workout lasted 4–6 hours and included 2 hours and 45 minutes of combined isotonic strengthening and cardiovascular conditioning exercises. Those in the B-200 group put in an additional 15 minutes a day, performing the B-200 Isostation exercises in 3 planes: sagittal, lateral, and rotation. All patients were tested before and 3 weeks after completion of the program.

Results.—The 2 treatment groups had few differences in the percentage of improvement on objective measurements of range of motion, isometric strength, and velocity of motion. However, the differences were greater between each treatment group, compared with the normal control group. There was a trend for the 2 patient groups to have a greater difference between the pretest and posttest parameters as opposed to the control group.

Conclusion.—The addition of exercise with the B-200 Isostation did not enhance the outcome of the standard work tolerance program. Although inclusion of the objective assessment dynamometer machine in the work tolerance program for nonsurgical exercise has been justified for testing purposes, the standard program appears to be sufficient for improving patients' functional capacity.

▶ Back pain rehabilitation programs—particularly those that stress work conditioning—vary widely in their emphasis on instrumentation as part of the evaluation and/or treatment procedures. These authors specifically evaluated the inclusion of the B-200 Isostation as part of the treatment program. However, I suspect that similar findings would have resulted from other types of equipment. Additional research with larger sample sizes and more attention to the process of change is needed, however, before it can be concluded that computerized instrumentation does not serve a unique role in at least some aspects of rehabilitating the patient with back pain.—T.E. Rudy, Ph.D.

A Stochastic Model of Trunk Muscle Coactivation During Trunk Bending

Mirka GA, Marras WS (Ohio State Univ, Columbus)

Spine 18:1396–1409, 1993 131-95-5–13

Background.—Occupation-related low back disorders are increasingly common in the industrialized world. Results of numerous studies suggest a link between injury during heavy work and the biomechanical stresses placed on the spine. Traditional biomechanical models of the spine assume that external moments imposed about the spine are countered by the activity of the trunk musculature. However, the large number of muscle groups within the trunk means that there is an infinite number of possible combinations of muscle forces that can satisfy the biomechanical balance requirement for a given condition. A stochastic (probabilistic) model of trunk muscle activation was, therefore, developed.

Methods.—The first part of the study consisted of collection of experimental data. Five male college students, all without a history of low back disorder, performed a variety of exertions using trunk muscles. The subjects had surface electrodes applied to their skin before being secured in the apparatus. The data on trunk muscle activity obtained from the experimental part of the study became the foundation on which the stochastic stimulation model was based.

The Stochastic Model.—The model, based on a simulation of the experimentally derived data, predicted the possible combinations of time-dependent trunk muscle coactivations that could be expected, given a set

Proportion of Actual Electromyographic Data Points Within the Range, as Predicted by the Simulation Model, Partitioned by Motion Type

	RLAT	LLAT	RES	LES	RAB	LAB	REX	LEX	RIN	LIN
Isometric	.995	.915	.921	.985	.929	.935	.951	.747	.833	.816
Isokinetic	.945	.991	.539	.910	.763	.855	.717	.729	.581	.644
Isoinertial	.901	.994	.851	.942	.628	.755	.637	.734	.926	.820

(Courtesy of Mirka GA, Marras WS: *Spine* 18:1396–1409, 1993.)

Moving?

I'd like to receive my ***Year Book of Pain*** without interruption.
Please note the following change of address, effective:

Name: ______________________________

New Address: ______________________________

____

City: ______________________ State: ________ Zip: ________

Old Address: ______________________________

____

City: ______________________ State: ________ Zip: ________

Reservation Card

Yes, I would like my own copy of ***Year Book of Pain***. Please begin my subscription with the current edition according to the terms described below.* I understand that I will have 30 days to examine each annual edition. If satisfied, I will pay just $61.95 plus sales tax, postage and handling (price subject to change without notice).

Name: ______________________________

Address: ______________________________

City: ______________________ State: ________ Zip: ________

Method of Payment

❍ Visa ❍ Mastercard ❍ AmEx ❍ Bill me ❍ Check (in US dollars, payable to Mosby, Inc.)

Card number: ______________________ Exp date: ____________

Signature: ______________________________

LS-0909

*Your *Year Book* Service Guarantee:

When you subscribe to the *Year Book*, we'll send you an advance notice of future volumes about two months before they publish. This automatic notice system is designed to take up as little of your time as possible. If you do not want the *Year Book*, the advance notice makes it quick and easy for you to let us know your decision, and you will always have at least 20 days to decide. If we don't hear from you, we'll send you the new volume as soon as it's available. And, of course, the *Year Book* is yours to examine free of charge for 30 days (postage, handling and applicable sales tax are added to each shipment.).

NO POSTAGE
NECESSARY
IF MAILED
IN THE
UNITED STATES

BUSINESS REPLY MAIL
FIRST CLASS MAIL PERMIT No. 762 CHICAGO, IL

POSTAGE WILL BE PAID BY ADDRESSEE

Chris Hughes
Mosby-Year Book, Inc.
200 N. LaSalle Street
Suite 2600
Chicago, IL 60601-9981

NO POSTAGE
NECESSARY
IF MAILED
IN THE
UNITED STATES

BUSINESS REPLY MAIL
FIRST CLASS MAIL PERMIT No. 762 CHICAGO, IL

POSTAGE WILL BE PAID BY ADDRESSEE

Chris Hughes
Mosby-Year Book, Inc.
200 N. LaSalle Street
Suite 2600
Chicago, IL 60601-9981

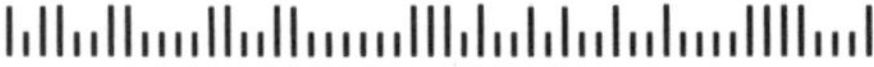

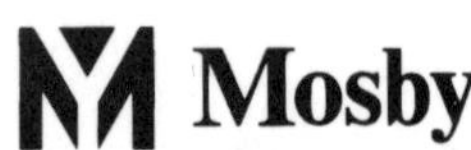

Dedicated to publishing excellence

of trunk-bending conditions. The magnitude and variability of the spine reaction forces were estimated when simulated muscle activities were used as input to an electromyographically assisted biomechanical model. Thus, the range of spinal loads expected with a specific task could be assessed. Each lifting activity was found to result in a significant variability in muscle activities. The variability in trunk muscle force had little effect on spinal compression variability but a considerable influence on both lateral and anteroposterior shear forces.

A validation study was performed with 2 different male subjects, 1 similar to the original 5 subjects and 1 who was significantly larger and stronger. The model's overall predictive ability (82.4%) was not significantly diminished by use of a subject different in size and strength from the original experimental group. The success rate was 83.1% for thc similar subject and 81.8% for the larger subject (table).

Conclusion.—This study shows that it is possible to predict the range of electromyographic activities that would be expected during a trunk-bending task, given adequate knowledge of the trunk motion and external loading conditions. The model developed could aid in understanding the muscle system activities and spinal loading associated with low back disorders.

▶ Biomechanical models of the lumbar spine have undergone substantial revisions in the past several years, in part as a result of the innovative work of these authors. Many more widely accepted biomechanical models are too static and restrictive to have much ecologic validity, i.e., to effectively translate to the clinic or job site. The findings of this paper help to narrow this gap, particularly in terms of repetitive lifting motions commonly performed in many occupations.—T.E. Rudy, Ph.D.

Acute and Chronic Low Back Pain: Cognitive, Affective, and Behavioral Dimensions

Hadjistavropoulos HD, Craig KD (Univ of British Columbia, Vancouver, Canada)

J Consult Clin Psychol 62:341–349, 1994 131-95-5–14

Introduction.—Patients who express medically incongruent back pain use more health care resources; have poorer response to surgery, rehabilitation, acupuncture, and outcome; and differ in their subjective reactions to pain from patients with congruent signs and symptoms of pain. Multidimensional assessments were used to compare cognitive, affective, behavioral, and demographic dimensions of acute, chronic congruent, and chronic incongruent pain.

Methods.—Three groups of 30 patients with low back pain were screened and assigned to a pain group. A physical impairment index was performed. The Oswestry Low Back Pain Disability, Coping Strategy,

Results of Discriminant Function Analysis Predicting Congruent and Incongruent Pain Groups

Predictor variables	Function 1	Univariate F (1.58)
Catastrophizing	0.58	9.35†
Emotionality	0.54	8.26†
Movement unpleasantness	0.51	7.23†
Compensation status	0.51	7.25†
Regular pain killers	0.50	6.93†
Socioeconomic status	−0.46	5.93*
Physical impairment	0.44	5.55*
Disability	0.43	5.21*
Daily unpleasantness	0.42	5.05*
Passive coping	0.39	4.33*
Canonical *R*	0.57	
Eigenvalue	0.48	

* $P < .05$.
† $P < .01$.
(Courtesy of Hadjistavropoulos HD, Craig KD: *J Consult Clin Psychol* 62:341–349, 1994.)

Pain Experience Scale, and Descriptor Differential Scale questionnaires were administered. Patients were asked to lift both legs 10 inches off the examining table. If unable to do so, they were asked to do single leg raises. With facial responses recorded by videotape, patients were asked to (1) express the pain or discomfort experienced while doing leg lifts; (2) try to mask the discomfort; and (3) exaggerate the pain or discomfort. Videotapes were scored for the presence or absence of 44 facial action units.

Results.—Patients in the chronic incongruent and acute pain groups were more likely to have negative reactions to pain; use passive coping strategies; report dysfunctional, catastrophizing cognitions; be on compensation; have a lower socioeconomic status; use opiates for pain; and report greater disability caused by pain than patients in the chronic congruent group (table).

Conclusion.—Expectations were that acute and chronic congruent group differences would be small compared to the chronic incongruent group. Actual findings indicate the need to revise attitudes, assessment, and treatment of patients with low back pain.

▶ Multidimensional assessment from an interdisciplinary perspective has become the accepted standard for evaluating patients with chronic low back pain. However, this comprehensive evaluation model generally has not been adopted for the evaluation of acute back pain. This paper provides new and important information suggesting that the duration of symptoms may be an arbitrary distinction in low back pain. If we accept that disability is a subjective, personalized reaction to one's physical or impairment condition that varies widely across individuals, it seems only appropriate to focus on this reaction rather than to assume that time alone leads to greater disability.—T.E. Rudy, Ph.D.

Clinical Practice Issues

Patterns in Low Back Pain Hospitalizations: Implications for the Treatment of Low Back Pain in an Era of Health Care Reform
Volinn E, Turczyn KM, Loeser JD (Univ of Washington, Seattle; Natl Ctr for Health Statistics, Hyattsville, Md)
Clin J Pain 10:64–70, 1994 131-95-5–15

Introduction.—The cost of treatment of back pain has been estimated to be as high as $24.3 billion compared with $10.3 billion for AIDS. In studies of geographic variation, rates of common health care practices vary widely from area to area. Regarding 2 treatments for back pain (spine surgery and nonsurgical hospitalization), rates vary among countries and hospital market areas in the United States.

Methods.—Patterns in surgical and nonsurgical hospitalizations for low back pain among geographic regions and through time were explored for the implications of these patterns for health care reform. Data (1979–1987) on surgical and nonsurgical hospitalizations for low back pain, obtained from the National Hospital Discharge Survey (conducted by the National Center for Health Statistics), were analyzed.

Results.—Rates for surgical and nonsurgical low back pain hospitalization varied among United States regions, and average lengths of stay varied considerably. The United States rate of surgery for low back pain increased sharply (by 49%) during the period covered by the study. Over the same period, the rate of nonsurgical low back pain hospitalization in the United States decreased by 33%, as did the average lengths of stay for both types of low back pain hospitalization (42% for surgical and 31% for nonsurgical). For surgical and nonsurgical low back pain hospitalization, rates were twice as high in the South as they were in the Northeast. The average length of surgical stays was 20% longer in the South than in the Midwest and West. The average length of nonsurgical stays was 29% longer in the Northeast than in the South.

Conclusion.—More research needs to be done on changing physician practice style, as indicated by the increasing rate of low back pain surgery. Savings in health care costs would be considerable if such research resulted in a reduction in low back pain hospitalization.

▶ Variability in clinical practices in the treatment of low back pain is understandable, even to be expected. What is not expected, however, is the magnitude of variability reported by these authors. Although the role of surgery in low back pain is frequently questioned and is often discouraged by leaders in the field, the treatment of this message appears to have had little impact on practitioners. What will change the current clinical practices of spine surgeons—national clinical practice guidelines, internal organizational standards developed by surgeons, or external pressures from third-party payers?—T.E. Rudy, Ph.D.

Physicians' Attitudes and Practices Regarding the Long-Term Prescribing of Opioids for Non-Cancer Pain

Turk DC, Brody MC, Okifuji EA (Univ of Pittsburgh, Pa)

Pain 59:201–208, 1994 131-95-5–16

Introduction.—The use of opioids in the management of noncancer chronic pain has been controversial. Information on the actual prescribing practices of physicians regarding opioids has been limited as the surveys have been on narrow populations. This study surveyed physicians regarding their beliefs and practices of prescribing long-term opioids for patients with chronic pain.

Methods.—A stratified random sample of 6,962 physicians in 2 states from each of the 5 regions of the United States and 7 medical specialties was surveyed. A total of 1,912 (27.46%) responded. The survey instrument included questions about years of practice, the total number of patients with chronic pain in their practice, opioid prescription frequency, and treatment goals as well as concerns about opioids, the adequacy of their education regarding pain control, and regulatory pressures.

Findings.—The use of opioids appears to be reasonably widespread. Physicians in the Midwest had the lowest prescribing frequency, whereas physicians in the Pacific region had the highest. Rheumatologists and general practitioners were most likely to prescribe opioids, and they emphasized that improvement in symptoms was an appropriate goal even if there was little functional improvement. Surgeons and neurologists were the least likely to prescribe opioids. There was little concern about addiction, tolerance and dependence being impediments to prescribing opioids. Regulatory pressures had little impact on the prescribing practices of this sample of physicians.

Conclusion.—Although less than 15% of these physicians thought that the use of opioids was a "legal and acceptable medical practice," most physicians had some patients receiving long-term opioid therapy. The identification of patients who will experience both symptomatic and functional improvement is unsettled. Because of the lack of definitive data on this topic, physicians lean on their own attitudes while patients are left to the biases of their physicians.

▶ Perhaps the most controversial and highly debated issue in pain management in recent years is the long-term use of opioids in the treatment of chronic noncancer pain. The findings of this study, despite the low response rate (27%), provide important insights into this debate. Interestingly, opioid prescribing practices showed regional differences, as did clinical practices for spine surgeries (see Abstract 131-95-5–15). The variability of prescribing practices across medical specialties found in this study is also quite interesting. Current practices and clinical opinions aside, to date there have not been any well-controlled clinical trials that evaluate the efficacy of the long-term use of opioids in patients with noncancer pain, particularly in terms of improved function.—T.E. Rudy, Ph.D.

The Americans With Disabilities Act: Issues for Back and Spine-Related Disability

Blanck PD (Univ of Iowa, Iowa City)

Spine 19:103–107, 1994 131-95-5–17

Introduction.—Effective implementation of the Americans with Disabilities Act (ADA) is endangered by criticism and lack of understanding. Title I of the act defines employment provisions. Economic and social costs of back- and spine-related injuries call for a closer examination of the ADA's effect on diagnosis, treatment, rehabilitation, and compliance strategies.

Overview of Title I of the ADA.—The ADA is considered a vehicle for social and cultural changes that will shape attitude and behavior toward persons with disabilities well into the next century. Communication regarding the act is essential for this paradigm shift. A person with a disability is substantially limited physically or mentally in the performance of major life activities. Employers must define essential functions and make reasonable accommodations that allow disabled employees to perform the job. Accommodations should not make undue hardship for the employer. The Equal Employment Opportunity Commission is responsible for enforcement.

Implications of Title I for Back- and Spine-Related Disability.—It is imperative that the act be understood as an effort to include and empower persons with disabilities. It is not intended as an affirmative action initiative. Unfounded fears exist concerning the ADA. To encourage informed and cost-effective compliance with the law, everyone concerned needs information about the costs and benefits of employing qualified persons with back- and spine-related disabilities. Disputes about ADA can be handled voluntarily by negotiation, mediation, and arbitration. Although the interests of those protected under the act should be represented, it is important that disputes be handled well to avoid undermining public support.

Conclusion.—The ADA is primarily a civil rights law. Persons with disabilities must be treated equally with everyone else. Recognition, education, and understanding are essential to success in meeting the challenges posed by the ADA.

▶ The most common type of ADA claim in the United States involves back impairments, which account for almost one fifth of all charges filed and represent more than twice as many charges as the next most common claim, mental disability. This article provides an excellent introduction to the ADA and should be of particular interest to practitioners involved in low back rehabilitation.—T.E. Rudy, Ph.D.

A Quality-Based Protocol for Management of Musculoskeletal Injuries: A Ten-Year Prospective Outcome Study

Wiesel SW, Boden SD, Feffer HL (Georgetown Univ, Washington, DC; Emory University, Atlanta, Ga; George Washington Univ, Washington, DC)

Clin Orthop 301:164–176, 1994 131-95-5–18

Introduction.—Musculoskeletal injuries are a major health problem in the workplace and account for significant disability, health care costs, and lost productivity. In most states, the workers' compensation system does not provide incentives for minimizing disability. It was hypothesized that workers' compensation patients were receiving care of widely varying quality and that using quality-based standardized protocols for diagnosis and treatment of industrial musculoskeletal injuries would both improve the quality and reduce the costs of care. The hypothesis was tested in a 10-year prospective study.

Methods.—More than 5,300 employees of a utility company were studied upon the institution of a surveillance program. Within 24 hours of an occupational musculoskeletal injury, the employee was seen by a company physician. Employees who lost time from work were evaluated within 1 week by an orthopedic consultant, who diagnosed the injury and recommended a course of management. Both the diagnosis and the recommended course of management were based on standardized algorithms developed for each anatomical site. The patients were reviewed weekly and, at the appropriate time, a physical therapist recommended rehabilitation exercises. Return to work was accomplished gradually, with medical surveillance.

Results.—Most of the musculoskeletal injuries involved the low back or the knee. New injuries to the low back declined by an average of 51% annually, and there was a 55% average decrease in work days lost because of low back injuries. The number of work days lost annually because of knee injuries decreased by an average of 40%. Low back surgical procedures decreased by 67%, and 90% of these patients returned to work. The costs of lost work time and replacement wages were reduced by an average of 59% with back injuries and 65% with knee injuries.

Discussion.—By implementing a program designed to reduce inappropriate variations in care and provide continuous feedback for quality improvement, quality care was provided at reduced cost. These findings support the hypothesized relationship between consistently high-quality care and cost reduction.

▶ The establishment of clinical algorithms, protocols, and practice guidelines is becoming increasingly important in the management of chronic pain, as in many other areas of medicine. However, the development of more standardized clinical procedures and practices, based on currently available scientific evidence, is a difficult task. This paper provides a comprehensive treatment of the complexities inherent in developing clinical algorithms for low back and knee pain. Its emphasis on establishing criteria for the effective use of costly diagnostic procedures and early restoration of patients' functional abilities is particularly noteworthy. Methodological issues related to the prospective study of clinical algorithms are also effectively addressed. Close inspection of this paper is highly recommended to all pain clinicians and clinical investigators.—T.E. Rudy, Ph.D.

Temporomandibular Disorders

Brief Group Cognitive-Behavioral Intervention for Temporomandibular Disorders

Dworkin SF, Turner JA, Wilson L, Massoth D, Whitney C, Huggins KH, Burgess J, Sommers E, Truelove E (Univ of Washington, Seattle)
Pain 59:175–187, 1994 131-95-5–19

Background.—The term "temporomandibular disorder" (TMD) refers to an interrelated set of conditions with signs and symptoms of the masticatory and related muscles of the head and neck, as well as the soft tissue and bony parts of the temporomandibular joint. In every major respect, TMD is fundamentally a chronic pain condition. Treatment of many common chronic pain conditions, particularly in pain clinics, includes cognitive-behavioral (CB) treatment methods. The effects of a minimal CB intervention for TMD were assessed in a randomized, clinical trial.

Methods.—The study included 139 patients with pain and related symptoms of TMD. Eighty-five percent were women and 96% were white; the average age was 37 years. Patients were randomly assigned to receive either a CB intervention before the usual dental treatment for TMD or the usual treatment alone. The small-group CB intervention consisted of two 2-hour sessions in which the patients were taught about TMD and received training in pain and stress reduction and physiotherapy exercises. The 2 groups were compared at 3 and 12 months for TMD pain and related physical and psychological variables to see whether the CB intervention enhanced the effects of the usual dental treatment. The study also sought to determine whether the patients' so-

Mean Values of Usual Treatment (*UT*) ($n = 73$) and Cognitive-Behavioral (*CB*) ($n = 66$) Groups for Clinical and Psychological Variables

Dependent variables	Baseline		3 Months		12 Months		*P*		
	UT	CB	UT	CB	UT	CB	Group	Time	Group × Time
Maximum assisted mandibular opening	46.5	43.1	46.9	45.2	46.9	45.6	n.s.	0.05	n.s.
Unassisted mandibular opening	36.4	35.1	38.9	38.1	38.5	39.2	n.s.	0.001	n.s.
Depression score *	0.26	0.12	−0.06	0.04	−0.20	−0.06	n.s.	0.001	n.s.
Somatization score *	0.75	0.86	0.54	0.59	0.44	0.44	n.s.	0.001	n.s.

* SCL-90-R scores age/sex-adjusted and standardized to population norms.
Repeated-measures analysis of variance (ANOVA) for group effects (CB vs. UT); time effects (baseline, 3-, and 12-month follow-ups); group × time interaction.
(Courtesy of Dworkin SF, Turner JA, Wilson L, et al: *Pain* 59:175–187, 1994.)

matization and psychosocial dysfunction classification would affect response to the CB intervention.

Results.—Long-term pain reduction was greater in the CB group than in the usual treatment group. The CB group also had a greater decrease in pain interference in daily activities. No differences were noted at the 3-month follow-up. However, at 12 months, the usual treatment patients were at about the same level of characteristic pain, whereas the CB patients had continued to improve. At the same time, the CB group also demonstrated a strong trend toward continued improvement in pain interference with activities. There were no differences between groups in depression, somatization, or jaw range of motion (table). Patients with psychosocial dysfunction did not appear to benefit from CB.

Conclusion.—A brief CB intervention before usual dental care can reduce the symptoms of TMD. The effects may be only modest, but they are long-lasting. The authors call for further studies to determine which components of the CB intervention are most potent. Like biomedical treatments, biobehavioral treatments are not equally effective for all patients with chronic pain.

▶ Historically, studies describing the diagnosis and treatment of TMD have appeared primarily in the dental medicine literature. More recently, however, there has been increased recognition that TMDs have many features that parallel other types of chronic pain conditions. These authors have been leaders in that cross-fertilization, and this study is no exception. Because patients with the same biomedical diagnoses display widely varying psychosocial and behavioral/functional reactions, it seems logical to assume that there would also be considerable response variances to more psychosocially based treatments. However, this issue has only received limited attention in the literature. This study contributes to that literature and, hopefully, will encourage other investigators in other areas of chronic pain research to address differential treatment response patterns based on psychosocial assessment findings.—T.E. Rudy, Ph.D.

First Onset of Common Pain Symptoms: A Prospective Study of Depression as a Risk Factor

Von Korff M, Le Resche L, Dworkin SF (Ctr for Health Studies Group Health Cooperative of Puget Sound, Seattle; Univ of Washington, Seattle)

Pain 55:251–258, 1993 131-95-5–20

Introduction.—Depression may be a factor that influences the development of chronic pain, irrespective of anatomical site. Many studies have examined the association of pain and depressive illness, but the nature of this complex relationship remains unclear. Whether depressive symptoms at baseline are associated with an increased risk of onset for 5 common pain symptoms was investigated in a prospective study of adult enrollees in a health maintenance organization (HMO).

Odds Ratios for First Onset of Selected Pain Symptoms Adjusted for Age, Gender, and Educational Attainment

	Back pain (%)	Severe headache (%)	Chest pain (%)	Abdominal pain (%)	TMD pain (%)
Age					
18–44	1.00	1.00	1.00	1.00	1.00
45–64	0.39*	0.14**	2.01	0.31	0.80
65–74	0.90	†	5.09**	0.99	0.65
Gender					
Male	1.00	1.00	1.00	1.00	1.00
Female	0.92	1.25	0.74	4.92**	1.49
Education					
High school or less	1.00	1.00	1.00	1.00	1.00
Some college	0.59	0.13***	0.84	1.17	1.33
College grad.	1.01	0.21***	0.38	0.63	0.83
Depression severity					
Normal	1.00	1.00	1.00	1.00	1.00
Moderate	0.23	5.02***	4.51**	0.47	1.17
Severe	0.28	1.68	4.62**	†	1.60
Number of pain conditions					
None	1.00	1.00	1.00	1.00	1.00
One or more	2.09**	4.29***	1.39	6.25**	3.69***

* $P < .10$.
** $P < .05$.
*** $P < .01$.
† Cells were combined because of the small number of cases.
(Courtesy of Van Korff M, Le Resche L, Dworkin SF: *Pain* 55:251–258, 1993.)

Methods.—Two interviews were conducted in a probability sample of this large HMO. The participants were asked about their lifetime history and their age at onset of back pain, severe headache, abdominal pain, chest pain, and temporomandibular (TMD) pain and whether they had experienced any of these pain conditions in the previous 6 months. They were reinterviewed 3 years later to measure site-specific first-onset rates in those reporting no current pain conditions at baseline. The depression scale of the Symptom Checklist 90–Revised was used at both interviews.

Results.—A total of 1,016 HMO enrollees were initially interviewed, and 803 took part in the second evaluation. The rates of first onset for the 5 symptoms during the 3-year follow-up interval were 17.7% for back pain, 4.2% for severe headache, 3% for chest pain, 3.1% for abdominal pain, and 6.5% for TMD pain. The onset rates of persistent pain and chronic pain dysfunction were substantially lower, but more than 1% of patients experienced the onset of chronic pain dysfunction for back pain and headache. There were no significant differences in the onset rates of back pain, abdominal pain, and TMD pain by severity or chronicity of depressive symptoms. Persons with moderate-to-severe depressive symptoms, however, were more likely to experience the onset of headache and chest pain during follow-up. When adjustments were made for age, gender, education, and severity of depression, persons with at least 1 pain condition at baseline were more likely to report the first onset of a new pain condition during follow-up. The odds ratios were highest for abdominal pain (6.3), headache (4.3), and TMD pain (3.7) (table).

Conclusion.—The effect of depression on the onset of pain was inconsistent across sites and did not become stronger with increasing severity of depression. Overall, the presence of a pain condition at baseline was a more consistent predictor of the development of a new pain condition. Clinical and epidemiologic data suggest that some persons may have a heightened response to both physical and psychological stressors.

▶ The link between pain and depression remains illusive and confusing, despite the multitude of studies. Most studies to date, however, have been retrospective or cross-sectional and, therefore, have serious interpretational limitations regarding cause-and-effect relationships. This study, which included not only patients with TMD but those with headache and low back pain as well, provided important prospective information that challenges the assumption held by some pain investigators that depression is causally linked to the development of painful conditions.—T.E. Rudy, Ph.D.

Tyramine Conjugation Deficit in Patients With Chronic Idiopathic Temporomandibular Joint and Orofacial Pain

Aghabeigi B, Feinmann C, Glover V, Goodwin B, Hannah P, Harris M, Sandler M, Wasil M (Eastman Dental and Univ College Hosps, London; Queen Charlotte's and Chelsea Hosp, London)

Pain 54:159–163, 1993 131-95-5–21

Introduction.—There may be a common biological predisposition to chronic pain and depression. Patients with these syndromes respond to antidepressive medications. Approximately 30% to 60% of patients with "nonorganic" chronic pain are depressed. Patients with endogenous unipolar depression excrete subnormal amounts of tyramine sulfate. Patients with chronic facial pain of varying causes were tested to determine whether chronic facial pain and depression were correlated with a tyramine conjunction deficit.

Methods.—Twenty-nine patients with chronic facial pain were given a capsule containing 100 mg of tyramine. Urine was collected for 3 hours, and tyramine-O-sulfate levels were determined. Patients had a structured clinical interview for the diagnosis of mental disorders and were screened with the Hospital Anxiety and Depression Questionnaire to determine current levels of anxiety and depression. Endogenous and neurotic depression were differentiated.

Results.—Three patients were experiencing a major depressive episode during testing, and 11 had a history of at least 1 major depressive episode. These patients had a significantly lower mean urinary 3-hour tyramine-O-sulfate output than the controls. Patients with a history of depression had a nearly significantly lower level than patients with no history of depression.

Conclusion.—A low tyramine sulfate level appears to be a marker for vulnerability to idiopathic orofacial pain and is independent of depression. Idiopathic facial pain and endogenous depression probably share a common metabolic vulnerability.

▶ Studies that attempt to find a common biological link between pain and depression are not new. This study extends that methodology to the study of patients with TMD. Although the sample size limits the conclusions and generalizability of the findings, this might be a fruitful area for further investigations.—T.E. Rudy, Ph.D.

The Efficacy of Oral Splints in the Treatment of Myofascial Pain of the Jaw Muscles: A Controlled Clinical Trial

Dao TTT, Lavigne GJ, Charbonneau A, Feine JS, Lund JP (Université de Montréal, Québec, Canada)

Pain 56:85–94, 1994 131-95-5–22

Introduction.—Oral splints are frequently used to treat temporomandibular disorders. They are widely assumed to have true therapeutic value, but the mechanisms involved are not clear.

Objective.—A randomized, controlled, blinded trial was done in 63 patients having a primary diagnosis of myofascial pain in the jaw muscles in an attempt to confirm the therapeutic value of occlusal splinting.

Study Design.—The patients, 53 females and 10 males 16–45 years of age, had experienced myofascial pain for a mean of 44 months. Thirty-one patients had not previously been treated for temporomandibular joint disease. The patients were randomly assigned to wear a full occlusal splint for 24 hours a day, a full occlusal splint for 30 minutes at each appointment, or a palatal splint 24 hours a day. The participants rated the intensity of pain on a visual analogue scale, at rest and after masticating, during 7 visits over a 10-week period. The 3 groups were similar in age and gender distribution.

Results.—In general, pain lessened during the treatment period, and the patients' quality of life improved. Pain and unpleasantness decreased by similar degrees in all groups. Patients whose initial pain scores were relatively high tended to retain higher-than-average scores after treatment. Pain from chewing on wax also was comparable in all groups at the end of the treatment period. All groups improved in quality of life, with a large majority of patients in each group reporting a better quality of life at the end of treatment than before treatment began. Responses to a gray stimulus, taken as a general measure of sensory state, remained stable.

Conclusion.—These results cast doubt on whether oral splints actually have therapeutic value for patients with myofascial pain. They, nevertheless, remain a conservative alternative to irreversible measures or long-term drug treatment until a more specific approach becomes available.

▶ A host of mechanisms have been proposed for the efficacy of oral splints in the treatment of patients with temporomandibular disorders. Although myogenic theories of temporomandibular disorder are popular and are used to explain the effects of oral splints, this well-controlled clinical trial challenges the hypothesized mechanism for the effectiveness of splints. Unfortunately, the sample sizes of this study may not have had the necessary power to detect statistical differences between the experimental groups.—T.E. Rudy, Ph.D.

Comparison of Psychologic and Physiologic Functioning Between Patients With Masticatory Muscle Pain and Matched Controls

Carlson CR, Okeson JP, Falace DA, Nitz AJ, Curran SL, Anderson D (Univ of Kentucky, Lexington)

J Orofac Pain 7:15–22, 1993 131-95-5-23

Background.—There has been a general consensus in the dental community that destructive oral habits are the primary cause of most temporomandibular disorders (TMDs). Some recent studies, however, have reported the presence of postural hyperactivity and elevated resting electromyogram (EMG) activity in patients with TMD. In an attempt to characterize the mechanisms that might account for TMD, patients with masticatory muscle pain were compared with age- and sex-matched normal controls.

Methods.—The study subjects were 34 patients and 18 normal controls. The patient sample of 32 women and 2 men had an average age of 34.1 years. They had experienced prolonged primarily masticatory muscle pain with no clinical evidence of joint pathology or dysfunction. All participants completed several standardized psychological tests and underwent evaluation of EMG activity, heart rate, and systolic and diastolic blood pressure under conditions of rest, mental stress, and relaxation. Skin temperature was also recorded.

Results.—Patients with masticatory muscle pain reported significantly more trait anxiety and state anxiety than did normal controls, indicating that the patients experienced significantly more cognitively oriented symptoms of anxiety. The patients also rated themselves as less confident of their ability to relax. At baseline, controls and patients were similar with regard to resting EMG activity at each of the 4 muscle sites examined, heart rate, blood pressure, and skin temperature. During the stress phase of the study, patients with masticatory muscle pain had higher heart rates and systolic blood pressure than the controls. Patients and controls did not differ, however, in EMG activity in the masseter regions during stress.

Conclusion.—Muscle hyperactivity has long been accepted as the primary cause of masticatory muscle pain, and a number of diagnostic and therapeutic approaches to this type of pain are based on increased EMG activity. Yet in this group of patients and controls, the increases in EMG activity associated with stress were similar. The etiology of masticatory muscle pain may have to be sought elsewhere, perhaps in the area of sympathetic overactivity.

▶ Although psychophysiologic models of TMD have been around for many years, few well-controlled studies have directly tested the assumptions of these models. A primary assumption of these models is that psychological stressors lead to hypermuscle activity in the muscles of mastication. The lack of significant EMG differences between patients and controls in this study appears to challenge that assumption. An important caveat, however, is that patients with TMD may not be a homogeneous group in terms of masticatory stress reactions. The large EMG variances observed for the TMD patient group evaluated in this study seems to support that conclusion.—T.E. Rudy, Ph.D.

Pain Behaviors

Interpersonal Stress and Pain Behaviors in Patients With Chronic Pain

Schwartz L, Slater MA, Birchler GR (Univ of Washington, Seattle; Univ of California, San Diego)

J Consult Clin Psychol 62:861–864, 1994 131-95-5–24

Introduction.—Learning theory recognizes that social context affects pain behavior. Responses from spouses are particularly believed to affect pain behavior. Men with chronic pain and their wives were assigned to a stress interview or to a neutral talking task. Then the amount of time the men persisted at demanding physical exercise was measured.

Methods.—Thirty-four men (average age, 51 years) with chronic low back pain (averaging 18 years' duration) and their wives participated. They had been married for an average of 22.5 years and rated their marriages as satisfactory. Couples were randomly assigned to a stress interview concerning difficult life issues or to a neutral talking task concerning black-and-white drawings. Blood pressure measurements were used to determine the stress of the interviews. Immediately after the interviews, the men rode a stationary bicycle while their wives helped them maintain a steady pace. Ending the exercise before the maximum time of 20 minutes was measured as inability to persist because of pain. Pain behavior was defined as lack of persistence.

Results.—Before the interviews, men in both groups had blood pressures of about 130/82. After the stress interviews, blood pressure significantly increased to about 150/90. In contrast, after the neutral talking task, blood pressures remained the same. About two thirds of the stressed men stopped bicycling prematurely. Only one third of the unstressed men stopped prematurely, significantly fewer. Significantly more men who had stopped prematurely reported pain, compared with those who completed the exercise.

Conclusion.—Pain behaviors are more likely under stressful conditions. Reacting to stressful interpersonal relationships with pain behavior might be costly for the patient's relationships. Therefore, treatments addressing relationship skills might help to reduce pain behaviors and promote patient's function. Research is needed to determine whether exhibiting pain behavior in response to stress reduces the adverseness of the situation or ends an uncomfortable interaction. Work is also needed to determine the effect of a spouse's presence on the extent of stress induced, and on the elicitation of subsequent pain behaviors.

Depression and Pain Behavior in Patients With Chronic Pain

Krause SJ, Wiener RL, Tait RC (St Louis Univ, Mo)

Clin J Pain 10:122–127, 1994 131-95-5–25

Background.—Increased attention has been given to the association between depression and pain. Previous studies suggest that in patients with chronic pain, those who are depressed demonstrate more pain behavior than their nondepressed counterparts. Possible causes of these observed differences were investigated.

Patients and Methods.—Thirty-seven inpatients enrolled in a chronic pain program were evaluated. Pain behavior was rated simultaneously by patients and trained observers twice weekly during a 9- to 25-day hospitalization period, using the Pain Behavior Scale. Discharge scores on the

Beck Depression Inventory Short Form were used to place patients into high depressive (HD) or low depressive (LD) groups.

Results.—Consistently lower frequencies of exhibitions of pain behavior were noted by trained observers, compared with the assessments of both the HD and LD groups. Significantly more pain behavior was self-reported by HD vs. LD patients, whereas nurse ratings did not significantly differ between groups.

Conclusion.—Cognitive factors may play a role in the depressed patient's self-rated pain, with reports reflecting a negative perceptual bias rather than observable behavioral differences. The association between depression and pain behavior requires further study, using both self-report and observer ratings.

Pain Behavior in Industrial Subacute Low Back Pain. Part I. Reliability: Concurrent and Predictive Validity of Pain Behavior Assessments

Öhlund C, Lindström I, Areskoug B, Eek C, Peterson L-E, Nachemson A (Univ of Göteborg, Sweden; Göteborgs Datacentral, Sweden; Volvo Co, Göteborg, Sweden)

Pain 58:201–209, 1994 131-95-5–26

Introduction.—Since pain is partly a learned response and pain behaviors form the basis for the social response governing disability support, it is important to have reliable and valid pain and disability assessments. Therefore, the predictive value of both overt and covert pain behaviors, as measured by a variety of assessment means, was compared against employee absenteeism among patients with subacute low back pain.

Methods.—All workers at a car manufacturing plant who were absent from work for more than 6 weeks because of nonspecific benign low back pain were assessed by an orthopedic surgeon and a social worker. The patients were videotaped, and observers scored the occurrence of guarding, bracing, rubbing, grimacing, and sighing. The patients were assessed by Waddell's Behavioral Signs, the UAB Pain Behavior Rating scale, and self-reported visual analogue scale (VAS). A negative cognitive score was derived from patients' answers to 2 questions about their back strength and general health, revealing covert behaviors. The reliability of these measures was assessed from test-retest scores and by concordance among tests. Predictive ability was also analyzed.

Results.—There was good inter-rater reliability among the observers, particularly with the most common pain behaviors: guarding, rubbing, and bracing. There was a high degree of concordance between Waddell's Behavioral Signs and the UAB scale. Correlations were strong between covert pain behavior and Waddell's Behavioral Signs, less strong between covert pain and the UAB score, and absent between covert pain and the VAS score. The VAS scores correlated with both Behavioral Signs and the UAB scale. The UAB scale and covert pain behaviors best predicted the return to work. Covert pain behaviors best predicted absenteeism of up to 2 years.

Conclusion.—These comparison data indicate that pain behavior can be reliably assessed and that these assessments have predictive validity. An understanding of the potential diagnostic implications of pain behaviors may be helpful in guiding both the rehabilitation and compensation processes.

▶ The study of behaviors associated with the experience of chronic pain remains an important area of study. This is, in part, because of the importance that learning theory has played in models of chronic pain and in continued vigilance and concern regarding the validity and accuracy of self-report information. It is of particular importance that more recently, the concepts of functional performance and pain behaviors have begun to be more closely associated. Many so-called objective tests of functional capacity have been appropriately reconceptualized as behavioral measures. However, without carefully designed studies that include asymptomatic control groups, the behaviors observed during functional testing procedures *cannot* be equated with pain behaviors.

The study by Schwartz et al. (Abstract 131-95-5–24) provides some novel insights into the association between interpersonal stress and the performance of physical tasks in chronic back pain patients. However, because a control group was not included, the conclusion that the interpersonal stress manipulation led to premature termination of the physical task may not be a finding that is unique to patients with back pain. Thus, I believe that labeling this response as a "pain behavior" is unwarranted because of the limitations of the experimental design.

The results of the study by Krause et al. (Abstract 131-95-5–25) are fascinating, but I was left wondering whether "construct contamination" had occurred. That is, perhaps methodological biases occurred for patients' self-reports so that depression and pain scores no longer were independent measures from a psychometric perspective. The study by Öhlund et al. (Abstract 131-95-5–26) highlights the heterogeneity among patients in terms of pain behaviors. Although pain behaviors were significantly correlated with return to work and absenteeism, the amount of total variance explained was small and, thus, these findings, cannot, in and of themselves, be used to build a reliable, accurate, and ethical prediction model that could be generalized to other patient samples.—T.E. Rudy, Ph.D.

Fibromyalgia and Arthritis

Long Term Follow-Up of Fibromyalgia Patients: Clinical Symptoms, Muscular Function, Laboratory Tests. An Eight Year Comparison Study

Bengtsson A, Bäckman E, Lindblom B, Skogh T (Univ Hosp, Linköping, Sweden)

J Musculoskel Pain 2:67–80, 1994 131-95-5–27

Background.—The concept of fibromyalgia is relatively new, and few long-term studies have been published. New criteria for the classification of fibromyalgia were proposed by the American College of Rheumatology (ACR) in 1990. Fifty-five patients were reexamined with respect to these criteria, and their clinical symptoms, tender points, muscle pain, muscle function, and laboratory tests were studied.

Patients and Methods.—The patients received a diagnosis of fibromyalgia between 1981 and 1986 and were followed routinely thereafter. Forty-eight agreed to participate in a special follow-up in 1991. All but 1 of the patients were women; the mean age of the group was 50 years, and the mean duration of symptoms was 13 years. All fulfilled the ACR criteria. A dolorimeter was used to examine tender points at 9 bilateral sites and 4 control sites. The pain was recorded on a visual analogue scale, and function was evaluated by a self-administered questionnaire. Thirty-one patients underwent muscle function testing, and the results were compared with those of 19 healthy women volunteers.

Results.—All patients were observed for at least 6 years, and 13 had been followed for 10 years or longer. The generalized muscle pain, present in all patients, was continuous in 44. Muscular stiffness, particularly in the morning, was prominent in 45 patients. Conditions that increased symptoms included cold, repetitive work, and stress; warmth, exercise, and rest commonly relieved pain and stiffness. Other common problems were sleep disturbance, anxiety, subjective swelling, and irritable bowel syndrome. Only 4 patients were working full time. The results of laboratory tests were generally normal. Five patients had slightly increased levels of creatine kinase, creatine kinase together with lactate dehydrogenase, aspartate aminotransferase, and alanine aminotransferase. Muscle strength was significantly reduced, compared with that of healthy controls, and all patients showed a significant decrease in muscular endurance over the course of their illness. One patient had rheumatoid arthritis during the follow-up period, and another became free of symptoms.

Conclusion.—The findings in these patients confirm that fibromyalgia is a chronic disorder characterized by muscle pain, fatigue, and stiffness. A reduction in muscle function has a considerable impact on the patient's work capacity. There is some evidence that pain in fibromyalgia is related to a disturbance in microcirculation.

Multi-Method Assessment of Experimental and Clinical Pain in Patients With Fibromyalgia

Lautenbacher S, Rollman GB, McCain GA (Univ of Western Ontario, London, Canada)

Pain 59:45–53, 1994 131-95-5–28

Introduction.—Patients with fibromyalgia have increased responsiveness to noxious pressure at designated tender points, as well as various other body sites. An investigation was done to compare pressure, heat, and electric pain responsiveness between 26 female patients with fibromyalgia and a pain-free control group. Nonpainful warmth, cold, and electric stimuli were also assessed.

Methods.—All patients with fibromyalgia had significant pain, so medication was not withdrawn. The duration and frequency of pain and other fibromyalgia complaints were ascertained by questionnaire (table). The McGill Pain Questionnaire and Localized Pain Rating scales for typical pain (LPR-T) and present pain (LPR-P) were administered. A nontender point on the inner forearm was designated the control point, and the test tender point was located on the upper edge of the trapezius muscle. Both sites were tested in both groups for responsiveness to thermal stimuli, warmth and cold thresholds, heat pain, electrocutaneous stimuli, pain threshold, and pressure pain threshold.

Means (± SD) of Age, Height, Weight, and of Scores of the Localized Pain Rating-P (LPR-P) as Well as the Prevalence of Functional Complaints in Patients With Fibromyalgia and Healthy Controls

	Fibromyalgia patients	Healthy controls
Age (years)	44.0 ± 11.6	42.7 ± 8.2
Height (cm)	162.1 ± 7.5	161.4 ± 7.3
Weight (kg) †,**	70.1 ± 12.5	60.6 ± 15.1
LPR-P †,***	31.8 ± 16.9	2.5 ± 3.5
Morning stiffness ‡,***	92.3%	26.9%
Fatigue ‡,***	92.3%	42.3%
Headache ‡,**	92.3%	53.8%
Sleep disturbance ‡,***	84.6%	30.8%
Irritable bowel ‡,***	69.2%	11.5%
Subjective finger swelling ‡,***	65.4%	11.5%
Depressive mood	57.7%	30.8%

There were 26 patients in each group.
† *t* test (1-tailed).
‡ Chi-square test.
** $P < .01$.
*** $P < .001$.
(Courtesy of Lautenbacher S, Rollman GB, McCain GA: *Pain* 59:45–53, 1994.)

Results.—Mean ratings for present pain LPR-P were significantly higher in patients with fibromyalgia compared with controls (table). Patients with fibromyalgia had increased pain responsiveness for pressure, heat, and electric current. The electric pain threshold was lower for the tender point, but not the control point in patients with fibromyalgia. Sensitivity for nonpainful stimuli was significantly lower only for cold stimuli in patients with fibromyalgia.

Conclusion.—Pain hyperresponsiveness and clinical pain are explicit fibromyalgia features. Persons who are hyperresponsive to pain who do not have clinical pain may be at risk for fibromyalgia.

▶ Recently, considerable attention has been devoted in the literature to the diagnosis and treatment of fibromyalgia. Progress, however, has been slow, given the many complexities and anomalies of this disorder. Abstracts 131-95-5–27 and 131-95-5–28 provide useful new information related to tender points, site-specific hyperresponsivity, and characteristics of frequently reported generalized muscle pain. The article by Bengtsson et al. (Abstract 131-95-5–27) is particularly noteworthy, because these authors addressed the potential link between subjective reports of fatigue and patients' work capacities. This article is also important because of its longitudinal aspects.—T.E. Rudy, Ph.D.

Are Patient Self-Report Measures of Arthritis Activity Confounded by Mood? A Longitudinal Study of Patients With Rheumatoid Arthritis

Ward MM (Stanford Univ, Palo Alto, Calif)

J Rheumatol 21:1046–1050, 1994 131-95-5–29

Introduction.—Only 2 previous studies have specifically examined the effect of mood on self-report measures of pain completed by patients with rheumatoid arthritis (RA), and in these studies different conclusions were reached. In a prospective, longitudinal study, the effect of mood, particularly depression, on self-report measures of functional disability, pain, and global arthritis status was determined in patients with RA.

Patients and Methods.—The study cohort included 22 women and 2 men with active RA at study entry. The median age of the patients was 46 years, and the median duration of RA was 3 years. Examinations were performed every 2 weeks for up to 60 weeks. Patients completed the Health Assessment Questionnaire and 2 scales that assessed positive and negative moods and depression. The clinical measures obtained at each examination included swollen and tender joint counts, duration of morning stiffness, grip strength, 50-foot walk time, and the Westergren erythrocyte sedimentation rate. Pooled time series regression models were used to determine the confounding effect of mood or depression on the self-report measures, while controlling for clinical measures.

Results.—The patients generally had positive moods and few depressive symptoms at study entry. During the course of the study, however, they experienced substantial changes in arthritis activity, together with changes in mood. There was a high level of correlation between changes in mood measures and changes in patient-reported functional ability, pain, and global arthritis status. After controlling for objective measures of arthritis activity and patient differences, the Profile of Mood States-B explained 2% or less of the variation in longitudinal changes in each of the self-report measures. Depression, as recorded by the Center for Epidemiologic Studies Depression Scale, explained 6% of the variation in changes in pain and 8% of the variation in global arthritis status but less than 2% of the variation in changes of functional disability.

Conclusion.—Patient self-reports of pain and global arthritis status appear to be somewhat confounded by depression. Functional disability, in contrast, was far less susceptible to confounding by depression. Measures of overall mood confounded self-reports of pain and global arthritis status to a minimal degree.

The Relative Importance of Pain and Functional Disability to Patients With Rheumatoid Arthritis

Ward MM, Leigh JP (Stanford Univ, Calif; San Jose State Univ, Calif)

J Rheumatol 20:1494–1499, 1993 131-95-5–30

Background.—The management of rheumatoid arthritis (RA) is a balance of patient and physician goals, which, if disparate, can eventually lead to a deterioration of the patient's health. Pain and functional disability are 2 major factors that influence the health status of the patient with RA. The relationship of pain and functional disability with arthritis status was investigated in patients who were followed for 9.5 years.

Methods.—The 305 patients made up a closed cohort. They filled out the Health Assessment Questionnaire every 6 months. Complete data (19 surveys) were obtained on 58% of the initial sample. The effect of pain and functional disability on global arthritis was estimated over time.

Findings.—At the onset of the study, moderate arthritis was present as indicated by a pain score of 1.1 (range, 0–3), functional disability score of 1.25 (range, 0–3) and global arthritis status of 35 (range, 0–100). With time, changes in both pain and disability were significantly related to global arthritis status. Changes in pain were slightly more important in the patient's assessment of arthritis status. Nonwhites were more likely to rate pain as the important feature of their arthritis status, whereas men rated disability to be the more important feature. The relative importance of pain and disability was not influenced by the duration of the RA.

Comment.—It appears that pain and disability are of comparable importance in the patient's assessment of global arthritis status. This relationship was unaffected by the duration of the disease. Clinical management of RA focused equally on pain relief and functional disability would be most effective in the treatment of the patient with RA.

▶ Similar to the study by Magni et al. (Abstract 131-95-5–38), Ward (Abstract 131-95-5–29) conducted an ambitious study that tracked patients with RA every 2 weeks for up to 60 weeks to evaluate the impact of mood on other pain-related self-report measures. A particularly interesting conclusion reached in this study is that self-reported functional disability is uncorrelated with self-reported mood and pain severity measures, but the latter 2 measures were significantly correlated over time. However, as in the study by Magni et al., the association between mood and pain was very weak at best. Using a larger data set, the longitudinal study by Ward and Leigh (Abstract 131-95-5–30) concludes that in patients with RA, equal therapeutic attention should be paid to patients' reports of pain and disability, in addition to their disease status. Patients will give us unique and important information that "disrupts" our existing or preferred models if we take the time to ask them!—T.E. Rudy, Ph.D.

Criteria for Clinically Important Changes in Outcomes: Development, Scoring and Evaluation of Rheumatoid Arthritis Patient and Trial Profiles

Goldsmith CH, for the Omeract Committee (McMaster Univ, Hamilton, Ont, Canada)

J Rheumatol 20:561–565, 1993 131-95-5–31

Background.—Just how much of a change is necessary for an effect to be clinically significant? This problem crosses all medical disciplines. At a conference of professional personnel, criteria were developed for the minimum effect for clinical improvement in patients with rheumatoid arthritis.

Methods.—Clinical information, such as swollen joint count and tender joint count among others, on patient profiles and drug trial participants formed the basis for discussion. The professionals (rheumatologists, statisticians, and methodologists, plus individuals from the regulatory, pharmaceutical, and biotechnology industries) met twice, once to review the patient profiles and once to review the responses to drug trials. After a structured discussion, a vote of no change or improvement was taken, with a 70% agreement being defined as consensus.

Results.—In the patient profiles session, a median improvement of 36% was considered clinically significant. For the drug trial patients, a median of 18% improvement was considered significant.

Conclusion.—In patients, an improvement of 36% would be deemed significant. For patients undergoing a drug trial, an improvement of 18%

over that of placebo would be important. This method offers a beginning for establishing less arbitrary criteria for clinical improvement.

▶ The important distinction between statistical and clinical significance in evaluating the success of clinical trials has been recognized for some time. However, explicit methodology for clarifying this distinction in the field of chronic pain treatment has been difficult, in part because of the many "players" involved. That is, success is in the eyes of the beholder, with definitions of success varying widely among patients themselves, the treating clinician, the referral source, insurance companies, the employer, and so forth. Although this paper presents some interesting results related to professional consensus on outcome criteria for arthritis treatment, the patient's perspective unfortunately was not considered.—T.E. Rudy, Ph.D.

Home Exercise in Rheumatoid Arthritis Functional Class II: Goal Setting Versus Pain Attention

Stenström CH (Kullbergska Hosp, Katrineholm, Sweden)

J Rheumatol 21:627–634, 1994 131-95-5–32

Introduction.—A 12-week aerobic home exercise program was conducted to evaluate the effects of exercise on physical capacity, self-efficacy, and pain perception in 42 patients with rheumatoid arthritis. The effects of goal-setting and advice on how to exercise with pain were also assessed.

Methods.—Forty-two patients were randomly assigned to either a goal-setting or pain attention subgroup. The patients were given personal exercises to perform 5 days a week. Arthritis Self-Efficacy Scales and Functional Disability Indexes were given at baseline and again at 12 weeks. Joint mobility, the Ritchie Articular Index, and 6 functional tasks were performed. Patients in the goal-setting subgroup were encouraged to increase exercise as tolerated. When they complained of pain, they were encouraged to continue the exercise and to reduce the work load on affected joints only if swollen. Patients in the pain attention subgroup were not asked to set specific goals and were told to decrease the work load and rest joints when pain was experienced.

Results.—Patients exercised 98% of the requested 5 days per week. Seventeen patients in the goal-setting subgroup increased exercise loads compared with 4 patients in the pain attention group. Significantly greater decreases in pain ratings were seen in the goal-setting group compared with the pain attention group. Otherwise, no significant differences were observed between the 2 groups. Significant improvements were found in all functional tasks in both subgroups, with the exception of maximum walking speed.

Conclusion.—Low compliance with a home exercise program may be expected in patients with chronic pain. Giving patients support can affect success, as evidenced by a 98% participation rate. Goal-setting was important in increasing exercise load.

► "Homework," including exercise, has always been a recommended component of cognitive-behavioral treatment interventions for chronic pain conditions. Compliance (I prefer the term "adherence") is a difficult hurdle to overcome. The high level of participation reported in this study deserves special attention; it is almost "too high" to be believable or generalizable to other patient populations.—T.E. Rudy, Ph.D.

Psychological Symptoms and Cognitions

Somatization Symptoms in Chronic Low Back Pain Patients

Bacon NMK, Bacon SF, Atkinson JH, Slater MA, Patterson TL, Grant I, Garfin SR (San Diego Veterans Affairs Med Ctr, San Diego, Calif; Univ of California at San Diego, La Jolla)

Psychosom Med 56:118–127, 1994 131-95-5–33

Introduction.—Because somatization has been associated with high use of health care services, a better understanding of the mechanism of somatic complaints may result in a more efficient treatment for patients with such complaints. Patients with chronic back pain have been found to frequently report multiple somatic symptoms. Chronic back pain has also been associated with mood disorders. Although patients with chronic back pain have been described as somatizers, the lifetime rate of diagnosis of somatization disorders in these patients is low. To assess the relationship between somatic symptoms and mood disorder, patients with chronic low back pain (CLBP) and matched controls were evaluated using psychiatric interviews and symptom assessment.

Methods.—One hundred male patients with CLBP seen at a general orthopedic clinic were included in the study. Control patients were matched to patients with CLBP by age and socioeconomic status. The Diagnostic Interview Schedule IIIA (DIS III-A), Beck Depression Inventory, the Hamilton Rating Scale for Depression, Sickness Impact Profile, Pain and Impairment Relationship Scale, McGill Pain Questionnaire, and Waddell Physical Impairment Index were administered to all study participants during a single assessment session. Differences in these measures of assessment between patients with CLBP and control patients, and within subgroups of patients with CLBP were determined.

Results.—No study participants met the DMS-III criteria for a lifetime diagnosis of somatization disorder. Compared with control patients, patients with CLBP were more likely to report somatic symptoms ($P < .001$). Of patients with CLBP, 22.7% reported a low frequency of lifetime symptoms (< 6 symptoms), 51.5% reported an intermediate frequency (7–11 symptoms), and 25.8% reported a high frequency (≥ 12 symptoms); rates for control patients were 87.8%, 8.2%, and 4.1%, respectively. Patients with CLBP were also more likely to report a wider

TABLE 1.—Somatization Symptoms Discriminating Patients From Controls That Are Attributed to Back Disease

Symptom	CLBP Patients (N = 97)			
	f	% Endorsing symptom	*f*	% Of those endorsing symptom who attribute symptom to back disease
Pain				
Back pain	97	100.0%	97	100.0%
Joint pain	73	75.2%	15	20.5%
Pain in arms or legs	68	70.1%	44	64.7%
Cardiopulmonary				
Chest pain	41	42.3%	3	7.3%
Shortness of breath	24	24.7%	1	4.2%
Palpitations	23	23.7%	1	4.3%
Gastrointestinal				
Gas	25	25.8%	0	0.0
Nausea	20	20.6%	1	0.1%
Pseudoneurologic				
Trouble walking	74	76.3%	63	85.1%
Unconscious	46	47.4%	3	6.5%

(continued)

range of symptoms than control patients. In addition to back pain, most patients with CLBP attributed only 6 other complaints to back disorder (Table 1). Patients with CLBP who reported several somatic symptoms were more likely to experience major depression or alcohol dependence. The Sickness Impact Profile measured greater impairment in physical ability, social performance, and psychological function in patients with CLBP who reported high and intermediate numbers of symptoms than in patients with CLBP who reported few symptoms. No correlation was found between the number of symptoms reported and pain intensity (Table 2).

Table 1 *(continued)*

Weakness	38	39.2%	32	84.2%
Paralyzed	29	29.9%	20	69.0%
Lost Voice	30	30.9%	0	0.0
Blindness	24	24.7%	1	4.2%
Lump in throat	16	16.5%	0	0.0
Deaf	14	14.4%	1	7.1%
Sexual Symptoms				
Pain during intercourse	32	33.0%	30	93.8%
Lifestyle				
Had to give up work	53	54.6%	47	88.7%
Nondiagnostic symptoms				
Headaches	57	58.8%	3	5.3%
Lost feeling in an extremity	51	52.6%	41	80.4%

Abbreviation: CLBP, chronic low back pain.
(Courtesy of Bacon NMK, Bacon SF, Atkinson JH, et al: *Psychosom Med* 56:118–127, 1994.)

Conclusion.—Patients with CLBP had a higher lifetime rate of depression than the control patients. However, in most patients, depression appeared after the onset of pain, and no increased risk for mood disorder was noted before chronic pain developed. Development of lifetime depression in patients who reported a low number of somatic symptoms was similar to that in control patients. No association between pain severity and psychiatric disorders was seen, suggesting that the relationship between pain and depression is complex.

▶ The association between emotional disorders and physical symptoms and complaints remains confusing and illusive, particularly when attempting to

TABLE 2.—Measures of Pain, Mood, and Impairment Across Chronic Low Back Pain Somatization Groups

Variables	CLBP Somatization Groups							
	0-6 Symptoms (N = 22)		7-11 Symptoms (N = 50)		12+ Symptoms (N = 25)		$F(2,94)$	P
	Mean	(SD)	Mean	(SD)	Mean	(SD)		
Pain measures								
Visual Analog Scale*								
Current pain intensity	38.45	(21.00)	44.56	(24.43)	41.68	(19.66)	0.58	NS
Typical pain intensity	50.54	(25.28)	55.24	(23.10)	48.44	(19.50)	0.84	NS
Pain Duration (months)	127.18	(134.00)	197.56	(167.90)	171.96	(106.20)	1.76	NS
McGill Pain Questionnaire								
MPQ Total Score	29.86	(15.40)	34.70	(16.32)	32.04	(13.68)	0.80	NS
MPQ Sensory Score	18.32	(8.46)	19.80	(9.21)	17.80	(7.16)	0.53	NS
MPQ Affective Score	3.32	(3.64)	4.48	(3.75)	3.64	(3.35)	0.95	NS
MPQ Evaluative Score	3.23	(1.82)	3.44	(1.60)	3.84	(1.46)	0.89	NS
MPQ Miscellaneous	5.00	(3.87)	6.98	(4.28)	6.76	(4.60)	1.71	NS

(continued)

disentangle their temporal correlation. The strength of this study is that comprehensive structured interviews were included, as was a control group of patients not referred for psychiatric or pain treatment. I find it particularly interesting that none of the patients with CLBP studied met the *DSM-III* criteria for the diagnosis of somatization disorder.—T.E. Rudy, Ph.D.

Table 2 *(continued)*

Mood measures								
Beck Depression Inventory	6.77	(6.17)	10.52	(7.34)	16.08	(9.52)	8.78	< 0.001†
Hamilton Depression Rating Scale	5.27	(7.64)	9.56	(6.70)	13.32	(8.73)	6.78	< 0.01‡
Impairment measures								
Sickness Impact Profile								
Overall Impairment	11.32	(8.93)	19.84	(13.07)	22.50	(12.08)	5.64	< 0.01§
Physical	7.62	(7.41)	15.35	(11.76)	15.50	(10.73)	4.52	< 0.01§
Psychological	9.67	(8.80)	18.27	(17.14)	26.58	(16.96)	6.87	< 0.01‡
Other	18.15	(13.52)	27.58	(15.38)	26.08	(13.54)	3.30	< 0.05‖
Pain and Impairment Relationship Scale	59.27	(18.32)	71.34	(14.50)	70.64	(16.35)	4.73	< 0.01§

* Visual analogue scale of intensity, 0–100, where 0 is no pain and 100 is the worst pain imaginable.
† Symptoms of groups 0–6 and 7–11 differed significantly from those of groups 12 plus.
‡ All 3 groups significantly differed.
§ Symptoms of groups 0–6 differed significantly from those of groups 7–11 and 12 plus.
‖ Symptoms of groups 0–6 differed significantly from those of groups 7–11.
Abbreviations: CLBP, chronic low back pain; *MPQ*, McGill Pain Questionnaire.
(Courtesy of Bacon NMK, Bacon SF, Atkinson JH, et al: *Psychosom Med* 56:118–127, 1994.)

Relationship of Pain-Specific Beliefs to Chronic Pain Adjustment

Jensen MP, Turner JA, Romano JM, Lawler BK (Univ of Washington, Seattle)
Pain 57:301–309, 1994 131-95-5–34

Introduction.—The Survey of Pain Attitudes and measures of adjustment were explored in a heterogeneous group of 241 patients with chronic pain. The moderating influences of pain intensity and duration were also considered.

Multiple Regression Analysis Predicting Sickness Impact Profile (SIP) Physical Dimension From Beliefs

Step and variable	Total R^2	R^2 change	F change	β to enter
Criterion: SIP Physical Dysfunction				
1 Demographics	0.04	0.04	5.44	
Age				0.19**
Gender				0.10
2 Pain-related variables	0.10	0.06	7.49***	
Pain intensity				0.23***
Pain duration				−0.05
3 Beliefs				
SOPA Disability	0.21	0.10	29.59***	0.34***
SOPA Control	0.24	0.03	10.01**	0.20**
SOPA Harm	0.28	0.04	12.03***	0.23***
4 Interactions				
Harm × Pain Duration	0.29	0.01	4.10*	−0.34*

* $P < .05$.
** $P < .01$.
*** $P < .001$.
(Courtesy of Jensen MP, Turner JA, Romano JM, et al: *Pain* 57:301–309, 1994.)

Methods.—The median time since pain onset was 4.2 years. Primary pain sites were low back in 35%, lower extremities in 17%, head in 18%, neck in 8%, shoulders/arms in 9%, thoracic region in 3%, abdomen in 5%, and other sites in 5% of patients completing self-reporting questionnaires. The Survey of Pain Attitudes was used to assess 7 pain-related beliefs. A new category was added for this investigation: Harm (belief that pain signifies damage and that activity should be restricted). The Sickness Impact Profile was used to evaluate degree of physical and psychological dysfunction. Pain intensity was measured using the 101-point numerical rating scale. Patients were asked to record the number of times they had visited physicians and emergency rooms for pain treatment in the previous 3 months.

Results.—Patients who believed they were more disabled and would be harmed by physical exertion reported greater physical dysfunction than those who did not endorse the belief that physical exertion was harmful and who saw themselves as less disabled (table). No belief was associated with number of physician visits in the previous 3 months. Patients who visited the emergency room for pain relief were more likely to support the belief that medications were appropriate treatments for pain than patients who did not endorse this belief. The belief that activity should be avoided because of pain was significant only in patients reporting pain duration of less than $2^1/_3$ years.

Conclusion.—Further research is needed to target chronic pain treatment approaches in ways that address patients beliefs. Doing so may improve patient functioning and, perhaps, decrease chronicity.

Pain Beliefs: Assessment and Utility

Williams DA, Robinson ME, Geisser ME (Georgetown Univ, Washington, DC; Univ of Florida, Gainesville; Univ of Michigan, Ann Arbor)

Pain 59:71–78, 1994 131-95-5–35

Background.—Beliefs about pain affect pain perception, function, and treatment response. When pain persists for no obvious reason, patients might abandon common, culturally shared beliefs about pain, replacing them with beliefs that are more consistent with their experiences.

Beliefs are better judged by how they enable the believer to function, rather than by their truth or falsity. Specialized scales have been developed to determine whether new beliefs help patients adapt better. For example, the Pain Beliefs and Perception Inventory (PBPI) has 3 scales labeled Time, Mystery, and Self-Blame. The Time scale assesses whether a patient believes that pain is enduring, in contrast to the culturally shared belief that pain is a warning signal that ends when all is well. The Mystery scale finds out whether a patient believes that pain is poorly understood, in contrast to the culturally shared belief that pain serves a useful function. The Self-Blame scale determines whether a patient believes that he or she is an appropriate target for blame. Patients who believe this are less likely to cooperate with physical therapy and psychotherapy. The usefulness of a modified PBPI was studied.

Methods.—One hundred eighty-seven adult patients with chronic pain (106 women) at 3 United States pain clinics were surveyed. The average age was about 40, and back pain was the most common complaint. The patients had experienced pain for 3–9 years. About one half were receiving workers' compensation. Two studies were factor analytic, to identify belief factors associated with the PBPI. The other 2 studies based scoring on 4 scales: Constancy, Permanence, Mystery, and Self-Blame. The 4 scales were correlated with important pain indexes, such as pain quality, psychological state, physical functioning, and coping strategies.

Results.—The 2 factor analytic studies agreed with other studies identifying 4 belief factors associated with the PBPI. The other 2 studies showed that each of the 4 beliefs has a unique association with pain, supporting the scoring of the PBPI with 4 scales. Thus, constancy is associated with greater self-report of pain, permanence is associated with anxiety, mystery is associated with distress, and self-blame is associated with depression.

Conclusion.—When experience or perception fails to support existing beliefs about pain, some patients adopt new beliefs consistent with their experience. Patients who adopt new beliefs appear to be in greater pain than those who do not. With 4 scales, the PBPI is a useful clinical tool for research on how patients' thinking about pain affects their perception, feeling, and other behaviors. Dividing the Time scale into Constancy and Permanence enabled greater interpretation of which time-associated beliefs were associated with greater pain ratings.

There are no current treatment strategies directed at changing PBPI beliefs. However, the PBPI can be used to measure a patient's readiness for cognitive and behavioral psychotherapy for pain management. Future research is needed to compare the distress in adopting new pain beliefs with the distress in maintaining preexisting beliefs.

Appendix.—Provided are clinical norms for PBPI use, and a revised scoring key.

▶ Pain practitioners have recognized for some time the important clinical implications of patients' attributions and beliefs about their condition, including perceived level of disability and causation notions about their symptoms. Unfortunately, most investigators have considered cognitions as "soft" and unmeasurable data. Abstracts 131-95-5–34 and 131-95-5–35 demonstrate that patients' beliefs can be systematically studied; however, it would be useful if assessment instruments designed to measure pain-related attitudes and beliefs included validation procedures with more "objective" behavioral/functional measures, besides their correlational structure with other self-report instruments.—T.E. Rudy, Ph.D.

Cognitive-Behavioral Classifications of Chronic Pain: Replication and Extension of Empirically Derived Patient Profiles

Jamison RN, Rudy TE, Penzien DB, Mosley TH Jr (Harvard Med School, Boston; Univ of Pittsburgh, Pa; Univ of Mississippi, Jackson)
Pain 57:277–292, 1994 131-95-5–36

Introduction.—The development of a reliable and meaningful classification system has been attempted to give a better understanding to the complex phenomenon of chronic pain. On the basis of analyses of scores from the Multidimensional Pain Inventory, Turk and Rudy characterized 3 distinct profiles for patients with pain. The classification system developed by Turk and Rudy was replicated in this study, using different measures validated by factor analytic and cluster replication methods.

Methods.—Two significantly different samples of patients with chronic pain—sample 1 (1A and 1B) selected from a university pain center and sample 2 selected from the private practices of rural physicians—were assessed using pain evaluation questionnaires and the Symptom

Checklist-90 Revised. An examining physician rated each patient in sample 1 for nervousness, depression, irritation, symptom dramatization, and exaggeration. A history of medication and health care use was obtained from patients in sample 2. Items from the pain questionnaire were selected to measure the following constructs: activity interference, emotional distress, pain intensity, and social support. Statistical analyses included confirmatory factor analysis, cluster analytic methods, and external validation.

Results.—On the basis of confirmatory factor analysis, the questionnaire items selected were found to be effective in measuring activity interference, emotional distress, pain intensity, and social support. A reliable classification strategy, which could be applied to both patient samples, was derived from the scores of these constructs. Kappa means cluster analyses computed from the scores for the constructs AI, ED, PI, and SS for patients in sample 1A indicated that a 3-cluster solution was optimal for describing the profile structure of patients' scores from the 4 constructs. Cluster I contained 42.1% of patients in sample 1A; cluster II, 31.7%; and cluster III, 26.2%. These clusters corresponded well to groups characterized previously as adaptive copers, interpersonally distressed, and dysfunctional. Cluster replication methods provided evidence for the reliability of the 3 patient profiles derived from the 4 constructs when applied to patients in sample 1B. Of patients in sample 1B, 35.9% were classified in cluster I, 36.5% in cluster II, and 27.6% in cluster III. Cross-validation of these 3 clusters in a significantly different patient sample (sample 2) was shown using the same cluster replication methods and resulted in similar assignment of classifications. Cluster validation on the external variables for patients in sample 1 showed significant differences between the clusters for variables other than demographics. Similarly, cluster validation for patients in sample 2 showed significant differences in measured variables.

Conclusion.—The classifications previously characterized by Turk and Rudy can be reliably replicated using different measures for the 4 constructs in significantly different samples of patients with chronic pain. The use of a larger sample size allowed for a more demanding cluster replication and application to dissimilar samples of patients with chronic pain. Confirmatory factor analyses showed similar responses to the questionnaire items in the 2 patient samples used to develop the profile classifications, thereby showing the reliability and quantitative suitability of the classification in diverse patient populations. Although similarities with the results of Turk and Rudy were found, notable differences were also observed. In this study, fewer patients were classified as dysfunctional, and less prominent differences were seen between patients classified as dysfunctional and interpersonally depressed.

▶ The empirically derived classification system developed by Turk and Rudy has received increasing attention in the chronic pain literature, in part because it proves the obvious, i.e., patients' psychosocial reactions to their condition are heterogeneous. A potentially serious limitation of this classification system, however, is that the patient profiles derived may be the result of the particular assessment instrument used. This study, which used a much larger patient population, demonstrates that similar profiles emerged from a conceptually related but different assessment inventory. Additionally, this study presents additional validity for psychosocially based patient profiles. Further research is needed to establish the clinical utility of the patient profiles described in this paper, particularly their relevance to patient outcomes.—T.E. Rudy, Ph.D.

The Relationship Between Perceived Stress, Social Support and Chronic Headaches

Martin PR, Soon K (Univ of Western Australia, Nedlands, Australia)
Headache 33:307–314, 1993 131-95-5–37

Introduction.—Previous investigations have indicated that headache patients tend to appraise stressful events more negatively and cope with them differently than headache-free controls. A group of 49 research subjects with migraine headaches and 13 with tension-type headaches was compared with a group of 64 controls regarding social support and perceived stress.

Methods.—The self-administered Interpersonal Support Evaluation List, Social Support Questionnaire, Perceived Stress Scale, and demographic information questionnaires were completed by both groups.

Results.—Twelve dependent variables were used to measure aspects of social support and perceived stress (table). The patients with headache had significantly lower scores in all 4 functional support measures: appraisal, esteem, belonging, and tangible support. No significant differences were found in the availability, number, or sources of social support. There were also no differences seen in marital status or other demographic measures. In patients with headache, the lowest measure of social support was found in the middle, not the beginning or latest period of headache history. Patients with headache scored significantly higher on perceived stress than did controls.

Conclusion.—Social relationships and social support do not differ between patients with headache and controls. However, patients with headache view all types of social support as less available and are less satisfied than controls with the support available to them. Treatment programs need to teach patients with headache how to mobilize social support. The focus should be on problem-solving modes of coping vs. palliative modes. The psychosocial and developmental context of headaches has been neglected by researchers and needs more attention.

▶ The role of social support in chronic pain conditions has not been adequately studied. This may be because of the difficulty in operationalizing and

Comparison of Headache and Control Groups in Terms of Mean Scores on Stress and Social Support Variables

Variable	Headache ($n=59$)	Control ($n=59$)	F ($d.f.=1,116$)
Social integration domain of social support			
Group membership	1.00 (1.17)*	0.86 (0.97)	0.47
Functional support domain of social support			
ISEL			
Appraisal support	23.70 (5.93)	26.32 (3.83)	8.18‡
Esteem support	19.41 (4.99)	22.46 (4.54)	12.07§
Belonging support	21.58 (6.14)	25.25 (4.52)	13.74§
Tangible support	25.52 (5.37)	27.17 (2.90)	4.28†
Perceived social support			
SSQ			
Availability of support	2.76 (1.53)	3.27 (1.83)	2.70
Adequacy of support	4.72 (0.89)	5.42 (0.69)	22.72§
Sources of social support			
SSQ			
Spouse	4.05 (3.67)	4.27 (3.82)	0.10
Immediate family	8.10 (7.24)	9.34 (8.62)	0.71
Friends	9.97 (9.86)	12.24 (10.62)	1.45
Others	2.85 (4.40)	3.27 (1.83)	0.64
Perceived stress			
PSS	26.42 (6.88)	22.02 (6.06)	13.64§

* Standard deviations included in parentheses.
† $P < .05$.
‡ $P < .01$.
§ $P < .001$.
(Courtesy of Martin PR, Soon K: *Headache* 33:307–314, 1993.)

measuring this broad and often highly individualized construct. This study nicely shows the important distinction between the availability of support and patients' interpretation of the adequacy of that support.—T.E. Rudy, Ph.D.

Prospective Study on the Relationship Between Depressive Symptoms and Chronic Musculoskeletal Pain

Magni G, Moreschi C, Rigatti-Luchini S, Merskey H (Hoffmann-La Roche, Ba-

sel, Switzerland; Univ of Padua, Italy; Univ of Western Ontario, London, Canada)
Pain 56:289–297, 1994 131-95-5–38

Introduction.—Depression and chronic pain often co-exist, but the nature of this relationship is uncertain, because existing data do not clarify the causal relationship between the 2 variables. The relationship has been studied both among patients with psychological problems and in the general population. The belief in a relationship between chronic pain and depression has led to 2 main hypotheses, which were examined: chronic pain is caused by an underlying depressive disturbance, and chronic pain causes the depressive symptoms found in these patients.

Methods.—A sample of 2,324 patients were evaluated for the presence of musculoskeletal pain and the presence of depression using the Center for Epidemiologic Studies Depression scale (CES-D) to test the hypotheses that depression causes pain and that pain causes depression. The patients were first examined in 1974 and 1975, using the National Health and Nutrition Survey of the United States National Center for Health Statistics and were followed from 1981 to 1984.

Results.—Depressive symptoms at year 1 significantly predicted the development of chronic musculoskeletal pain at year 8 with an odds ration of 2.14 for the depressed patients compared with the nondepressed patients. No sociodemographic variable alone predicted the persistence of pain in patients who had pain present at baseline; however male sex and white race with 2 items of the CES-D predicted the persistence of pain. For the prediction of depression on regression analysis, chronic pain was the most powerful variable. Other significant factors included low education level, being unemployed, female sex, and living in areas containing up to 250,000 inhabitants. The odds ratio for the prediction of depression by chronic pain was 2.85.

Discussion.—The evidence supports the views that depression promotes pain and pain promotes depression, with the latter being more evident than the former. However, both accounted for a small proportion of the variance. The extent of this relationship was very weak, and it only explained an extremely low percentage of the variance; nevertheless depressive symptoms were the only variables that predicted pain, particularly restless sleep and lack of drive. Among the different localizations, neck-back and hip pain showed a significant relationship with respect to the development of depression.

▶ Magni and colleagues have substantially contributed to our understanding of pain and depression during the past several years by providing careful analyses of national epidemiologic databases. The longitudinal analyses reported in this study should be of interest to clinical investigators who may want to apply similar methodology with clinic samples during the follow-up phases of treatment outcome studies. The bidirectionality of their findings, combined with the small amount of variance accounted in the longitudinal pain-depression models, indicates that the debate of which comes first is not soon to be resolved, if ever.—T.E. Rudy, Ph.D.

Coping With Long-Term Musculoskeletal Pain and Its Consequences: Is Gender a Factor?

Jensen I, Nygren Å, Gamberale F, Goldie I, Westerholm P (Karolinska Inst, Stockholm; Natl Inst of Occupational Health, Stockholm)

Pain 57:167–172, 1994 131-95-5–39

Introduction.—Most studies of neck, shoulder, and back pain have been focused on men. But there are differences in the responsibilities and daily activities of men and women, and these differences might affect reactions to pain. Men and women were compared for pain coping strategies and for psychological consequences of pain.

Methods.—One-hundred twenty-one Swedish adults (71 women) referred to an orthopedics department were studied. The average age was 40 years, and two thirds were married. The patients worked in various unskilled and skilled occupations, and more than 80% were on sick leave. Patients had experienced intractable pain in the neck, shoulder, or back for over 6 years. They rated their pain intensity as 53–60 on a scale of 0–100, and their pain severity as about 4 on a scale of 0–6. After measuring their ability to perform daily tasks, the extent of disability was calculated to be over 40 on a scale of 0–100.

The Coping Strategies Questionnaire was used to measure 8 different coping strategies for pain, such as diverting attention, praying and hoping, catastrophizing, and increased behavioral activities such as shopping and socializing. The Multidimensional Pain Inventory was used to measure pain-related psychological consequences, such as affect on mood and on daily activities.

Results.—Men and women had different coping strategies and psychological consequences in response to pain. Women catastrophized significantly more often. They increased their behavioral activity more than men did. In contrast, women were less inclined to use cognitive coping strategies, such as reinterpreting or ignoring pain. Women had significantly higher distress than men, and pain significantly interfered more with the general daily activities of women than with men.

Conclusion.—Current treatment and rehabilitation for long-term disabling pain are the same for men and women. However, the sex of the patient should be considered. Clinical trials and epidemiologic studies are needed to better elucidate sex differences and to improve preventive and rehabilitative strategies for long-term pain.

▶ The need to develop and/or test existing pain-related measurement unbiased by external factors has received limited attention in the pain literature. This article reports on many gender differences in frequently used pain assessment measurements. The authors' conclusions are based on mean scale score differences between men and women. However, before accepting that gender differences exist in measurements of coping and daily activities, it seems important to show that the items in these scales function in similar ways before inferring differences in mean effect. Recent advances in psychometrics, namely the Item Response Theory, provide a definitive methodology to test for item bias.—T.E. Rudy, Ph.D.

Treatment Outcome

Return to Work/Work Retention Outcomes of a Functional Restoration Program: A Multi-Center, Prospective Study With a Comparison Group

Burke SA, Harms-Constas CK, Aden PS (Univ of Colorado, Denver; HealthSouth Rehabilitation Corp, Birmingham, Ala)

Spine 19:1880–1886, 1994 131-95-5–40

Introduction.—Participation in functional restoration programs is known to improve functional capacity and return-to-work rates. However, as yet there has been no prospective, multicenter study of the benefits of functional restoration programs in low-back–treatment populations. Data obtained from patients at early follow-up times (6 and 12

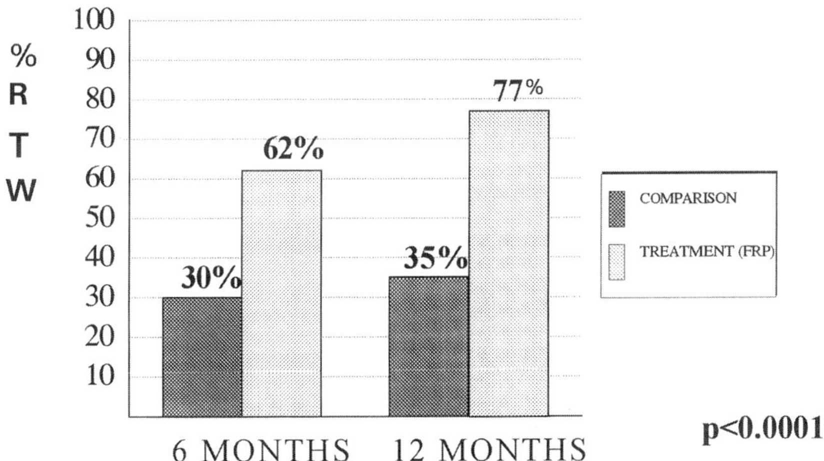

Fig 5–2.—The return-to-work rate for the treatment functional restoration program (*FRP*) group vs. the comparison group. (Courtesy of Burke SA, Harms-Constas CK, Aden PS: *Spine* 19:1880–1886, 1994.)

months) were used to assess the direct effects of such a program on working status.

Methods.—These patients with low back pathology were from 11 centers in 7 states. All had been referred for a work capacity assessment—an evaluation administered by an occupational therapist, a physical therapist, and an exercise physiologist. Those recommended for the functional restoration program were unable to perform essential job functions but did not require further medical intervention. The treatment group consisted of 303 patients, and the comparison group included 94 patients who were also recommended for the functional restoration program but whose entrance was denied by the physician or insurance company. The 2 groups were quite similar in age, sex, race, physical demand levels, and other recorded variables.

Results.—At both the 6- and 12-month follow-up, the treatment group had a much higher return to work rate than the comparison group (Fig 5–2). At 1 year, 98% of those in the treatment group who had been working at 6 months were still working, compared with only 62% of the comparison group. The return-to-work rates were higher in the treatment group than in the comparison group for all 3 status categories: postfusions, postlaminectomies, and nonsurgical management. The discharge recommendations of the functional restoration team were found to be quite accurate. At 12 months, 87% of those recommended for work were actually working, whereas only 33% of those not recommended for return to work were working.

Conclusion.—Patients with low back pathology who participated in a functional restoration program had a much higher return-to-work rate at 6 and 12 months than did patients who did not complete such a program. This improved status was achieved by both surgical and nonsurgical patients. In addition to functional and physical reconditioning, the program appeared to increase workers' confidence levels and lower their likelihood of reinjury.

Physical Progress and Residual Impairment Quantification After Functional Restoration: Part III. Isokinetic and Isoinertial Lifting Capacity

Curtis L, Mayer TG, Gatchel RJ (Productive Rehabilitation Inst of Dallas for Ergonomics; Univ of Texas, Dallas)

Spine 19:401–405, 1994 131-95-5–41

Introduction.—Chronic low back pain (CLBP) ranks as the leading cause of disability and loss of normal activities of daily living. The functional capacity of patients with CLBP in response to rehabilitation has been poorly documented. This functional capacity was determined in 4 separate groups of patients with CLBP.

Methods.—Patients were assessed at 3 time periods: initial evaluation, admission to an intensive rehabilitation program, and 12-week follow-up. A total of 193 patients were divided into 4 groups: postdiskectomy men (n = 26), nonsurgical CLBP men (n = 91), postdiskectomy women (n = 17) and nonsurgical CLBP women (n = 59). Tests included an isokinetic lifting task and the progressive isoinertial lifting evaluation.

Results.—All 4 groups improved significantly in both lifting tasks. Postdiskectomy patients achieved higher isokinetic scores, but not progressive isoinertial lifting evaluation scores, than the nonoperative patients.

Summary.—Lifting capacity can be improved in patients with CLBP, regardless of sex or surgical status. The study also demonstrates the utility of objective measures in following the restoration of function in the patient with CLBP.

▶ "Feeling better"—that is, less pain, improved mood, a more positive outlook on life, and so forth—although important, is not enough in pain rehabilitation. Increasing patients' quality of life includes increasing their functional abilities. Abstracts 131-95-5–40 and 131-95-5–41 provide important outcome information regarding the degree to which rehabilitation programs can produce functional changes. As suggested earlier in this chapter, I prefer to reconceptualize "functional abilities" as behaviors under the control of the patient and influenced by many cognitive and environmental factors.

The work of Burke et al. (Abstract 131-95-5–40), with its emphasis on return to work and the use of a control/comparison group, is noteworthy. However, this study, like previous studies of this nature, has experimental design problems, particularly in relation to the definition and selection of study groups. The comparison group consisted of patients referred for treatment but who were denied entry by either the physician or the insurance company. Thus, randomization did not occur. Methodologically, therefore, it is important to recognize that traditional statistical analyses contained in most software packages are inappropriate because they assume that randomization—that is, no systematic biases—exists between groups. Without complex statistical adjustments/corrections for nonrandomization, conclusions based on routine analyses are suspect and inconclusive.—T.E. Rudy, Ph.D.

Correlates of Improvement in Multidisciplinary Treatment of Chronic Pain

Jensen MP, Turner JA, Romano JM (Univ of Washington, Seattle)

J Consult Clin Psychol 62:172–179, 1994 131-95-5–42

Introduction.—Patients with chronic pain can benefit from multidisciplinary pain programs, showing improvement in psychological and physical functioning. Little is known, however, about which specific compo-

Zero-Order Correlation Coefficients Between Changes in Outcome and Changes in Beliefs and Coping Strategies, Pretreatment to Follow-Up

Belief/coping change scores	Outcome measure change scores: SIP Physical Dysfunction	BDI	Physician visits
SOPA subscales (beliefs)			
Medical Cure	−.15	−.35*	−.22
Solicitude	−.22	−.20	−.16
Medication	−.16	−.44*	−.13
Harm	−.34*	−.39*	−.09
Disability	−.37*	−.40*	−.15
Pain Control	.28*	.40*	.18
CSQ subscales (coping)			
Catastrophizing	−.19	−.30*	−.26*
Pray/Hope	−.16	−.33*	−.29*
Divert Attention	.02	.08	−.17
Ignore Pain	.14	.20	.09
Coping Self-Statements	.16	.18	.11
Coping ratings			
Rest	−.08	−.03	.00
Opioid medication use	−.10	−.16	−.13
Aerobic exercise	−.08	.09	−.02
Stretching exercise	.04	.14	.11
Keeping busy	.02	.05	.03
Muscle strengthening exercise	.07	.25*	.17
Relaxation	.03	.01	.00

Notes: Change scores were calculated by subtracting follow-up measure scores from pretreatment measure scores. Therefore, positive coefficients indicate that an increase in the predictor (process) variable is positively associated with improvement, and negative coefficients indicate that a decrease in the predictor variable is associated with improvement in the outcome variables. These correlations and significance levels are presented for descriptive purposes. The significance levels should be interpreted with caution given the large number of correlations performed on related variables.

Abbreviations: SIP, Sickness Impact Profile; *BDI,* Beck Depression Inventory; *SOPA,* Survey of Pain Attitudes; *CSQ,* Coping Strategy Questionnaire.

(Courtesy of Jensen MP, Turner JA, Romano JM: *J Consult Clin Psychol* 62:172–179, 1994.)

nents of the programs and which patient characteristics are associated with treatment efficacy. The hypothesis, derived from cognitive-behavioral theory, that improvement in physical and psychosocial functioning after multidisciplinary treatment is associated with changes in pain-related beliefs and coping strategies was tested.

Methods.—The study participants were 94 patients with chronic pain. Sixty percent of the patients were female, and the mean patient age was 42 years; the mean duration of pain was 5.26 years. Low back pain was the most common problem, affecting 46% of patients. To evaluate the relationship between treatment and outcome and changes in patient beliefs and coping strategies, patients completed measures of physical and psychological functioning, utilization of health care services, pain beliefs, and the use of pain-coping strategies. Physical disability was assessed with the use of the Physical Dysfunction scale of the Sickness Impact Profile, and psychological functioning was evaluated with the Beck Depression Inventory. The patients were asked to complete follow-up questionnaires 3 months after completing the 3-week inpatient multidisciplinary pain program.

Results and Conclusion.—The study hypothesis was confirmed, indicating that changes in pain-related beliefs and cognitive coping strategies were associated with an improvement in chronic pain after multidisciplinary treatment (table). A second major finding of the study was not anticipated. Significant amounts of improvement were not explained by coping strategies specifically targeted, including increases in aerobic exercise, stretching, relaxation, keeping busy, and decreases in pain-contingent rest and opioid medication use. Such coping strategies should not be discontinued, however, for they may require longer follow-up for their benefits to be apparent. Overall, the changes in what patients think about their pain may be more important than the changes in what they do about it.

Empirically Derived Chronic Pain Patient Subgroups: The Utility of Multidimensional Clustering to Identify Differential Treatment Effects

Sanders SH, Brena SF (Pain Control and Rehabilitation Inst of Georgia, Decatur)

Pain 54:51–56, 1993 131-95-5–43

Introduction.—Studies of the treatment of chronic pain require the identification of subgroups of patients with this problem. An ideal grouping model would be multidimensional, incorporating the medical-physical pathology data with psychosocial, behavioral, and general functioning measures. Such measures were applied to a group of 180 patients who were evaluated before and after participation in an outpatient interdisciplinary pain rehabilitation program.

Patients and Methods.—The study sample had a mean age of 42.75 years and was 56.57% female. The average duration of pain was 5.25 years. Many patients had a primary complaint of low back pain (42%), and 43% were receiving some kind of compensation for their pain problem. Ninety of the 157 patients who completed the pain rehabilitation treatment program were available for follow-up assessment. The measurement instruments included the Sickness Impact Profile (SIP), the Medical Examination and Diagnostic Information Coding System (MEDICS), patient self-reports of pain with the use of a visual analogue scale, the Medication Quantification Scale, and the Beck Depression Inventory. The interdisciplinary program consisted of an average of 12 treatment days over 6 weeks.

Results.—Four replicable subgroups were identified by multidimensional cluster analyses using SIP and MEDICS data. Cluster A was highly dysfunctional with moderate levels of physical pathology; cluster B had moderate dysfunction and moderate levels of physical pathology; cluster C was highly functional with low levels of physical pathology; and cluster D was highly dysfunctional with low levels of physical pathology. Patients in clusters A and D had significantly higher levels of depression, more medication usage, and less activity and were less likely than patients in the other clusters to be working at pretreatment. Cluster A and D patients also had the greatest improvement in subjective pain intensity, medication usage, activity level, and return to work after treatment. Cluster B patients had the least improvement from the program overall and failed to show any significant improvement in work status after treatment. The 4 cluster groups did not differ significantly in the median cost of treatment. The observed differences among the groups were not primarily a function of age, sex, depression, or the intensity, location, or duration of pain.

Conclusion.—A multidimensional clustering process that included psychosocial and medical-physical findings was able to distinguish 4 distinct subgroups of patients with chronic pain. A knowledge of the different responses of these groups to treatment may be helpful in customizing rehabilitation programs to achieve optimal benefits.

▶ Predicting treatment outcomes is an important and pressing issue in pain treatment. With the shrinking health care dollar combined with increased accountability of health care delivery systems, practitioners are being asked to make predictions about what types of patients or diagnostic groups are best treated by their specific programs. This goes against traditional medical perspectives that adhere to the belief that this question cannot be answered until patients are provided with an "adequate clinical trial."

From my perspective, our current scientific knowledge regarding predicting treatment success *a priori* (i.e., just based on pretreatment evaluation findings) is inadequate, and such prediction may result in substantial injustices to our patients. Our clinical "crystal balls" are not very accurate, and the same can be said for our statistical models. Nonetheless, to some degree we probably will have limited choices in this matter; therefore, additional studies similar to these (Abstracts 131-95-5–42 and 131-95-5–43) that begin to characterize factors that *may be* associated with outcomes are urgently needed. Let us not delude ourselves, however, that statistically significant associations lead to building adequate prediction models, that we know and/or can measure all of the important factors related to outcomes, or that describing high "correct classification rates" derived from a specific sample generalizes to other samples.—T.E. Rudy, Ph.D.

Is TENS Purely a Placebo Effect? A Controlled Study on Chronic Low Back Pain

Marchand S, Charest J, Li J, Chenard J-R, Lavignolle B, Laurencelle L (Université du Québec en Abitibi-Témiscamingue; Université de Bordeaux II, France; Université du Québec à Trois-Rivières, Canada)

Pain 54:99–106, 1993 131-95-5–44

Introduction.—Studies of the effectiveness of transcutaneous electric nerve stimulation (TENS) in the treatment of chronic pain have yielded contradictory results. One problem encountered in such investigations has been a lack of sensitive measures of pain. It is also important to recognize that placebo responses account for 20% to 30% of the clinical improvement in trials of analgesia. In this study of patients with chronic low back pain, separate visual analogue scales were used to measure the sensory-discriminative and motivational-affective components of their pain.

Patients and Methods.—All patients had chronic low back pain of more than 6 months' duration. Fourteen were randomly assigned to TENS, 12 to placebo-TENS, and 16 to a control group with no treatment. The groups were comparable in sex distribution, mean age, diagnosis, and pain severity. Treatment was administered twice weekly for 10 weeks. No current passed to the electrodes in the placebo-TENS procedure. The short-term effects of therapy were measured with visual analogue scale pain ratings taken before and after each treatment session. To assess long-term effects, patients rated their pain at home every 2 hours throughout a 3-day period before and 1 week, 3 months, and 6 months after the treatment sessions.

Results.—Home ratings of pain intensity before treatment were similar for the 3 groups. The TENS and placebo-TENS groups both had significantly reduced intensity and unpleasantness of chronic low back pain when ratings were made immediately before and after the treatment sessions, but the reduction in intensity of pain was significantly greater for the TENS group than for the TENS-placebo group. An additive effect over repetitive treatment sessions was obtained only with TENS. The evaluations at home showed an advantage for TENS in the measure of pain intensity 1 week after the end of treatment. There was no difference at any evaluation period in pain unpleasantness, and no significant difference between the 2 groups in pain intensity at 3 months and 6 months. Untreated controls experienced no significant change in pain intensity or pain unpleasantness, indicating no improvement with the mere passage of time.

Conclusion.—Transcutaneous electric nerve stimulation was found to be more effective than placebo-TENS as a short-term analgesia for low back pain. Its additive effect over time recommends its repetitive use over a short period of time. Although TENS reduces both the sensory-discriminative and motivational-affective components of low back pain, a placebo may be involved in the reduction of the affective component. The short-term reduction in pain allows the patient more physical activity, an important aspect of low back pain treatment.

▶ Better controlled studies, such as this one, that evaluate the "believed" efficacy of commonly used single-modality treatments for chronic pain conditions are imperative. Temporary relief is important; however, maintenance of change needs to be a long-term goal of every treatment intervention. Although this study focused on TENS, similar findings have occurred, or I believe will occur, for many other single modality interventions for chronic pain. Unfortunately, not enough pain practitioners are yet "enlightened" regarding the necessity of interdisciplinary treatment approaches. Thus, these types of studies remain necessary. However, I remain rather cynical about how much impact these studies will have on clinical practice.—T.E. Rudy, Ph.D.

Comparison of the Efficacy of Electromyographic Biofeedback, Cognitive-Behavioral Therapy, and Conservative Medical Interventions in the Treatment of Chronic Musculoskeletal Pain

Flor H, Birbaumer N (Univ of Tübingen, Germany)

J Consult Clin Psychol 61:653–658, 1993 131-95-5–45

Introduction.—A number of psychological treatments have been reported to be effective in chronic pain. Most studies, however, have not compared the various psychological treatment modalities in patients with different diagnoses. The efficacy of electromyographic biofeedback (BFB), cognitive-behavioral therapy (CBT), and conservative medical treatment (MED) were compared in 2 types of chronic musculoskeletal pain.

Patients and Methods.—Ninety patients with chronic back pain and 30 with chronic temporomandibular pain and dysfunction (TMPDS) entered the study and were randomized to the 3 treatment groups. The exclusion criteria were an inflammatory cause of pain, neurologic complications, duration of pain of less than 4 months, pregnancy, coincidence of chronic back pain and TMPDS, and major psychiatric illness. Sixty percent of the 57 patients with chronic back pain and the 21 with TMPDS who completed the study were women. Two thirds were employed, indicating a lack of severe impairment by the pain problem. The average duration of pain was 9.4 years. The MED treatment consisted of the best currently available medical interventions. Patients received various therapies, including analgesic agents, tranquilizers, physical therapy, and massages. The CBT group received instruction in pain and stress management, and in the BFB group exercises in tension perception and tension reduction were used.

Results.—Follow-up was conducted at 6 and 24 months. All 3 treatment groups showed improvement relative to baseline immediately post treatment, with the most substantial change recorded for the BFB group.

At both follow-up periods, only the BFB group maintained significant reductions in pain severity, interference, affective distress, pain-related use of the health care system, and stress-related reactivity of the affected muscles, and an increase in active coping self-statements. The chronicity of the pain problem was the best predictor of treatment outcome across all groups; the longer the history of chronic pain, the less change the patients experienced. Patients who practiced relaxation and distraction benefited most from BFB. The somatic findings did not correlate well with the therapeutic change, countering the assumption that only patients without somatic findings can profit from psychologically oriented treatments for chronic pain.

Conclusion.—Biofeedback proved to be superior to CBT and MED treatment in relieving chronic musculoskeletal pain. The differential treatment effects became apparent only at follow-up assessments conducted at 6 and 12 months.

► Being an "equipment freak" and having studied electromyographic BFB in TMPDS over the past 10 years, I must confess that I have always "believed" in the unique contributions of biofeedback in the treatment of chronic pain disorders. Therefore, I like the results obtained in this study. As noted in Abstract 131-95-5-44, however, I do not believe that biofeedback as a single modality is adequate to treat the complexities and many psychological and physical complications of chronic pain.—T.E. Rudy, Ph.D.

A Controlled Study of the Effects of an Early Intervention on Acute Musculoskeletal Pain Problems

Linton SJ, Hellsing A-L, Andersson D (Örebro Med Ctr, Sweden; Laxå Primary Care Ctr, Sweden)

Pain 54:353–359, 1993 131-95-5-46

Introduction.—Early intervention for acute musculoskeletal pain is beneficial in preventing chronic pain problems. Two investigations were made to evaluate an early intervention program for patients with back and neck pain.

Methods.—Study I consisted of patients who had a history of musculoskeletal pain during the past 2 years but had not been sick-listed in the most recent 3 months. In study II, patients had not been sick-listed for musculoskeletal pain during the previous 2 years. Within the 2 study groups, 106 patients were randomized to receive usual treatment and 134 to receive early activation. Patients completed treatment-satisfaction questionnaires, treatment-outcome questionnaires, and visual analogue scales during their first appointment and at 6- and 12-month intervals. Waiting times for physician evaluation, physical therapy, and education were considerably lower in the early activation groups than in the usual treatment groups. Well behavior and function were emphasized in the early activation groups.

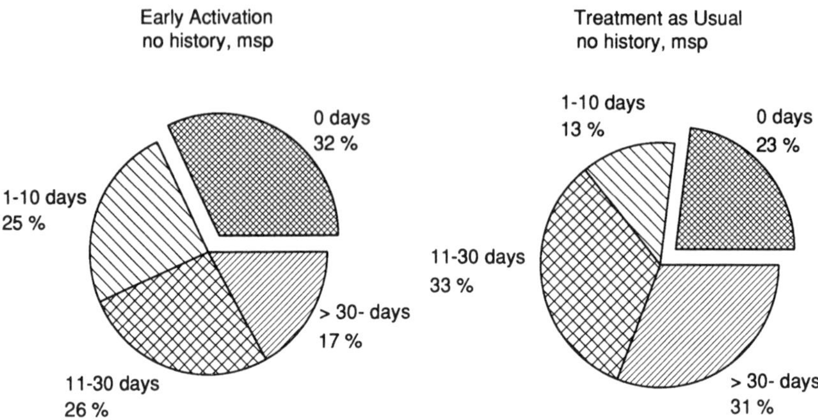

Fig 5–3.—The distribution of sickness absenteeism for musculoskeletal pain during the 1-year follow-up for the patients receiving early activation and those receiving usual treatment in study II. The group receiving early activation had more patients with 0 days and fewer patients with more than 30 days than the patients receiving usual treatment. (Courtesy of Linton SJ, Hellsing A-L, Andersson D: *Pain* 54:353–359, 1993.)

Results.—In study I, patients in the usual treatment and early activation groups had significant improvement in all indices assessed compared with controls. No significant differences were observed between the groups. Patients in study II also showed significant improvement in all assessments. There was also a significant decrease in sickness absenteeism in the early activation group compared with the usual treatment group (Fig 5–3).

Conclusion.—The risk for developing chronic pain was 8 times less, and the number of sick days was significantly decreased in the early activation group. In patients with neck and back pain, a focus on acute care may be worthwhile in terms of the human and financial costs of sick leave and chronic pain.

▶ Some of us (well, maybe just me) working in chronic pain rehabilitation facilities would not mind putting ourselves out of business. It is well established that the probability of returning patients to gainful employment decreases rapidly as the duration of pain conditions increases. Conducting prospective outcome studies of early intervention strategies, however, is difficult, and the studies are "high risk," which probably explains why so few have appeared in the literature. These authors are to be applauded for their efforts and the importance of their findings.—T.E. Rudy, Ph.D.

6 Anesthesiology

Acute and Perioperative Pain

A Comparison of Lumbar Epidural and Intravenous Fentanyl Infusions for Post-Thoracotomy Analgesia

Baxter AD, Laganière S, Samson B, Stewart J, Hull K, Goernert L (Ottawa Gen Hosp, Ont, Canada; Bureau of Drug Research, Ottawa, Ont, Canada)

Can J Anaesth 41:184–191, 1994 131-95-6–1

Background.—If the analgesic efficacy of epidural fentanyl is caused by systemic absorption rather than a direct spinal mechanism, there may be no advantage to the epidural route of administration over the IV route. The analgesic efficacy, respiratory effects, side effects, and pharmacokinetic disposition of lumbar and IV infusions of fentanyl were compared using the same dosage regimen in post-thoracotomy patients.

Methods.—Fifty patients undergoing elective thoracotomy were studied in a double-blind, randomized fashion. After a standard low-dose alfentanil and isoflurane general anesthetic, patients received continuous lumbar epidural or IV infusions of fentanyl (1.5-μg/kg bolus, then 1 μg/kg per hour) for postoperative analgesia. Patients received either epidu-

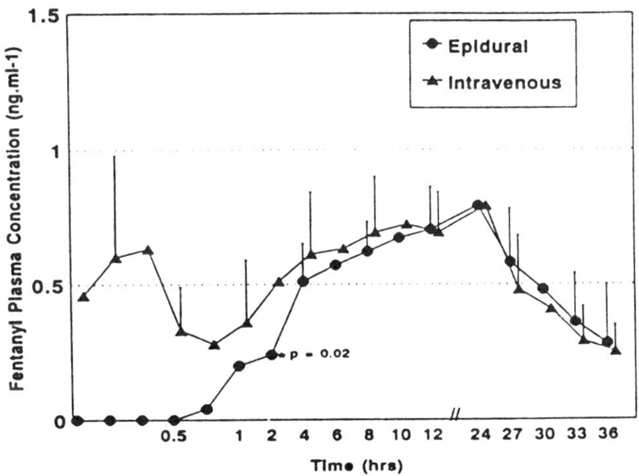

Fig 6–1.—Plasma concentration vs. time profile. Fentanyl was not detectable in plasma in epidural group before 2 hours, its plasma concentration was lower at 2 hours ($P = .002$), and plasma concentrations (mean ± SD) were similar in the 2 groups thereafter. (Courtesy of Baxter AD, Laganière S, Samson B, et al: *Can J Anaesth* 41:184–191, 1994.)

ral fentanyl and IV normal saline or IV fentanyl and epidural normal saline.

Results.—The amount of supplemental morphine self-administered by patient-controlled analgesic pump was the same in both groups. For the groups as a whole, visual analogue pain scores were lower in the epidural group only at 2 hours postoperatively. In those patients who did not receive naloxone, mean visual analogue pain scores were lower in the epidural group throughout the study. Pain relief in the epidural group during the first few hours appeared to be caused by a mainly spinal analgesic effect because fentanyl was not detectable in their plasma until 2 hours after bolus injection. By 4 hours, the plasma levels of fentanyl were similar in the 2 groups (Fig 6–1). Ten patients in the IV group and 7 patients in the epidural group received naloxone for an arterial blood partial pressure of carbon dioxide > 50 mm Hg. Irrespective of naloxone therapy, indices of respiratory function, spirometry, hemodynamic variables, morbidity, and other side effects were similar in both groups.

Conclusion.—Post-thoracotomy patients who do not require naloxone have better analgesia with epidural than with IV fentanyl. This advantage does not result in better pulmonary function or lower morbidity.

▶ To justify the expense and risk of a medical procedure, a difference in outcome must result from the intervention. These investigators should be commended for showing the relative lack of advantage of epidural vs. IV fentanyl for postoperative pain control. Furthermore, they show that despite small changes between subjects in a subjective measurement such as visual analogue scale, it is difficult to demonstrate differences in objective measurements such as respiratory or hemodynamic function. Large studies will be required to determine whether epidural fentanyl analgesia is advantageous when compared with IV analgesia.—E. Lang, M.D.

The Effect of Low-Dose Bupivacaine on Postoperative Epidural Fentanyl Analgesia and Thromboelastography

Benzon HT, Wong CA, Wong HY, Brooke C, Wade L (Northwestern Univ, Chicago)

Anesth Analg 79:911–917, 1994 131-95-6–2

Background.—In addition to other benefits, postoperative infusion of epidural fentanyl has been shown to decrease hypercoagulability as measured by thromboelastography (TEG) in patients undergoing vascular surgery. Fentanyl is often infused in combination with bupivacaine to improve postoperative analgesia. To test the effectiveness of this drug combination, various concentrations of bupivacaine were combined with epidural fentanyl to evaluate their analgesic effect and to determine whether increasing concentrations of bupivacaine produced postoperative numbness and hypotension or affected blood pressure. The TEG changes were measured to determine whether bupivacaine affects TEG and decreases hypercoagulability in patients undergoing extensive abdominal or genitourinary surgery.

Methods.—A total of 120 patients undergoing abdominal or genitourinary surgery were assigned randomly to 1 of 4 groups of 30. The epidural fentanyl was administered to patients in the postanesthesia recovery room according to their assignment. A concentration of 10μg/mL of fentanyl was administered in combination with bupivacaine in various concentrations (group II, .1%; group III, .15%; group IV, .2%) or with preservative-free saline (group I). Patients were evaluated 6 times in 24 hours for analgesia, sedation, respiratory rate, and pain relief using a visual analogue scale and a visual rating scale. Forced vital capacity measurements were made preoperatively and 24 hours postoperatively. The TEG measurements were determined on blood drawn preoperatively, in the postanesthesia recovery room, and 24 hours postoperatively.

Results.—No significant differences among the 4 groups were shown by the mean visual analogue scale score, the visual rating scale and total pain relief scores, or changes in the TEG values. There was also no statistical difference in the postoperative forced vital capacity values of sedation scores among the 4 groups or in the incidence of postoperative side effects such as nausea, vomiting, or pruritis.

Conclusion.—The addition of bupivacaine in any concentration to an epidural fentanyl infusion does not improve analgesia significantly in patients undergoing extensive abdominal or genitourinary surgery. Bupivacaine also does not affect the postoperative hypercoagulable state in these patients. This deficiency may be caused by the lack of specificity or sensitivity of the TEG measurement itself.

▶ This is an interesting study. If the addition of bupivacaine does not enhance analgesia in these patients, it is probably not advantageous to add it. On the other hand, if fentanyl provides analgesia through systemic uptake, as many studies suggest, epidural administration of fentanyl may not be necessary.—E. Lang, M.D.

Bupivacaine 0.125% Improves Continuous Postoperative Epidural Fentanyl Analgesia After Abdominal or Thoracic Surgery

Badner NH, Bhandari R, Komar WE (Univ of Western Ontario, London, Canada)

Can J Anaesth 41:387–392, 1994 131-95-6–3

Background.—Some authors have recently recommended using a narcotic combined with a local anesthetic in the management of postoperative pain. Effective local anesthetic-narcotic combinations with minimal side effects have yet to be determined, however.

Methods.—Thirty-nine patients undergoing abdominal or thoracic surgery were enrolled in a prospective, randomized, double-blind trial.

Bupivacaine, .125% and .25%, was added to continuous postoperative epidural infusions of fentanyl in a 10-μg/mL concentration. The patients were given an initial bolus of .1 mL of the study solution per kg and an infusion of 6 mL/hr, titrated to maintain analgesia. Pain, pulmonary function, and bowel function were assessed periodically until the second postoperative day.

Findings.—Analgesia in the 3 groups differed significantly over time, with fentanyl alone producing less analgesia than .125% bupivacaine. No differences were found in mean infusion rates, postoperative pulmonary function, or bowel function. Adverse effects—including somnolence, nausea and vomiting, and pruritis—were also comparable among groups. Fewer patients given .125% bupivacaine than those given .25% had transient sensory loss to pinprick and ice. Four patients in both bupivacaine groups had leg weakness.

Conclusion.—In patients undergoing abdominal or thoracic surgery, the addition of bupivacaine .125% to epidural infusions of fentanyl provided improved analgesia compared with fentanyl alone. Other outcome variables did not differ. Three of 13 patients had sensory changes, and 4 of 13 had minor motor weakness.

▶ These investigators found results different from those of the previous authors. The double-blind design of the study is important. Further research into the relative advantages of different medications infused through epidural catheters will be necessary.—E. Lang, M.D.

Prophylactic Antiemetic Therapy With Patient-Controlled Analgesia: A Double-Blind, Placebo-Controlled Comparison of Droperidol, Metoclopramide, and Tropisetron

Kaufmann MA, Rosow C, Schnieper P, Schneider M (Univ of Basel, Switzerland; Harvard Med School, Boston)

Anesth Analg 78:988–994, 1994 131-95-6–4

Introduction.—Opioid-induced nausea remains a major problem for patients using a patient-controlled analgesia (PCA) system for severe postoperative pain. In a placebo-controlled trial, 3 prophylactic antiemetic regimens were compared for their effects on postoperative nausea and vomiting (PONV) during the use of PCA with morphine.

Patients and Methods.—The eligible patients were adults scheduled for major orthopedic surgery. All had American Society of Anesthesiologists physical status I or II and were candidates for postoperative PCA. The anesthetic regimen varied according to the type of surgery. Group 1 controls (67 patients) received only morphine from the PCA device; group 2 (71 patients) received metoclopramide mixed with morphine in the PCA syringe; group 3 (70 patients) received droperidol mixed with morphine; and group 4 (78 patients) received tropisetron, not in the

Incidence of Postoperative Nausea and Vomiting

	Group 1: NaCl 0.9% (n = 67) (%)	Group 2: metoclopramide (n = 71) (%)	Group 3: droperidol (n = 70) (%)	Group 4: tropisetron (n = 78) (%)
Day of operation, 1–9 h	36	25	10*	17‡
First night, 10–18 h	26	17	7†	12‡
First postoperative day, 19–36 h	24	13	7†	22
Incidence				
1–18 h	48	30‡	11*	22†
1–36 h	54	40	17†	33‡

* $P < .001$, compared with control.
† $P < .01$, compared with control.
‡ $P < .05$, compared with control.
(Courtesy of Kaufmann MA, Rosow C, Schnieper P, et al: *Anesth Analg* 78:988–994, 1994.)

PCA device but as a single IV dose. After operation, patients were assessed for the frequency and severity of PONV, the need for rescue, side effects of the antiemetics, and overall patient satisfaction. A symptom-severity score based on intensity and duration measured the severity of PONV.

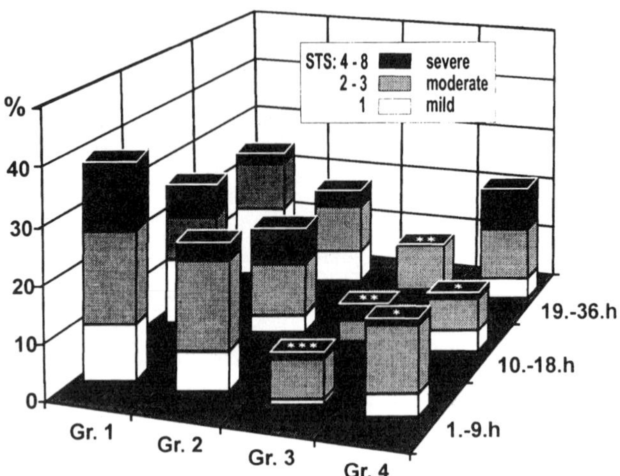

Fig 6–2.—The incidence (%) and severity (symptom therapy scores [*STS*]) of postoperative nausea and vomiting in the 4 experimental groups over time. The results are shown for the day of operation (1–9 h), the postoperative night (10–18 h), and the postoperative day (19–36 h). The incidence was significantly lower for the droperidol and tropisetron groups. The mean STS for droperidol and tropisetron were significantly lower than for placebo during hours 1–9, but the difference remained significant only for droperidol at later times. (Courtesy of Kaufmann MA, Rosow C, Schnieper P, et al: *Anesth Analg* 78:988–994, 1994.)

Results.—The average total doses of the antiemetics were 53.8 mg of metoclopramide, 5.99 mg of droperidol, and 6.1 mg of tropisetron. The incidence of PONV over the initial 36-hour postoperative period was 54% in controls, 40% in group 2, 17% in group 3, and 33% in group 4 (table). The severity of PONV over time is shown in Figure 6–2. Droperidol (group 3) significantly reduced both the incidence and severity of PONV for the entire 36-hour study period. Although tropisetron (group 4) also had a significant antiemetic effect, a single bolus was effective for only 18 hours. The effects of metoclopramide were only marginally significant. Only droperidol decreased the need for rescue medication, but patients receiving this agent tended to be sleepier and to recall somewhat more anxiety. The 3 antiemetic prophylaxis groups had similar side effects and satisfaction scores.

Conclusion.—The administration of opioids with a PCA system for postoperative pain can aggravate PONV. The addition of droperidol to PCA morphine was effective in reducing the incidence and severity of PONV. Tropisetron was also a useful antiemetic in this series of patients, but more than 1 dose was required during the 36-hour postoperative study period.

► Postoperative nausea and vomiting has emerged as a significant morbidity in the era of same-day surgery. Kaufmann et al. verify the efficacy of droperidol, but their study also illustrates its shortcomings with respect to sedation and anxiety. Newer antiemetics show promise with PONV; high acquisition costs may impede their general use, except as rescue medications.—D.A. Van Alstine, M.D.

Comparison of the Efficacy of Epidural Morphine Given by Intermittent Injection or Continuous Infusion for the Management of Postoperative Pain

Rauck RL, Raj PP, Knarr DC, Denson DD, Speight KL (Wake Forest Univ, Winston-Salem, NC; Natl Pain Inst, Atlanta, Ga; Univ of Cincinnati, Ohio; et al)

Reg Anesth 19:316–324, 1994 131-95-6–5

Background.—Research on the use of epidural opioids for the management of pain after surgery has focused on the efficacy of various agents. However, the method of delivery of epidural drugs may be equally important. A commonly used epidural agent, morphine sulfate, was used to determine whether postoperative outcome, analgesia, or adverse effects were a function of the method of administration.

Methods.—By random assignment, 30 patients undergoing upper abdominal surgery received morphine sulfate through a thoracic epidural catheter by 1 of 2 delivery techniques. Patients in group 1 were given an initial bolus of morphine, .07 mg/kg, at the end of surgery, followed by

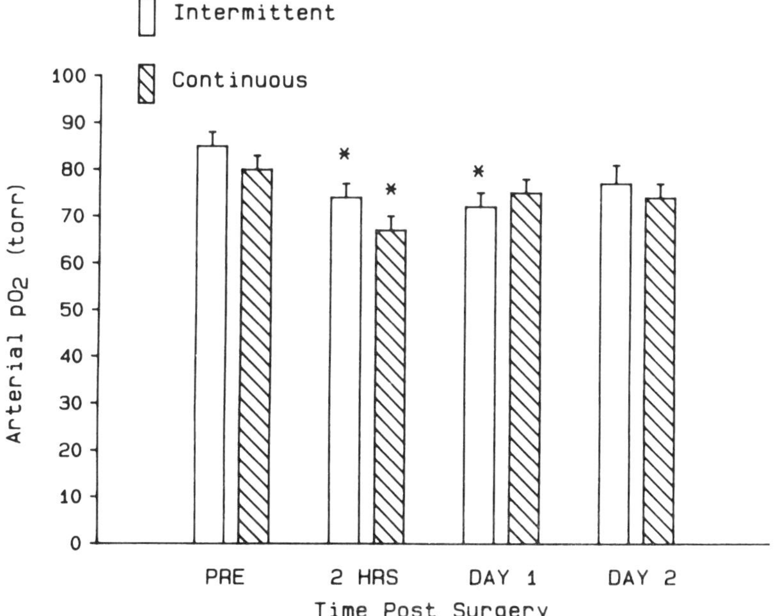

Fig 6–3.—Arterial oxygen pressure (pO_2) values for both groups. Significant decreases from the preoperative values were noted at 2 hours and on day 1 for group 1 and at 2 hours for group 2. * $P < .05$. (Courtesy of Rauck RL, Raj PP, Knarr DC, et al: *Reg Anesth* 19:316-324, 1994.)

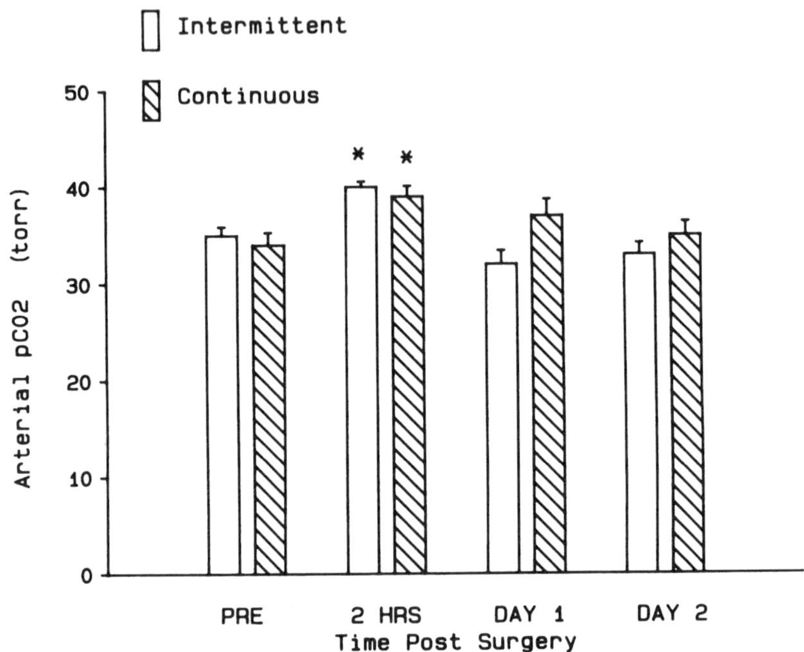

Fig 6–4.—Arterial carbon dioxide pressure (pCO_2) results for both groups. Significant increases were noted for both groups only for the 2-hour measurement, at 2 hours after the operation. * $P < .05$. (Courtesy of Rauck RL, Raj PP, Knarr DC, et al: *Reg Anesth* 19:316–324, 1994.)

injections of 2 to 5 mg of morphine into the epidural catheter on demand. Group 2 patients were given an initial bolus of .03 mg of morphine per kg during surgical peritoneal closure, then were immediately started with an infusion of .01% morphine at 5 mL/hr. Depending on side effects, the infusion dose was titrated from .2 to 1 mg/hr.

Findings.—The 2 groups were comparable in forced vital capacity, forced expiratory volume in 1 second, and arterial blood gas measures (Figs 6–3, 6–4, and 6–5). Adverse effects were also similar in the 2 groups. Respiratory depression did not occur in either group. Patients in group 2 reported significantly better analgesia than those in group 1 on the first 2 days after surgery. Group 1 peak plasma morphine levels were significantly greater than the steady-state plasma morphine levels in group 2.

Conclusion.—Both groups had similar pulmonary function studies, arterial blood gases, and side effects, with no incidences of respiratory depression. The continuous infusion of morphine was associated with analgesia superior to that of intermittent bolus injection given on demand.

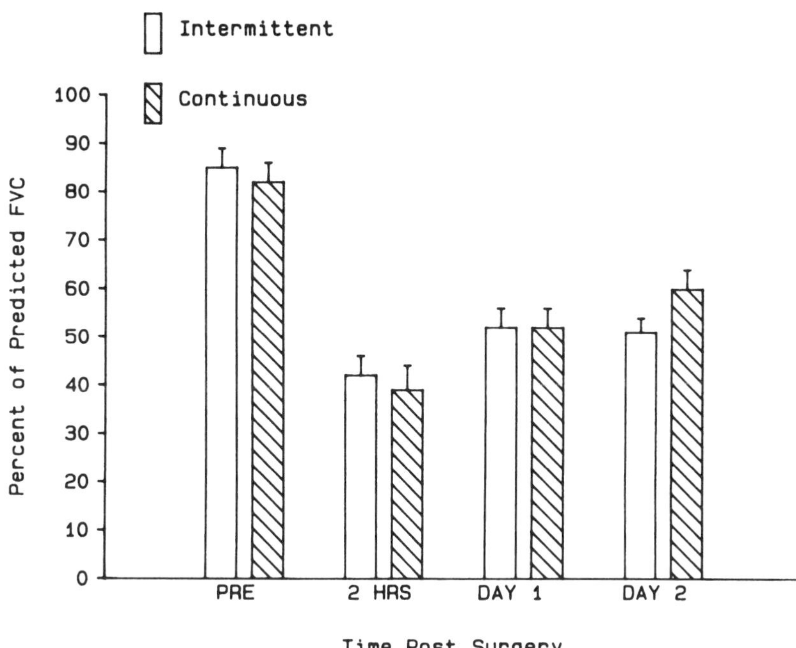

Fig 6–5.—Forced vital capacity (*FVC*) measurements for both groups showing significant decreases from the preoperative values at all the postoperative times studied. (Courtesy of Rauck RL, Raj PP, Knarr DC, et al: *Reg Anesth* 19:316–324, 1994.)

▶ Continuous infusion for epidural analgesics has been the most common technique on most acute pain services. It is important to have evidence that this method provides superior pain control in most patients, with no difference in side effects. In comparison, continuous delivery of narcotics IV by using basal rates on patient-controlled analgesia has generally been shown to provide no improvement in pain control, with an increase in side effects. Replication of this study with a larger patient population would be important to validly show that effectiveness and side effect incidence are unchanged by constant infusion. Unfortunately, the total 24-hour dose of morphine for each group was not reported.—D.A. Van Alstine, M.D.

Video-Assisted Thoracoscopic Placement of Paravertebral Catheters: A Technique for Postoperative Analgesia for Bilateral Thoracoscopic Surgery

Soni AK, Conacher ID, Waller DA, Hilton CJ (Freeman Hosp, Newcastle upon Tyne, England)

Br J Anaesth 72:462–464, 1994 131-95-6–6

Objective.—Patients with a history of bilateral pneumothoraces are treated by parietal pleurectomy, usually by staged bilateral thoracotomy or median sternotomy. Now, video-assisted thoracoscopy (VAT) may offer a minimally invasive alternative. Pleural stripping is still painful, however, so a good form of analgesia is needed. A new approach to the insertion of paravertebral catheters under thoracoscopic vision for post-VAT analgesia was attempted.

Case Report.—Woman, 30, was undergoing VAT for recurrent, bilateral pneumothoraces. After the 10-mm video thoracoscope was inserted, bilateral paravertebral catheters were placed through a 16-gauge Tuohy needle under direct video control. Catheter advancement was facilitated by injection of saline to dissect the pleura. The indwelling paravertebral catheters were used to infuse .125% bupivacaine and to administer bolus doses of morphine after surgery. Infusion continued for 48 hours, after which the catheters were removed. Although initial pain scores were high, they decreased to 0 after the second bolus dose at 6 hours. Peak expiratory flow rates improved at this time as well. Hypotension was anticipated in the postoperative period but did not occur. Pain was initially less severe on the left side, probably reflecting the spread of local anesthetic in the left paravertebral gutter.

Conclusion.—Bilateral placement of paravertebral catheters during VAT is easily accomplished. These catheters allow for continuous postoperative infusion of local anesthetics, which are effective and well tolerated. Catheter insertion may be a routine part of surgery for patients undergoing bilateral procedures, especially if their respiratory function is less than optimal.

▶ This article was chosen because it describes a novel method of providing analgesia for thoracoscopic surgery.—E. Lang, M.D.

Prolonged Analgesia After Epidural Injection of a Poorly Soluble Salt of Fentanyl

Randell TT, Östman PLG, Flanagan DR, Perng C-Y, Hardy J (Univ of Iowa, Iowa City)

Anesth Analg 79:905–910, 1994 131-95-6–7

Purpose.—Fentanyl citrate (FC) is commonly used for postoperative epidural analgesia. The onset of action of epidural FC is rapid, but its duration is short. The analgesic effect of some parenterally administered drugs can be increased by using poorly soluble salts of the drugs. Whether the analgesic effect of epidural fentanyl can be prolonged by using fentanyl pamoate (FP), which is a poorly soluble fentanyl salt, was examined.

Methods.—The dose-response relationship and duration of analgesic action of FC and FP were studied in white male Sprague-Dawley rats. Fentanyl citrate and FP were administered epidurally in equianalgesic doses. Visceral and nociceptive stimulation were used to evaluate the analgesic effects of the drugs. Three epidural doses of each drug were studied.

Results.—Epidurally administered FC was approximately 10 times more potent than epidurally administered FP. The analgesic effect was not prolonged when the FC dose was increased, but it was markedly prolonged when the FP dose was increased. When equianalgesic large doses of FC and FP were used, the analgesic effect of FP lasted significantly longer than that of FC.

Conclusion.—The analgesic effect of epidural fentanyl can be prolonged by administering the drug as a poorly soluble salt.

▶ Alternative formulations of medications already on the market—such as liposomal bupivacaine and poorly soluble salts of fentanyl—may expand our analgesic armamentarium while maintaining the benefit of using agents whose properties and side effects are already well understood.—D.A. Van Alstine, M.D.

Do Agents Used for Epidural Analgesia Have Antimicrobial Properties?

Feldman JM, Chapin-Robertson K, Turner J (Temple Univ, Philadelphia; Univ of South Alabama, Mobile; Yale Univ, New Haven, Conn)

Reg Anesth 19:43–47, 1994 131-95-6–8

Objective.—There is a low incidence of infection resulting from catheter placement in the epidural space, possibly because the local anesthetics used have anti-infective properties. The capability of lidocaine and bupivacaine in combination with fentanyl and sufentanil to inhibit bacterial growth was evaluated.

Methods.—Cultured specimens from epidural catheters yielded 53 bacterial isolates (table). Isolates were grown for 24 hours on Mueller-Hinton agar alone or in the presence of 2%, 1.5%, and 1% lidocaine; .5%, .25%, and .125% bupivacaine; .125% bupivacaine plus 2 mcgs/mL fentanyl; .125% bupivacaine plus 3 mcgs/mL sufentanil; and 5 mcgs/mL fentanyl, 2 mcgs/mL fentanyl, and .3 mcgs/mL sufentanil.

Results.—Significantly fewer isolates grew in the presence of all concentrations of lidocaine and bupivacaine, although there was a significant increase in bacterial growth with decrease in lidocaine or bupivacaine concentration. Neither opioid inhibited bacterial growth, and neither opioid plus bupivacaine significantly inhibited bacterial growth when compared with bupivacaine alone.

Conclusion.—Anesthetics appear to decrease the already low risk of infection from epidural catheters. More studies need to be done to de-

Number of Isolates by Species That Grew in the Presence of the Study Agents

	Catheter Isolates								**Noncatheter Isolates (sterile sites)**
	Staph. Coagulase (−)	*Staph. aureus*	*Strep.* spp.	*Micrococcus*	*Coryn*	*Bacillus* spp.	Fastidious GNR	Growth Total	*Staph. aureus*
Agar alone	38	1	2	2	1	8	1	53	11
Lido 2%	0	0	0	0	0	0	0	0	0
Lido 1.5%	4	0	0	0	0	2	0	6	2
Lido 1.0%	15	1	0	1	1	4	0	22	6
Bup 0.5%	2	0	0	0	0	0	0	2	0
Bup 0.25%	2	1	0	0	0	0	0	3	6
Bup 0.125%	32	1	0	0	1	3	0	37	6
Bup 0.125% plus Fent 2	35	0	0	0	0	3	0	38	6
Bup 0.125% plus Sufent 0.3	32	0	0	0	0	3	0	35	6
Fent 5	38	1	2	2	1	8	1	53	11
Fent 2	38	1	2	2	1	8	1	53	11
Sufent 0.3	38	1	2	2	1	8	1	53	11

*Abbreviations: **Bup**,* bupivacaine; *Coryn, Corynebacterium; **Fent**,* fentanyl; GNR, gram-negative rod; *Lido,* lidocaine; *Staph, Staphylococcus; Strep, Streptococcus; **Sufent**,* sufentanil.
(Courtesy of Feldman JM, Chapin-Robertson K, Turner J: *Reg Anesth* 19:43–47, 1994.)

termine whether anesthetics can decrease the risk of infection for at-risk patients.

▶ The severe consequences of infections of the epidural space make it important to maximize our understanding of all the factors that predispose to infection or those factors that are protective. The low incidence of infection relative to central lines is fortunate but poorly understood. At the doses typically used for postoperative and cancer pain management, the bacteriostatic properties of local anesthetics appear minor. Opioids do not appear to be bacteriostatic at all.—D.A. Van Alstine, M.D.

Quantitative Sensory Examination of Epidural Anaesthesia and Analgesia in Man: Dose-Response Effect of Bupivacaine

Brennum J, Nielsen PT, Horn A, Arendt-Nielsen L, Secher NH (Gentofte Hosp, Denmark; Rigshospitalet, Denmark; Aalborg Univ, Denmark)

Pain 56:315–326, 1994 131-95-6–9

Background.—Epidurally applied local anesthetics induce a semiselective inhibition of somatosensory and motor functions, with pain and temperature perception inhibited more easily than tactile stimuli perception and motor function. Analgesia, with a minimal effect on motor function, is frequently provided by administration of low doses of epidural local anesthetics, often in combination with other analgesic drugs such as opioids. The effects of a series of epidural doses of bupivacaine on selected sensory and motor functions were determined.

Methods.—Ten volunteers each received epidural injections of 15 mg, 25 mg, 50 mg, and 100 mg of bupivacaine in a volume of 20 mL on 4 separate days separated by at least 1 week. Sensory and motor functions were assessed before anesthesia and every hour for 8 hours afterward.

Results.—Nonpainful stimuli were blocked differentially. The order of blockade was warmth > cold > electric. A similar differential blockade of prolonged painful stimuli occurred in the order of heat > mechanical > electric. Mechanical and electric stimuli were blocked at a lower dose when the stimuli were brief than when they were prolonged. Motor function, judged by knee extension strength, was not reduced by 15 or 25 mg bupivacaine but it was decreased by 42.8% by 50 mg, with recovery occurring in 3 hours. A decrease of 83.5% with a 6-hour recovery was induced by 100 mg.

Conclusion.—Differential blockade of painful and nonpainful stimuli is induced by epidural administration of bupivacaine. Hypoalgesia with no or minimal blockade of motor function can be induced by 20 mL of

.125% bupivacaine (25 mg), indicating that it is a suitable dose for treatment of pain alone or combined with opioids such as morphine.

▶ These authors were able to demonstrate, in a clinically relevant paradigm, a differential blockade of somatosensory perceptions, including pain. The finding that bupivacaine produced better analgesia for both mechanical and electrical stimuli as opposed to prolonged stimuli is consistent with the comment after Abstract 131-95-6–57 with regard to incident vs. rest pain. In this study, the short-duration stimuli more closely resemble incident pain, for which local anesthetic is quite effective. The design of this study is such that it makes it difficult to infer mechanisms.—J.D. Haddox, D.D.S., M.D.

Interpleural Block for Patients With Multiple Rib Fractures: Comparison With Epidural Block

Shinohara K, Iwama H, Akama Y, Tase C (Fukushima Med College, Japan)

J Emerg Med 12:441–446, 1994 131-95-6–10

Background.—Pain control in patients who have multiple rib fractures is essential because pain interferes with respiration, which can lead to pneumonia or atelectasis. Epidural block (EB) is commonly used for trauma patients with rib fractures. Interpleural block (IPB) has been used for the same purpose in patients undergoing thoracotomy or laparotomy. The effectiveness of IPB for pain control of rib fractures was compared with EB.

Methods.—Seventeen adult patients who sustained unilateral rib fractures constituted the cohort. All patients had severe pain, a hemopneumothorax that required a chest drain, and no other trauma. An IPB catheter and a chest drain were inserted and left in place. Both EB and IPB were instituted with an infusion of 10 mL of 1% lidocaine. An original pain scale was used to gather pain relief data. Each patient's respiratory rate, heart rate, blood pressure, blood gas, and range of thermohypesthesia were determined after each procedure. A venous plasma lidocaine concentration was collected 30 minutes and 120 minutes after each block. An analysis of variance for repeated measures was used to analyze the information.

Results.—No hypesthesia was shown in 4 patients with IPB, but it was shown in 2 patients with EB. The IPB and EB relieved intolerable pain to the same degree; pain lasted longer than 2 hours with both methods. The heart rate declined and blood pressure fell after EB but not after IPB. There were no significant differences in the respiratory rate, the plasma lidocaine concentration, or the blood gas results between the 2 blocks. There were no toxic reactions with lidocaine, and no other complications, such as infection, were noted.

Conclusion.—An EB applied to the upper thoracic region relieves the pain of multiple rib fractures adequately with 10 mL of 1% lidocaine.

Provided patients undergo careful observation, IPB may be a better choice for control of pain in trauma patients than EB because of its unilateral, narrow effect.

▶ The conclusion that IPB with 1% lidocaine may be a better choice than EB may not be justified. Adequate thoracic epidural analgesia is usually possible with lower concentrations of local anesthetic than those used in this study. Furthermore, analysis of plasma lidocaine concentrations is not routinely used for patient follow-up. After surgery or trauma, a patient might systemically absorb larger doses of local anesthetic, leading to toxic plasma lidocaine concentrations. In the following article, the investigators have reached different conclusions.—E. Lang M.D.

Prospective Evaluation of Epidural Versus Intrapleural Catheters for Analgesia in Chest Wall Trauma

Luchette FA, Radafshar SM, Kaiser R, Flynn W, Hassett JM (State Univ of New York, Buffalo)

J Trauma 36:865–870, 1994 131-95-6–11

Objective.—Blunt chest trauma can cause serious ventilation problems and a great deal of chest pain. Studies have shown that nerve blocks are more effective than systemic narcotics at reducing pain. Subjective pain relief and pulmonary function improvement experienced by patients

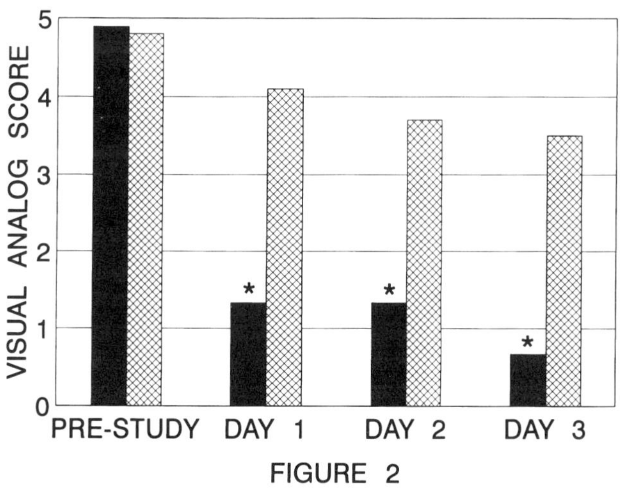

Fig 6–6.—Pain with movement or coughing was significantly less throughout the study in the epidural group. *Analysis was performed with paired Student's *t* tests and significance of $P < .05$. (Courtesy of Luchette FA, Radafshar SM, Kaiser R, et al: *J Trauma* 36:865–870, 1994.)

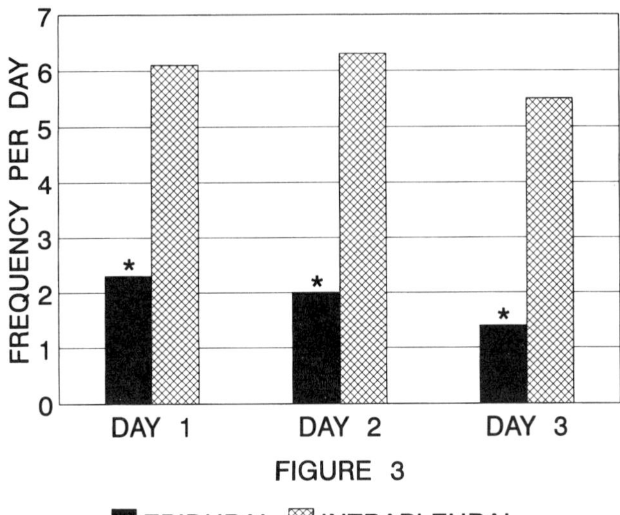

Fig 6–7.—Parenteral narcotic use was significantly less with epidural bupivacaine administration compared with the intrapleural group. *Analysis was performed with paired Student's *t* tests and significance of $P < .05$. (Courtesy of Luchette FA, Radafshar SM, Kaiser R, et al: *J Trauma* 36:865–870, 1994.)

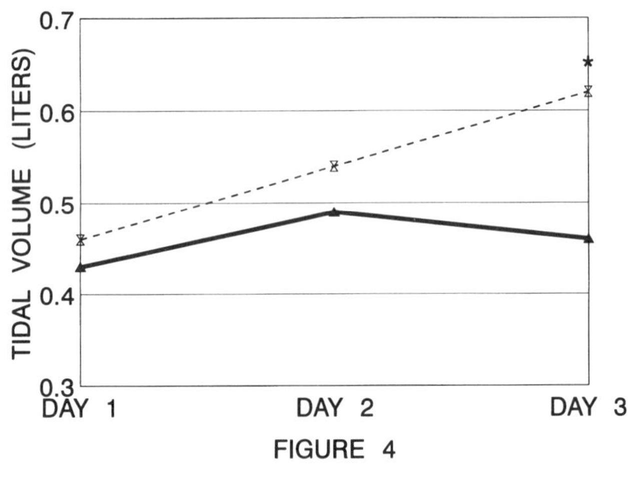

Fig 6–8.—Tidal volume was significantly greater in the epidural group by day 3. *Analysis was performed with analysis of variance and significance at $P < .05$. (Courtesy of Luchette FA, Radafshar SM, Kaiser R, et al: *J Trauma* 36:865–870, 1994.)

with blunt chest trauma receiving local anesthetics through epidural or intrapleural catheters were evaluated.

Methods.—Nineteen patients aged 18 to 80 were admitted with multiple injuries including chest trauma. They received either bupivacaine or lidocaine.

Results.—Ten received intrapleural catheters and 9 received epidural catheters. All had similar treatment histories. Both groups had better pain relief with bupivacaine. The epidural group had significantly less pain (Figs 6–6 and 6–7). Tidal volume and negative inspiratory pressure were significantly greater for the group receiving epidural bupivacaine (Fig 6–8). Frequently, these patients initially experienced mild-to-moderate hypotension, which was easily corrected.

Conclusion.—Local anesthesia delivered by the epidural route is preferred over the intrapleural or systemic route.

▶ Epidural analgesia has repeatedly been shown to be an effective and versatile pain control option in the treatment of acute thoracic pain. Misperceptions about the risk and difficulty of epidural catheter insertion in the thoracic region have been slow to abate.—D.A. Van Alstine, M.D.

Interpleural Analgesia for Postoperative Pain Relief in Renal Surgery Patients

Kaukinen S, Kaukinen L, Kataja J, Kärkkäinen S, Heikkinen A (Tampere Univ, Finland)

Scand J Urol Nephrol 28:39–43, 1994 131-95-6–12

Background.—After major upper abdominal surgery, good analgesia promotes early mobilization and adequate ventilatory function. Because centrally acting opioids can cause excessive sedation and hypoventilation, different regional analgesic methods have been explored. The feasibility of interpleural bupivacaine analgesia for relief of pain after transabdominal renal surgery by anterior subcostal incision was compared with that of IM oxycodone.

Methods.—Sixteen adults were enrolled in the study. Ten patients received 20 mL of bupivacaine plain, 5 mg/mL, and 6 patients received the same dose of bupivacaine with epinephrine, 5 μg/mL. The agents were injected through epidural catheters into the pleural space of the operated side 3 times per 24 hours maximally. Oxycodone was given IM as additional pain medication was needed. Oxycodone was the only medication given for pain in 10 control patients.

Findings.—Among patients receiving interpleural bupivacaine plain, postoperative pain relief was excellent in 4, moderate in 4, and poor in 2. These patients received a mean of 2.1 injections of oxycodone over 3 days for supplemental pain relief. The patients in the control group received 11.6 injections of oxycodone. Pain relief was excellent in 6 of these patients and moderate in 4. The median duration of interpleural analgesia was 6 hours in those receiving bupivacaine plain and 7 hours in those receiving bupivacaine with epinephrine. The mean peak serum levels were 1,868 ng/mL for bupivacaine plain and 1,312 ng/mL for bupivacaine with epinephrine. There were no complications.

Conclusion.—Interpleural analgesia is safe and efficient in relieving postoperative pain after transabdominal renal surgery when the dose of 10 mL of bupivacaine, 5 mg/mL maximally 3 times a day, is not exceeded. Adding epinephrine reduces the peak concentrations of serum bupivacaine. Parenteral opioids are a feasible choice when additional pain relief is needed.

▶ The investigators compared interpleural bupivacaine with IM oxycodone to evaluate analgesia after renal surgery. The weaknesses of the article include the fact that relief of pain was not evaluated with a visual analogue scale, and that although respiratory function was discussed in the article, it was not measured in the patients. The authors state that interpleural bupivacaine decreases both the dose requirements of opioids and complications such as excessive sedation. However, from a clinician's standpoint, if the patient is allowed to titrate the opioid dose with a patient-controlled analgesia, excessive sedation is unlikely.—E. Lang, M.D.

Interpleural or Thoracic Epidural Analgesia for Pain After Thoracotomy: A Double Blind Study

Brockmeier V, Moen H, Karlsson BR, Fjeld NB, Reiestad F, Steen PA (Ullevål Univ, Oslo, Norway)

Acta Anaesthesiol Scand 38:317–321, 1993 131-95-6–13

Introduction.—Epidural analgesia using bupivacaine is often used to control pain after thoracotomy. However, serious complications can be associated with this approach. Although information regarding interpleural analgesia is limited, it may offer adequate analgesic effect with a lower risk than epidural analgesia. Interpleural and epidural analgesic effects after thoracotomy were compared in a double-blind, placebo-controlled investigation.

Methods.—Interpleural and epidural catheters were placed in 32 patients undergoing elective thoracotomy. Patients were randomized to receive either interpleural or epidural analgesia. The 16 patients in the interpleural group received bupivacaine, 5 mg/mL, with 5 μg of epinephrine as a 30-mL interpleural bolus. Drainage tubes were clamped during and 15 minutes after the bolus injection. The epidural group of 16 patients received bupivacaine, 3.75 mg/mL, with 5 μg of epinephrine as a 5-mL epidural bolus. Pain intensity was graded using the Prince-Henry pain scale.

Results.—Although not significant, there was a tendency toward faster analgesic effect in the interpleural group. There was no significant difference in pain scores between the 2 groups. No significant difference was observed in the need for increased infusion rates of analgesic or the need for additional morphine in either group. One patient in the epidural group experienced an epidural hematoma, which was removed. However, the patient experienced complete paralysis below the T5 level resulting from an unacceptable delay in diagnosis and treatment.

Conclusion.—There was no difference in analgesic effect between the interpleural and epidural groups. Interpleural analgesia is recommended because the catheter can be quickly and easily positioned, and it is not associated with the serious side effects that are associated with epidural analgesia.

▶ It is important to note that epidural catheter placement can have serious, albeit rare, complications. The authors did not investigate the plasma concentrations of local anesthetic, an important consideration for interpleural analgesia. The double-blinded design of this study should be commended.—E. Lang, M.D.

Interpleural Infusion of 2% Lidocaine With 1:200,000 Epinephrine for Postthoracotomy Analgesia

Raffin L, Fletcher D, Sperandio M, Antoniotti C, Mazoit X, Bisson A, Fischler M (CMC Foch, Suresnes, France; Hôpital de Bicêtre, France)

Anesth Analg 79:328–334, 1994 131-95-6–14

Background.—Interpleural administration of local anesthetics after thoracotomy may be beneficial because this method does not induce respiratory depression or change thoracic sympathetic tone when combined with opiates. However, the efficacy and toxicity of this procedure have been questioned. Interpleural analgesia with lidocaine and its effect on thoracostomy drainage were evaluated. In addition, the effectiveness of this therapy on pain, pulmonary function, and IV morphine requirements was assessed.

Methods.—Plasma concentrations of lidocaine after interpleural administration were measured in a group of 14 patients undergoing pneumonectomy or lobectomy. Seven patients had pneumonectomy without thoracostomy drainage (group TD−), and 7 had a lobectomy with thoracostomy drainage (group TD+). All patients received general anesthesia during surgery. A catheter was placed in the pleural cavity, and patients were connected to a patient-controlled analgesia pump that delivered morphine in a bolus of 1–1.5 mg on request. A 2% lidocaine solution combined with 1:200,000 epinephrine was administered upon the first report of postoperative pain. A bolus of 3 mg/kg was injected during a 5-minute period, and then it was infused continuously for the next 48 hours. Blood samples were drawn at intervals in relation to the bolus and after the infusion was completed. A second group of 16 patients undergoing lobectomy was divided equally into 2 groups: group L received 2% lidocaine combined with 1:200,000 epinephrine; group P received normal saline as a placebo. A .15-mL/kg bolus of solution was injected during 5 minutes; it was then infused continuously for 48 hours. Visual analogue scale (VAS) pain scores were recorded hourly for 6 hours, and then every 6 hours for 48 hours. Arterial blood gases and pulmonary function tests were conducted. The amount of morphine requested and actually used by this group was noted. Data were analyzed with 2-way analysis of variance, Scheffe's test, and the Mann-Whitney *U*-test.

Results.—No severe toxicity was noted in any group despite the high levels of lidocaine measured in many patients 24 hours after the first infusion. A high concentration of lidocaine is the result of a low clearance rate that is masked in the thoracic drainage group because the drug is lost through the chest tubes. The plasma concentration of lidocaine after 24 hours was lower in the TD+ group than the TD− group, but elimination of the drug was approximately the same in both groups. Initially, VAS pain scores were higher in the placebo group, but after 6 hours, the scores were about the same in groups P and L. Morphine requirements were nearly the same in groups P and L, but no patient in this study reported consistent analgesia. Little clinical effect on pain, arterial blood gas, or pulmonary function test was noted.

Conclusion.—Interpleural administration of lidocaine does not diminish morphine requirements significantly. Because of the high level of drug that accumulates in the interpleural space, interpleural analgesia is unsafe in patients undergoing pneumonectomy without thoracic drainage.

▶ It is interesting how different investigators come to different conclusions in their studies. In this case, the authors stress the potential for local anesthetic toxicity despite not having had problems with it in their study. In any event, they did not find interpleural lidocaine to be beneficial.—E. Lang, M.D.

Effect of Intraoperative Ketorolac on Postanesthesia Care Unit Comfort

Valdrighi JB, Hanowell LH, Loeb RG, Behrman KH, Disbrow EA (Univ of California at Davis, Sacramento)
J Pain Symptom Manage 9:171–174, 1994 131-95-6–15

Background.—Previous studies have found that ketorolac is an effective analgesic for patients with moderate postoperative pain. However, it is not as effective as morphine for managing severe pain in the immediate postoperative period. The effectiveness of combined intraoperative ketorolac and opioid analgesics has not been well studied. The effects of

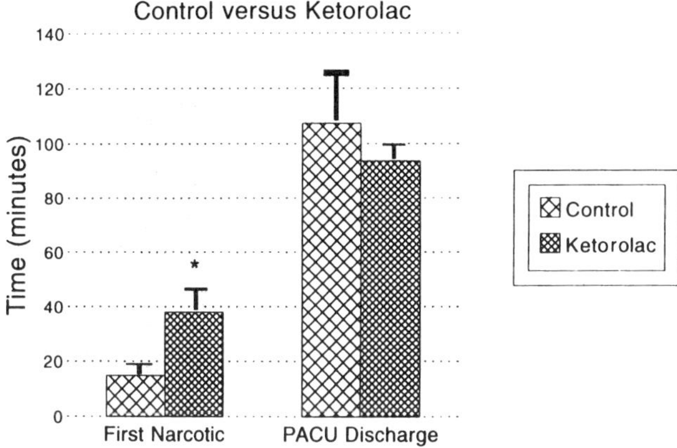

Fig 6–9.—Times to first opioid supplementation and postanesthesia care unit (*PACU*) discharge. The time to the first required dose of opioids in the PACU was greater in the ketorolac group vs. the control group ($P < .01$). The time to discharge from the PACU was not different between groups. (Courtesy of Valdrighi JB, Hanowell LH, Loeb RG, et al: *J Pain Symptom Manage* 9:171–174, 1994.)

intraoperative ketorolac on patient comfort in the postanesthesia care unit (PACU) were assessed.

Methods.—The prospective, randomized, double-blind study included 30 patients undergoing general anesthesia for orthopedic or lower abdominal surgical procedures. All patients received equivalent doses of intraoperative opioids. At the time of surgical closure, 1 group received 60 mg of ketorolac IM, and the other received 2 mL of normal saline. The patients were followed for up to 2 hours in the PACU; at 1 hour after PACU admission, pain was measured on a 100-point visual analogue scale.

Results.—Patients in the control group needed opioids more often and earlier than those in the ketorolac group. Time to first opioid dose in the PACU was 22 vs. 76 minutes, respectively (Fig 6–9). There was no significant difference in total dosage of postoperative opioids. Pain scores at 1 hour were 36 in the ketorolac group vs. 64 in the control group; there was no difference in time to PACU discharge.

Conclusion.—Intraoperative ketorolac appears to be an effective adjunct in the management of postoperative pain. It is possible that the analgesic properties of ketorolac are additive to those of morphine. Because ketorolac acts peripherally, independent of central opioid receptors, it may act synergistically with opioids to interrupt pain transmission.

▶ Not all studies have shown a benefit from intraoperative ketorolac. The timing of administration relative to the end of the procedure may be important.—D.A. Van Alstine, M.D.

Preoperative Naproxen Sodium Reduces Postoperative Pain Following Arthroscopic Knee Surgery

Code WE, Yip RW, Rooney ME, Browne PM, Hertz T (Royal Univ Hosp, Saskatoon, Saskatchewan)

Can J Anaesth 41:98–101, 1994 131-95-6–16

Introduction.—Although arthroscopy offers a number of advantages compared with open orthopedic surgical procedures, there are few reports of postarthroscopic pain. Some studies have suggested that nonsteroidal anti-inflammatory drugs (NSAIDs) may decrease the inflammation associated with arthroscopic procedures, probably through inhibition of prostaglandin synthesis. The efficacy of preoperative naproxen sodium in reducing postoperative pain and length of day surgery stay in patients undergoing arthroscopic knee surgery was investigated in a randomized, double-blind trial.

Methods.—The subjects were 66 American Society of Anesthesiologists (ASA) I and II patients undergoing outpatient arthroscopic knee surgery. Twenty-six patients received two 275-mg capsules of naproxen sodium, and the other 40 received placebo. Outcome measures included preoperative and postoperative visual analogue pain scores, postoperative analgesic requirements before discharge and 24 hours afterward, and length of day surgery stay.

Results.—Postoperative pain decreased with naproxen, both in the hospital and after discharge. The groups did not differ in their need for in-hospital postoperative analgesics or time to discharge. However, 71% of the placebo group required analgesics after discharge, compared with 30% of the naproxen group.

Conclusion.—A single preoperative dose of naproxen sodium, 550 mg, can reduce postoperative pain in patients undergoing arthroscopic knee surgery. Significant pain reductions are noted both before discharge and for up to 24 hours afterward.

▶ The effectiveness of this simple intervention was fascinating. It remains unclear how the concepts of preemptive analgesia and "wind-up" fit into the acute postoperative pain control techniques we routinely use. The potential for bleeding problems from a single dose of naproxen sodium is small, but it probably should have been addressed in this article.—D.A. Van Alstine, M.D.

The Effects of Perioperative Ketorolac Infusion on Postoperative Pain and Endocrine-Metabolic Response

Varrassi G, Panella L, Piroli A, Marinangeli F, Varrassi S, Wolman I, Niv D (L'Aquila Univ, Italy)

Anesth Analg 78:514–519, 1994 131-95-6–17

Objective.—Ketorolac is a nonsteroidal anti-inflammatory drug that has potent analgesic properties. The effectiveness and safety of infusing ketorolac in the perioperative period was examined in 95 patients undergoing cholecystectomy with a subcostal incision.

Study Plan.—Forty-eight patients received IM ketorolac in a dose of 30 mg at the time of premedication, followed by a continuous infusion of 2 mg/hr for 24 hours. Forty-seven patients received a bolus of physiologic saline followed by a continuous infusion of 2 mL/hr. Morphine was available by patient-controlled analgesia.

Results.—Patients who were given ketorolac had better relief of pain than the control patients, and they had significantly lower sedation scores. Ketorolac-treated patients required less morphine postoperatively, but the difference was not significant. The ketorolac group had significantly lower plasma cortisol levels at 2 and 6 hours postoperatively. There were no significant group differences in plasma catecholamine or glucose, and ketorolac did not alter hemostasis or renal function. Adverse effects were substantially less frequent in the patients given ketorolac. Two controls had clinically evident respiratory depression.

Conclusion.—Ketorolac given perioperatively to patients having major abdominal surgery safely reduces pain in the immediate postoperative period and also limits the need for opioid treatment.

▶ This paper was selected because it investigated the novel method of ketorolac administration as well as endocrine effects. Although the effect on cortisol was not overwhelming, it was clinically significant, suggesting that this may be one more means of ameliorating stress response in selected patients. Interestingly, despite many surgeons' fears, no problems with renal function or coagulation were noted.—J.D. Haddox, D.D.S., M.D.

Ketorolac as a Component of Balanced Analgesia After Thoracotomy

Power I, Bowler GMR, Pugh GC, Chambers WA (Royal Infirmary of Edinburgh, Scotland; City Hosp, Edinburgh, Scotland)

Br J Anaesth 72:224–226, 1994 131-95-6–18

Rationale.—Patients undergoing thoracotomy may receive an intercostal nerve block and patient-controlled morphine to relieve postoperative pain. Many patients are not satisfactorily relieved, however, and they may require a repeat block. Accordingly, a double-blind, placebo-controlled study was planned to learn whether adding IM ketorolac to the basic regimen enhances patient comfort.

Study Plan.—Seventy-five adult patients (age range, 18–75 years) requiring elective pneumonectomy or lobectomy (or, in 10 cases, segmental resection) for cancer were assigned to receive either ketorolac or a placebo at the end of surgery. Anesthesia included an intercostal nerve block with bupivacaine. Ketorolac was given IM in a dose of 10 or 30 mg every 6 hours, starting before anesthesia was discontinued and continuing for 50 hours. The use of patient-controlled morphine was monitored, and pain was rated on a visual analogue scale.

Results.—Inadequate analgesia was more frequent in placebo recipients than in patients given either dose of ketorolac. The higher dose conferred no apparent advantage. The placebo recipients used 15 mg more morphine on average in the first 48 hours than the ketorolac-treated patients.

Conclusion.—Ketorolac improved analgesia after thoracotomy when added to the basic regimen of intercostal nerve block and patient-administered morphine.

▶ This article demonstrates the efficacy of using ketorolac in addition to patient-administered morphine and intercostal block. The study size is comparatively large. It is interesting to note that the higher dose of ketorolac did not confer any additional benefit. Could this be because of the age of the patients? In many institutions, patients in this age range receive doses that are lower than "normal" because of presumed lower renal clearance of the drug, which would allow these patients to achieve reasonable tissue levels of ketorolac at lower doses. Unfortunately, serum levels of ketorolac were not measured. The small amount of morphine savings is not clinically significant. Rather, the improved comfort is more important, in my opinion. Also, no unusual side effects were noted. This is one more paper to justify the use of this drug as part of a "balanced analgesic" scheme for the postoperative patient.—J.D. Haddox, D.D.S., M.D.

Indomethacin as Adjunct Analgesia Following Open Cholecystectomy

Turner GA, Gorringe J (Royal Perth Hosp, Australia)

Anaesth Intensive Care 22:25–29, 1994 131-95-6–19

Objective.—Because nonsteroidal anti-inflammatory drugs (NSAIDs) are increasingly used to relieve postoperative pain, it was determined whether indomethacin, in suppository form, can limit the need for opioid after open cholecystectomy.

Study Design.—Fifty patients who were scheduled for elective cholecystectomy were anesthetized in a standard manner and were randomly assigned to receive indomethacin or placebo suppositories. Two 100-mg suppositories were given before anesthesia was reversed, followed by 100 mg given twice daily for 3 days. Meperidine was given as needed by patient-controlled analgesia (PCA).

Results.—Patients given indomethacin suppositories required significantly less opioid than placebo recipients at all postoperative intervals. They also had lower pain scores at rest and on movement. Less than half as much opiate was used by indomethacin-treated patients in the first 3 postoperative days. Nausea and indigestion were comparably frequent in the 2 groups. Two NSAID-treated patients had symptoms of proctitis. There was no difference in peak serum creatinine values.

Conclusion.—The use of indomethacin suppositories for 3 days after major abdominal surgery can reduce the need for PCA meperidine by as much as half and, at the same time, enhance pain relief.

▶ This is yet one more study that demonstrates the efficacy of NSAIDs in the treatment of postoperative pain. This is one of the few studies to use indomethacin. The only significant side effect was proctitis, the result of the route of administration. Indomethacin is available for IV pediatric use for patent ductus arteriosus closure, but it has not been used, to my knowledge, in the management of postoperative pain.—J.D. Haddox, D.D.S., M.D.

A Placebo-Controlled Comparative Evaluation of Diclofenac Dispersible Versus Ibuprofen in Postoperative Pain After Third Molar Surgery

Bakshi R, Frenkel G, Dietlein G, Meurer-Witt B, Schneider B, Sinterhauf U (Ciba-Geigy Limited, Basel, Switzerland; Centre for Dental, Oral and Maxillo-Facial Diseases, Frankfurt, Germany)

J Clin Pharmacol 34:225–230, 1994 131-95-6–20

Introduction.—Diclofenac is a potent nonsteroidal anti-inflammatory drug (NSAID) that is chiefly used to treat rheumatic disorders, but these drugs have increasingly been used to treat other types of painful conditions. They exert a rapid analgesic effect through inhibiting cyclooxygenase and, thereby, the production of prostaglandin. Diclofenac is now available as an oral solution.

Objective.—The analgesic value of single doses of liquid diclofenac was compared with that of ibuprofen and a placebo in a randomized, double-blind study of 245 adults who had severe pain after undergoing extraction of an impacted lower third molar.

Methods.—A double-dummy, parallel-group, placebo-controlled design was used to compare single 50-mg doses of liquid diclofenac with 400 mg of ibuprofen. Only patients whose visual analogue scores indicated severe or very intense pain after extraction were included in the study.

Results.—Both diclofenac and ibuprofen significantly reduced pain 1 hour after the start of treatment, compared with placebo, and both active treatments led to a sustained reduction in mean pain intensity scores over the 6-hour study. Diclofenac was significantly better than ibuprofen only at 20 minutes after intake. Two thirds of the placebo recipients and only about one fourth of those who were actively treated required additional analgesia. Adverse effects were infrequent in all groups.

Conclusion.—Severe pain from extraction of an impacted molar may be rapidly relieved by diclofenac solution. This agent also may be useful for patients, such as those having tonsillectomy, who cannot easily swallow solid medication.

▶ This article was chosen to highlight the applicability of different forms of NSAIDs to various clinical situations. Although the results are not earth-shattering, it is, nonetheless, an interesting formulation of drug that may have widespread potential. Interestingly, oral administration of parenteral ketorolac appears to be quite effective in patients who are unable to swallow pills. Naprosyn is currently available in a liquid form in the United States.—J.D. Haddox, D.D.S., M.D.

Low-Dose Intra-Articular Morphine Analgesia in Day Case Knee Arthroscopy: A Randomized Double-Blinded Prospective Study

Dalsgaard J, Felsby S, Juelsgaard P, Froekjaer J (Aarhus Univ, Denmark)

Pain 56:151–154, 1994 131-95-6–21

Background.—Some studies have shown a significant effect of low-dose morphine injected into the knee joint after arthroscopy; other studies have revealed no significant effect. The analgesic effect of low-dose intra-articular morphine on the first postoperative day in patients undergoing knee arthroscopy with lidocaine infiltration analgesia was evaluated.

Methods.—Fifty-two healthy adult patients were double-blindly randomized to receive either 1 mg of morphine chloride (.2 mg/mL, 5 mL) or a saline placebo (5 mL). Infiltration analgesia was done with lidocaine (10 mg/mL) with epinephrine, 20 mL into the skin and joint capsule and

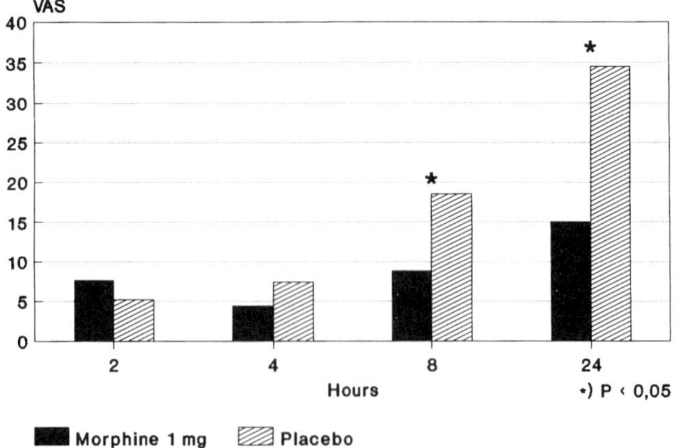

Fig 6–10.—Visual analogue scale score (mean) in patients given intra-articular morphine or placebo after knee anthroscopy. (Courtesy of Dalsgaard J, Felsby S, Juelsgaard P, et al: *Pain* 56:151–154, 1994.)

10 mL within the joint. Postoperatively, irrigation fluid was drained from the knee and 5 mL of blinded project medicine injected intra-articularly. At 2, 4, 8, and 24 hours after arthroscopy, the patients recorded their pain on a standard visual analogue scale. At discharge, the patients were requested to record their acetaminophen consumption.

Results.—The visual analogue scale scores were similar in the 2 groups at 2 and 4 hours after surgery. However, the scores at 8 and 24 hours were significantly lower in the morphine group (Fig 6–10). Between 8 and 24 hours after surgery, the consumption of acetaminophen was significantly lower in the morphine group. The maximal effect of morphine occurred 24 hours postoperatively. Because any central effect of 1 mg of intra-articular morphine must be negligible, the hypothesis that intra-articular opiate receptors exist was supported. Analgesia was more effective after transarthroscopic surgery than after purely diagnostic arthroscopy, consistent with a local anti-inflammatory effect of morphine. The intra-articular lidocaine provided analgesia for the first few postoperative hours.

Conclusion.—After knee arthroscopy, 1 mg of intra-articular morphine gives efficient analgesia for more than 24 hours. When combined with lidocaine used as anesthesia, the combination offers effective and long-lasting pain relief without side effects.

▶ This article suggests that opioid receptors exist peripherally in humans. Intra-articular morphine after arthroscopy may provide analgesia, as this study suggests. It is important that the investigators differentiated between the multitude of procedures that are done arthroscopically. Not all studies have done this.—E. Lang, M.D.

Intraarticular Morphine for Pain Relief After Knee Arthroscopy Performed Under Regional Anaesthesia

Niemi L, Pitkänen M, Tuominen M, Björkenheim J-M, Rosenberg PH (Helsinki Univ, Finland)

Acta Anaesthesiol Scand 38:402–405, 1994 131-95-6–22

Background.—After arthroscopic knee surgery in patients receiving general anesthesia, low doses of intra-articular morphine have an analgesic effect. The analgesic effect of low-dose, intra-articular morphine after arthroscopic surgery done under 2 types of regional anesthesia—spinal and local—was examined.

Methods.—Eighty adult patients undergoing knee arthroscopy were divided into 2 groups—40 patients for the spinal anesthesia study and 40 patients for the local anesthesia study. Patients in the spinal anesthesia study (overnight-inpatients) received 3 mL of hyperbaric .5% bupivacaine in the subarachnoid space at the L3–4 interspace. The patients were randomized into 2 groups of 20 patients each. Postoperatively, in double-

Need for Postoperative Analgesics in the Study Patients

	Morphine	Control
Spinal anaesthesia		
- Oxycodone requirement		
- No. of patients	10/20	10/20
- No. of doses	17	27
- Ketoprofen requirement		
- No. of patients	9/20	9/20
- No. of doses	12	13
- Initial analgesia time (min) [range]	426 [250–1200]	375 [230–535]
Local anaesthesia		
- Need for ketoprofen		
- No. of patients	14/20	18/20
- No. of doses	22*	39*
- Initial analgesia time (min) [range]	590 [15–1110]	412 [60–990]

* $P < .05$.

(Courtesy of Niemi L, Pitkänen M, Tuominen M, et al: *Acta Anaesthesiol Scand* 38:402–405, 1994.)

blind fashion, the surgeon injected intra-articularly either 1 mg of morphine or .5 mL of saline (both to a total volume of 10 mL). A numeral pain scale was used to assess pain postoperatively at 1, 3, 6, and 24 hours. Side effects and need for supplemental medications were recorded. The other group of 40 patients (day surgery) received local anesthesia with 1% lidocaine plus epinephrine. They were randomized into 2 groups of 20 patients each. Postoperatively, they received either 1 mg of morphine in 10 mL of saline or 10 mL of saline intra-articularly in a double-blind fashion. Postoperative pain was assessed at 1 and 3 hours after the intra-articular injection. On discharge from the hospital, the patients were asked to record their use of ketoprofen for 24 hours postoperatively.

Results.—In the spinal anesthesia group, there were no significant differences in the pain scores or in the requirement for rescue medication between patients who received intra-articular morphine and those who did not (table). The median pain scores assessed at the predetermined time points were similar in both local anesthetic groups, but the group that received intra-articular morphine needed significantly less postoperative ketoprofen.

Conclusion.—Postoperative analgesia in patients undergoing knee arthroscopy under local anesthesia is improved by the intra-articular injection of 1 mg of morphine at the end of the procedure. Intra-articular injection of morphine in patients receiving bupivacaine spinal anesthesia for arthroscopy has no apparent analgesic effect postoperatively.

▶ It is noteworthy that these authors did not find a correlation between the degree of pain/consumption of supplemental analgesics and the surgical procedure. The conclusion that patients undergoing knee arthroscopy while receiving bupivacaine anesthesia had no benefit from intra-articular morphine could be the result of spinal analgesia with bupivacaine that outlasted the intra-articular morphine. Repeating this study with lidocaine spinal analgesia would be interesting.—E. Lang, M.D.

Intra-Articular Morphine and Bupivacaine Analgesia After Arthroscopic Knee Surgery

Haynes TK, Appadurai IR, Power I, Rosen M, Grant A (Univ Hosp of Wales, Cardiff; Prince of Wales Hosp, Pentyrch, Wales)

Anaesthesia 49:54–56, 1994 131-95-6–23

Background.—Authorities disagree on the value of intra-articular bupivacaine injection after arthroscopy. The efficacy of intra-articular morphine, intra-articular bupivacaine, and a combination of the 2 in the first 24 hours after arthroscopic knee surgery was assessed.

Methods and Findings.—Forty patients undergoing arthroscopic knee surgery were enrolled in the double-blind, randomized, controlled trial. Facilitation of mobilization, reduction of postoperative pain, and analgesic requirement for 24 hours after surgery were noted. Compared with placebo, all treatments were more effective in enabling earlier mobilization and reducing postoperative pain as assessed on a visual analogue scale. Morphine alone provided the best analgesia. This agent significantly reduced analgesic consumption for 24 hours after surgery.

Conclusion.—In patients who have had arthroscopic knee surgery, 1 mg of morphine delivered intra-articularly effectively relieves pain and reduces postoperative analgesia requirements. Adding bupivacaine is less effective and is not cost-effective.

▶ The authors found that the addition of bupivacaine to intra-articular morphine was less effective than morphine alone. They suggest that this may be caused by the patients feeling a change as the bupivacaine wears off. A fascinating idea!—E. Lang, M.D.

Analgesic Effect of Intraarticular Morphine, Bupivacaine, and Morphine/Bupivacaine After Arthroscopic Knee Surgery

Boden BP, Fassler S, Cooper S, Marchetto PA, Moyer RA (Temple Univ, Philadelphia)

Arthroscopy 10:104–107, 1994 131-95-6–24

Background.—Some studies have shown that intra-articular bupivacaine is an effective analgesic. The effects of intra-articular bupivacaine were compared with those of morphine and a combination of morphine and bupivacaine.

Methods.—Thirty-eight patients were enrolled in the double-blind, randomized trial. The patients were divided into 4 groups and given intra-articular injections of different agents after arthroscopic surgery. The 7 patients in group 1 were given saline; the 10 in group 2, morphine; the 10 in group 3, bupivacaine; and the 11 in group 4, combined morphine and bupivacaine. Pain levels were documented at regular intervals, and patient requests for supplemental IV morphine postoperatively were recorded.

Findings.—The mean consumption of supplemental analgesia was lowest in the group receiving combined morphine and bupivacaine. Pain scores differed significantly between the saline group and the other 3 groups in the early postoperative period. No significant differences were found among the 3 active treatment groups.

Conclusion.—Intra-articular injection of analgesics after surgery effectively reduces pain levels. The combination of morphine and bupivacaine appears to be best, as patients receiving this injection had the lowest mean consumption of supplemental analgesia.

▶ In this study, the authors found that patients receiving a combination of intra-articular bupivacaine and morphine required less supplemental analgesia than the other groups. The visual analogue scale was statistically similar in all groups, except those receiving intra-articular saline. This contrasts with results from the previous study.—E. Lang, M.D.

Addition of Morphine to Intra-Articular Bupivacaine Does Not Improve Analgesia After Day-Case Arthroscopy

Laurent SC, Nolan JP, Pozo JL, Jones CJ (Royal United Hosp, Bath, England; Leicester Royal Infirmary, England)

Br J Anaesth 72:170–173, 1994 131-95-6–25

Introduction.—Effective control of postoperative pain will affect the outcome of day-case surgery. Surgeons frequently inject bupivacaine into the knee joint after knee arthroscopy to reduce postoperative pain; however, results are variable. Recent reports suggest that intra-articular morphine provides more effective and longer-acting analgesia than expected from the same dose given systemically. Three studies have suggested that a mixture of morphine and bupivacaine may be the optimal analgesia.

Methods.—A randomized, double-blind, controlled study was conducted in patients undergoing day-case knee arthroscopy to evaluate the analgesic effect of intra-articular morphine, 2 mg or 5 mg, added to .25% bupivacaine and to compare the analgesic effect with .25% bupivacaine alone. Twenty patients received .25% bupivacaine, 40 mL, with morphine, 5 mg (group BM5); 20 patients received .25% bupivacaine, 40

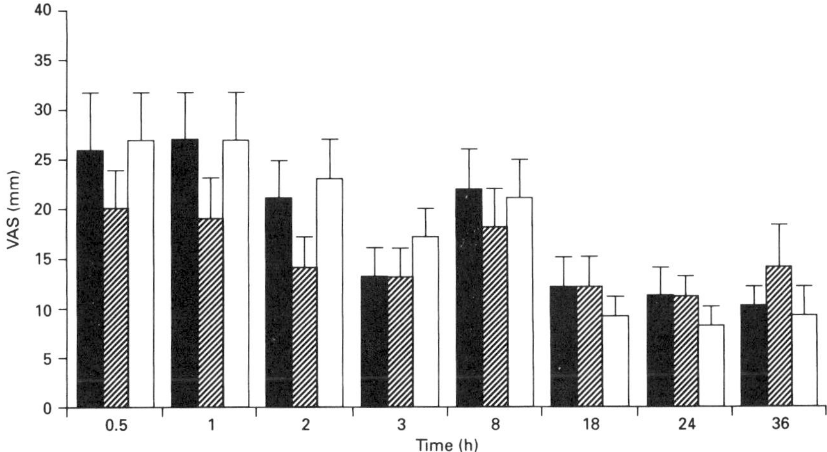

Fig 6–11.—Visual analogue scores (VAS) (mean [SEM]), with the knee at rest, with time after tourniquet release. Group BM5 (*filled square*), *n* = 20; group BM2 (*striped square*), *n* = 20; group B0 (*open square*), *n* = 18. (Courtesy of Laurent SC, Nolan JP, Pozo JL, et al: *Br J Anaesth* 72:170–173, 1994).

mL, with morphine, 2 mg (group BM2); and 18 patients received .25% bupivacaine, 40 mL only (group B0). Pain was assessed before and after the operation for 36 hours, at rest and with movement, using a 100-mm visual analogue scale.

Results.—There were no significant differences in pain scores, in consumption of additional analgesia, or in the time to first request for analgesia between any of the groups (Fig 6–11). A difference was detected with 80% certainty in the visual analogue scale of 12 mm at rest and 16 mm on movement. None of the patients experienced side effects that required inpatient admission. One patient required medication for nausea.

Conclusion.—No additional analgesic effect is seen by the addition of morphine to intra-articular bupivacaine after day-case knee arthroscopy.

▶ The authors found no benefit in using intra-articular bupivacaine and morphine as opposed to using bupivacaine alone. Clearly, further research on the subject of intra-articular morphine will be required before the clinical importance of this technique is fully determined.—E. Lang, M.D.

Pre-Emptive Analgesia From Intravenous Administration of Opioids: No Effect With Alfentanil

Wilson RJT, Leith S, Jackson IJB, Hunter D (York District Hosp, England)
Anaesthesia 49:591–593, 1994 131-95-6–26

Objective.—Whether IV alfentanil given before the surgical incision reduces the postoperative need for opioid analgesia compared with administering the same dose after surgery begins was determined.

Methods.—Forty American Society of Anesthesiologists class I or II patients (25 to 65 years of age) were scheduled for total abdominal hysterectomy via a transverse lower abdominal incision. All patients received temazepam as premedication and propofol for induction. The patients were assigned to receive either alfentanil in a dose of 40 μg/kg (study group) or physiologic saline (control group) at the time of induction. Anesthesia was maintained with 1% to 2% enflurane in oxygen and 65% to 70% nitrous oxide. The control patients received the same 40-μg/kg dose of alfentanil 1 minute after surgical incision, and patients in both groups received morphine, .1 mg/kg, at this time. Patient-controlled analgesia with morphine was used postoperatively.

Results.—There were no significant group differences in the amount of morphine used during surgery, in the recovery room, or as long as 24 hours postoperatively. At 24 hours, control patients had significantly lower visual analogue pain scores at rest, but scores on movement were identical in the 2 groups.

Conclusion.—Preemptive analgesia, using conventional doses of parenteral opioid, was not found to be clinically useful.

▶ This is an interesting article. It is possible that preemptive analgesia cannot be provided with systemic opioids. Possibly, sufficient doses of systemically administered opioids cannot be achieved in the dorsal horn to effect neuroplasticity. Perhaps administration of the opioid must begin some time before the surgery, as has been reported with regional preemptive analgesia. This certainly warrants further study.—E. Lang, M.D.

Interactions Between Fluoxetine and Opiate Analgesia for Postoperative Dental Pain

Gordon NC, Heller PH, Gear RW, Levine JD (Univ of California, San Francisco; Kaiser Found Hosp, Hayward, Calif)

Pain 58:85–88, 1994 131-95-6–27

Objective.—The role of serotonergic mechanisms in opiate analgesia was investigated in a double-blind, placebo-controlled study comparing the analgesic efficacy of combinations of fluoxetine, a serotonergic tricyclic antidepressant, with either the μ-opiate morphine or the κ-opiate pentazocine.

Methods.—Seventy patients who were to have impacted third molar teeth extracted participated. The patients were randomly assigned to receive either fluoxetine in an oral dose of 10 mg or a placebo each day for 1 week before surgery. Pain was recorded on a visual analogue scale, and when pain of at least one quarter (2.5 cm) was recorded (but no sooner than 80 minutes after the onset of local anesthesia), the patients received a single-blind open IV injection of either 6 mg of morphine sulfate or 45 mg of pentazocine.

Results.—Placebo recipients experienced a peak reduction in pain of about 2 cm on the visual analogue scale. Morphine analgesia lasted 2–3 hours, whereas pentazocine analgesia lasted about 1.5 hours. Pretreatment with fluoxetine did not affect pentazocine analgesia, but it significantly lessened the analgesic effect of morphine. After 90 minutes, patients given fluoxetine and morphine had more pain than at baseline.

Interpretation.—The attenuating effect of fluoxetine on μ-opiate analgesia probably reflects an alteration in the serotonergic circuits that modulate pain.

▶ There are reports of fluoxetine being a useful agent in some chronic pain states. Its apparent attenuation of the analgesic effect of morphine is fascinating and serves to emphasize the concept that acute and chronic pain are often very different entities that share the final common end point of perception of pain by the patient.—D.A. Van Alstine, M.D.

Immediate and Prolonged Effects of Pre- Versus Postoperative Epidural Analgesia With Bupivacaine and Morphine on Pain at Rest and During Mobilisation After Total Knee Arthroplasty

Dahl JB, Daugaard JJ, Rasmussen B, Egebo K, Carlsson P, Kehlet H (Hvidovre Univ, Denmark; Univ Hosps in Århus, Denmark)

Acta Anaesthesiol Scand 38:557–561, 1994 131-95-6–28

Introduction.—Some recent studies have suggested that preoperative induction of analgesia may improve postoperative control of pain, but the results of comparative trials have varied. The immediate and prolonged analgesic effects of preoperative initiation vs. immediate postoperative initiation of intensive epidural administration of bupivacaine and morphine were compared.

Methods.—Thirty-two patients undergoing total knee arthroplasty were randomly assigned to receive identical epidural blockades initiated either 30 minutes before incision or during surgical closure. The patients assessed their pain using both a visual analogue scale and a verbal scale at rest and during elevation of the limb. Pain scores and requests for additional pain medication during a 7-day observation period were compared for the 2 groups.

Results.—There were no significant differences between the 2 groups in either visual analogue or verbal scale pain scores. The need for additional morphine or ketobemidone/morphine was comparable in the 2 groups throughout the 7 days. Only the use of postoperative fentanyl differed, with more patients in the postoperative epidural block group receiving fentanyl.

Discussion.—Immediate and prolonged pain control did not significantly differ between the group receiving preoperative initiation and the group receiving postoperative initiation of the epidural blockade.

▶ The notion of preemptive analgesia has received a great deal of interest in the literature. With our present understanding of spinal cord mechanisms, it seems to make intuitive sense. This study, however, is one of several that have demonstrated that, using conventional techniques, the timing of analgesia does not appear to make a significant difference in outcome in the postoperative period. Also, as noted in the figures accompanying the original article, continuous epidural infusion of .125% bupivacaine plus .005% morphine was insufficient to completely treat incident pain in the immediate postoperative period.—J.D. Haddox, D.D.S., M.D.

Sciatic Nerve Block: A Comparison of Single Versus Double Injection Technique

Bailey SL, Parkinson SK, Little WL, Simmerman SR (Naval Hosp, Portsmouth, Va)

Reg Anesth 19:9–13, 1994 131-95-6–29

Introduction.—The sciatic nerve, almost 2 cm wide, is the largest nerve in the body. Its 2 major components are the tibial and common peroneal branches. Because the nerve is so large, more than 1 injection may be better than a single injection. Two techniques for blocking the sciatic nerve, single vs. double injection, were prospectively evaluated for onset and efficacy in 50 adult patients undergoing lower extremity surgery.

Methods.—Twenty-five patients received a single injection of 20 mL of an amide-ester solution (1% lidocaine/.2% tetracaine) with epinephrine 1:200,000 when either component of the sciatic nerve (tibial or peroneal) was identified using a peripheral nerve stimulator. Twenty-five patients received two 10-mL injections of the same solution, with the tibial and peroneal components of the sciatic nerve being identified and injected separately. The tibial, common peroneal, and posterior femoral cutaneous nerves were evaluated up to 45 minutes after the initial injection of local anesthetic. To assess the block of the tibial and common peroneal nerves, motor function was used, whereas the pinprick response was used to assess block of the posterior femoral cutaneous nerve.

Results.—The double-injection group showed a faster onset and better efficacy ($P < .05$) at all time intervals (5–45 minutes). No complications were seen in any of the 50 patients tested.

Discussion.—The double-injection technique has a more rapid onset and increased efficacy of block than the single-injection technique for sciatic nerve block. A working knowledge of the anatomy of the sciatic

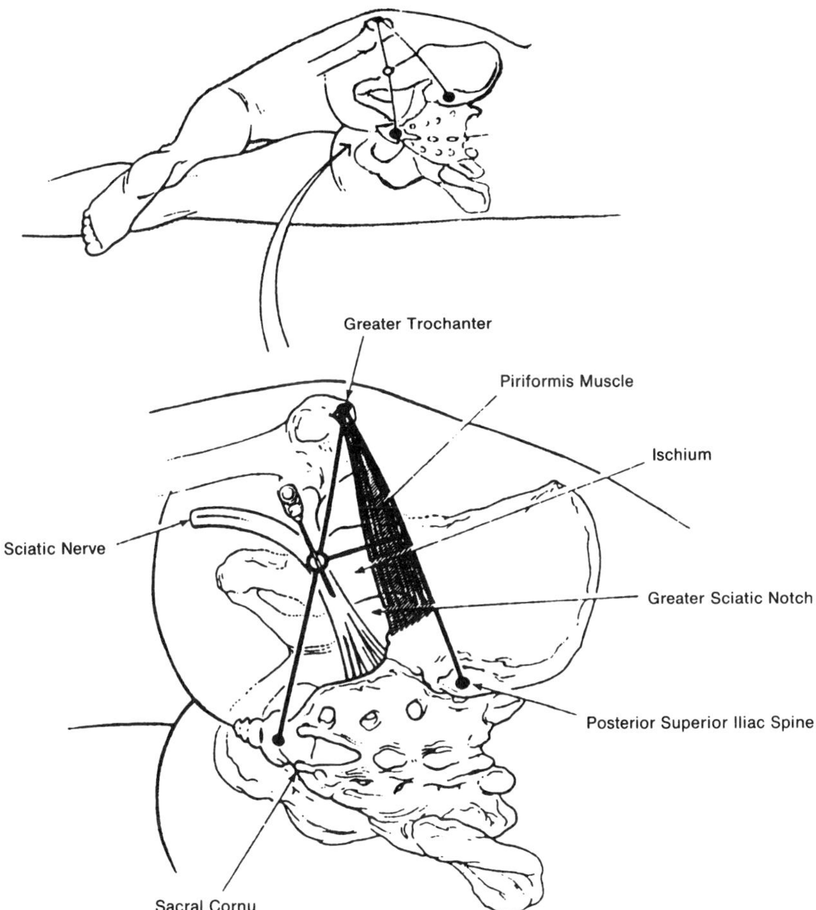

Fig 6–12.—Landmark anatomy for sciatic nerve block via Labat's approach. (From Bailey SL, Parkinson SK, Little WL, et al: *Reg Anesth* 19:9–13, 1994. Courtesy of Cousins MJ, Bridenbaugh PO: *Neural Blockade in Clinical Anesthesia and Management of Pain*, ed 2. Philadelphia, JB Lippincott, 1988, pp 424–426.)

nerve is required. The approach was a modification of Labat's classical approach. Lines were drawn from the greater trochanter to the posterior superior iliac spine and to a point about 1 cm below the sacral hiatus. From the midpoint of the superior border, a perpendicular line was drawn, and the needle was placed at the intersection of the perpendicular line and the inferior border (Fig 6–12).

▶ Many clinicians do not perform lower extremity nerve blocks because of lack of knowledge and fear of failure. This article was chosen because it describes an effective technique for blocking the sciatic nerve and increasing the chance of getting a good block with 2 injections.—E. Lang, M.D.

Brachial Plexus Block: A Comparison of the Supraclavicular Lateral Paravascular and Axillary Approaches

Fleck JW, Moorthy SS, Daniel J, Dierdorf SF (Indiana Univ, Indianapolis; Richard L Roudebush VA Med Ctr, Indianapolis, Ind)

Reg Anesth 19:14–17, 1994 131-95-6–30

Introduction.—Injuries to adjacent structures of the brachial plexus have been associated with anesthesia of the brachial plexus. Completion of the surgical procedure can be hindered by only partial block of the upper extremity. An effective, safe, recently proposed alternative to the traditional approaches to brachial plexus anesthesia is the supraclavicular lateral paravascular (SCLP) approach to brachial plexus anesthesia.

Methods.—In a randomized, prospective study, it was determined whether the SCLP approach was as effective as the transarterial axillary approach, the most common brachial plexus block used. Forty adult patients scheduled for upper extremity surgery were randomly assigned to receive brachial plexus block with either the SCLP or the axillary approach. Sensory function was assessed every 15 minutes.

Results.—The 2 groups did not differ with respect to age, weight, or type of surgery; however, 33 of the 40 patients were men. Eighty percent

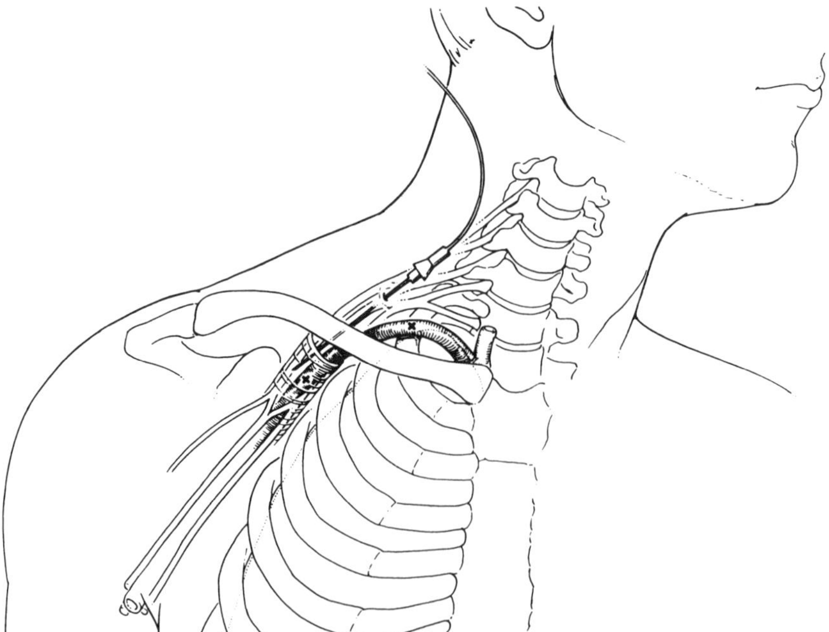

Fig 6–13.—In the supraclavicular lateral paravascular approach to brachial plexus block, the needle is directed caudally, posteriorly, and laterally toward the axilla and parallel to the subclavian artery. (Courtesy of Fleck JW, Moorthy SS, Daniel J, et al: *Reg Anesth* 19:14–17, 1994.)

of SCLP blocks (16 of 20) were good, and 65% (13 of 20) of axillary blocks were also good. The success rate was 95% with the SCLP approach and 90% with the axillary approach. There were no serious complications in either group.

Discussion.— In the SCLP approach to brachial plexus block, the needle is directed caudally, posteriorly, and laterally toward the axilla and parallel to the subclavian artery (Fig 6–13). The SCLP approach objectively identifies the brachial plexus and minimizes the risk of complications from brachial plexus block. The SCLP approach is as effective as the axillary approach.

► This article was chosen because it describes an effective technique for blocking the brachial plexus that has potentially fewer complications than the axillary approach.—E. Lang, M.D.

The Addition of Triamcinolone Acetonide to Bupivacaine Has No Effect on the Quality of Analgesia Produced by Ilioinguinal Nerve Block

McCleane G, Mackle E, Stirling I (Craigavon Area Hosp, County Armagh, Northern Ireland)

Anaesthesia 49:819–820, 1994 131-95-6–31

Background.—Although postoperative analgesia induced by local infiltration, nerve block, or epidural has the advantage of being nonsedating, it has the disadvantage of short duration. Local anesthetics bolstered by the addition of a steroid have been found to prolong analgesic effects through several mechanisms. The quality and duration of postoperative pain were evaluated in 30 men undergoing elective inguinal hernia repair. Patients who received bupivacaine alone were compared with patients who received bupivacaine in combination with triamcinolone acetonide.

Methods.—Thirty men scheduled for elective herniorrhaphy were randomly assigned to receive an ilioinguinal nerve block with either .5% bupivacaine alone or .5% bupivacaine supplemented with 40 mg of triamcinolone acetonide. Pain was assessed by the patients using a visual analogue scale and a patient rating scale at various intervals for 14 postoperative days. The amount of morphine delivered through a patient-controlled analgesia device was recorded for 24 hours after surgery. The Mann-Whitney *U*-test and the Wilcoxon rank sum test were used to analyze results.

Results.—The mean visual analogue scale scores showed no significant differences between groups, and there were no significant differences in the patient rating scales. Morphine consumption in the bupivacaine-only group and the bupivacaine/triamcinolone group was similar.

Conclusion.—The combination of 40 mg of triamcinolone acetonide with .5% bupivacaine administered as an ilioinguinal nerve block offers no advantage compared with the use of bupivacaine only with regard to the quality and duration of pain after inguinal hernia repair.

▶ It is not surprising that the addition of a steroid did not confer any advantage. A weakness of this study is that the investigators did not demonstrate that the ilioinguinal nerve block was useful in decreasing postoperative morphine requirements in their cohort. A third control group that received a block with saline would have been useful for this purpose. Repeating studies of this nature with better controls would be very worthwhile.—E. Lang, M.D.

Role of Psychological Factors in Postoperative Pain Control and Recovery With Patient-Controlled Analgesia

Perry F, Parker RK, White PF, Clifford PA (Stanford Univ, Palo Alto, Calif; Tufts Baystate Med Ctr, Medford, Mass; Univ of Texas Southwestern Med Ctr, Dallas)

Clin J Pain 10:57–63, 1994 131-95-6–32

Background.—According to patient reports, postoperative patient-controlled anesthesia (PCA) does not provide substantially improved pain relief compared with that achieved by IM injection of analgesics. Psychological variables may contribute to the perception of postoperative pain and the varied effectiveness of PCA. The effect of demographic and psychologic variables on the degree of postoperative pain, morphine usage, and the recovery profile was examined. The variables studied included age, ethnicity, preoperative anxiety level, preoperative expectation of pain, and the patient's need to be in control.

Patients.—A questionnaire was administered before surgery to 99 women undergoing abdominal hysterectomy who had no known cancer. The 5-question instrument measured preoperative anxiety level, expectations of pain, and the perceived need to be in control. All patients received standard anesthesia during surgery with thiopental and fentanyl for induction, then isoflurane and nitrous oxide for maintenance. In the recovery room, patients were connected to a PCA pump that infused morphine in a 2-mg bolus on demand. The number of milligrams of morphine actually infused postoperatively as well as the number of requests for the drug were recorded. The McGill Pain Questionnaire was administered to evaluate sensory and affective pain quality and to determine pain location and intensity. Visual analogue scales and the 5-point Likert scale measured the overall pain level. Recovery information was gleaned from patient records. A postoperative questionnaire was administered before discharge. Data were analyzed using Pearson product-moment correlation and multiple linear regression techniques.

Results.—The majority of women were satisfied with their PCA pain management, and 60% described their postoperative pain as moderate. Patients who had anticipated a great deal of pain and patients who reported a strong need to be in control of their pain reported a high degree of postoperative pain. Although older patients reported less pain, they required the same amount of morphine as other patients. The number of requests for morphine and the doses of morphine varied widely. Preoperative anxiety correlated positively with postoperative pain and predicted time to discharge. Anxious patients experienced more postoperative pain and were released from the hospital earlier than others; older patients were discharged later. Patients who had anticipated more pain overall indicated less pain on pain rating index scales.

Conclusion.—Psychological factors, such as the preoperative level of anxiety and demographic variables such as age, are significant predictors of postoperative pain. These factors influence the control of pain with PCA therapy and the time to hospital discharge.

▶ This article is important in that it shows how psychological considerations can determine the degree of postoperative pain that patients experience. The practitioner who is managing patients with postoperative pain needs to be aware of these factors.—E. Lang, M.D.

A Survey of the Intended Management of Acute Postoperative Pain by Newly Qualified Doctors in the South West Region of England in August 1992

Gould TH, Upton PM, Collins P (Derriford Hosp, Plymouth, England)

Anaesthesia 49:807–810, 1994 131-95-6–33

Purpose.—Many medical schools do not adequately teach the management of postoperative pain. The ability of newly qualified house staff to order and provide safe and effective postoperative analgesia was assessed.

Methods.—A questionnaire was sent to 203 medical and surgical house physicians. The questionnaire asked physicians to prescribe analgesia for 4 patients who had undergone various operations, to consider the appropriateness of prescribing nonsteroidal anti-inflammatory drugs (NSAIDs) for 6 patients with various medical conditions, and to manage pain in a hypotensive patient with epidural analgesia after a gastrectomy.

Results.—Only 54 (27%) completed questionnaires were received. Only 7 physicians (13%) would have prescribed the correct postoperative analgesia for all 4 patients, 16 (30%) would have prescribed NSAIDs for a patient with renal disease, 10 (18%) would have prescribed an NSAID for a patient receiving warfarin, and only 2 (4%) would have known how to correctly manage pain with an epidural infusion.

Conclusion.—The responses to this questionnaire indicate that most house physicians lack the required knowledge and skills to manage postoperative analgesia.

▶ In the face of ample evidence that most postoperative pain can be well controlled with easily learned techniques, the continued failure to teach medical students and house staff the basic elements of pain medicine represents a disconcerting lack of priorities in medical education.—D.A. Van Alstine, M.D.

Failure of Pain Relief After Surgery: Attitudes of Ward Staff and Patients to Postoperative Analgesia

Oates JDL, Snowdon SL, Jayson DWH (Royal Liverpool Univ Hosp, England)

Anaesthesia 49:755–758, 1994 131-95-6–34

Purpose.—Because postoperative pain management is often inadequate, many hospitals have instituted an acute pain service to manage postoperative analgesia. In a 3-part study, the severity of postoperative pain was assessed, the reasons why patients with pain did not receive more of the pain medication prescribed for them were examined, and why patients are reluctant to accept the analgesics prescribed for them was determined.

Methods.—During a 2-week period, 206 patients underwent a wide variety of elective operations and stayed in the hospital for at least 24 hours after. At 24 hours after surgery, patients were asked to rate the severity of their pain on a 10-point visual analogue scale. All analgesics prescribed and administered were recorded. For the second part of the study, 176 nursing and medical staff members were asked to complete a questionnaire to determine why patients who were in pain did not receive more of their prescribed analgesics. For the last part of the study, 200 patients completed a questionnaire between 11 hours and 3 days after surgery to determine why they were reluctant to accept analgesia.

Results.—Thirty patients (14.6%) reported no pain, and 105 (51%) rated their pain as mild, 52 (25.2%) as moderate, and 19 (9.2%) as severe. Patients with moderate and severe pain received only 36% of the pain medication prescribed for them. The most common reasons given by staff for not administering more of the prescribed analgesics were that patients did not ask for pain relief, were too sleepy, or refused the dose. Less common reasons were concerns about respiratory depression or addiction. The most common reason given by patients for not asking for pain relief was dislike or fear of injections.

Conclusion.—The hospital stay of many surgical patients could be improved by increasing staff awareness of the problems of postoperative pain and by encouraging patients to ask for pain relief more freely.

▶ The variability of patient and health care provider responses to questions about pain control reveals some of the underlying complexity that this "simple" issue actually contains. Given the options of IV, rectal, and even sublingual routes to deliver analgesics, we should be able to eliminate the fear of IV injections as a barrier to acceptable pain control.—D.A. Van Alstine, M.D.

Pre-Operative Analgesia for Acute Surgical Patients: No Place for Complacency

Fung ASY, Bentley TM (East Birmingham Hosp, England)

Ann R Coll Surg Engl 76:11–12, 1994 131-95-6–35

Purpose.—Because of concern that surgical patients may often fail to receive adequate relief of pain, the prescribing of preoperative analgesia was surveyed for 2 weeks at a district hospital in England that admits acute general surgery patients. Fourteen physicians who first treated these patients were asked about how and when they prescribe analgesics. A total of 139 patients were admitted on an emergency basis during the study.

Findings.—Opioid analgesia was believed to be appropriate preoperatively in 61 (44%) patients. Opinions about the need for analgesia in a given case differed, as did the perceived analgesic need and the actual provision of analgesia. Both under- and overprescribing were observed. All the physicians agreed that, when analgesia is thought to be needed, it is best given where the patient is first seen. Only 13% of patients, however, received analgesia before being taken to a ward. The mean time of treatment was 5 hours after arrival. More than one fourth (28%) of the patients received no analgesia before being operated on.

Conclusion.—For a variety of reasons, patients frequently fail to receive adequate analgesia preoperatively or must wait for an undue period. There is an urgent need to audit analgesic practices and optimize the provision of analgesia to acute surgical patients.

▶ When one looks at the distribution of cases in this study, it is a sad commentary that only 2 of 4 patients with peritonitis, 2 of 5 with an incarcerated hernia, 11 of 16 with appendicitis, and 2 of 3 with limb ischemia leading to amputation were given preoperative analgesics. Those of us who practice pain medicine must do everything in our power to heighten the sensitivity of our surgical and medical colleagues to this current epidemic of needless pain.—J.D. Haddox, D.D.S., M.D.

Intraperitoneal Bupivacaine for the Relief of Pain Following Day Case Laparoscopy

Loughney AD, Sarma V, Ryall EA (Royal Victoria Infirmary, Newcastle upon Tyne, England; North Tees Gen Hosp, Stockton on Tees, Cleveland, England)

Br J Obstet Gynaecol 101:449–451, 1994 131-95-6–36

Purpose.—Abdominal and shoulder tip pain are common after laparoscopic surgery. However, such pain might not be given sufficient attention in women outpatients. The severity and duration of postlaparoscopic pain were recorded, and the analgesic effectiveness of intraperitoneally infused bupivacaine was evaluated.

Methods.—Forty-seven women (age range, 18–55 years) underwent elective diagnostic laparoscopy because of intermittent pelvic pain or dyspareunia. None had presurgical pain. All patients received the same presurgical medication; laparoscopies were performed by one surgeon, and anesthetic was administered by one anesthetist. At the end of the procedure, 22 patients received saline solution and 25 received 17 mL of 0.25% bupivacaine instilled abdominally through the laparoscopic cannula and injected around the incision site. Subsequently, patients recorded the severity of pain.

Results.—Of the 22 women who received saline solution, 20 had abdominal pain, 6 had shoulder tip pain, 12 required papaveretum for pain relief, and 16 were discharged on the same day. In significant contrast, of the 25 given bupivacaine, only 15 had abdominal pain, and none had shoulder tip pain. Furthermore, up to 4 hours postoperatively, pain was significantly less severe than in the group given saline solution. Only 6 women in the bupivacaine group needed papaveretum, and 24 were discharged on the same day. Age and body mass index did not predict postoperative pain. Efficacy of bupivacaine was undiminished in overweight women. Bupivacaine was not beneficial for long-term pain relief.

Conclusion.—Infusion of bupivacaine into the peritoneal cavity significantly reduced postsurgical abdominal pain but was not beneficial for long-term pain relief. The use of bupivacaine and similar local anesthetics deserves further investigation.

▶ I chose this paper because it appeared to describe an extremely simple, comparatively safe intervention that would greatly enhance immediate postoperative comfort, thereby allowing earlier discharge from an ambulatory surgical unit. In the current climate, the cost of one bottle of bupivacaine is negligible compared with the cost of delaying the patient's discharge from the ambulatory care unit by even 1 hour. This should be suggested to our obstetric colleagues.—J.D. Haddox, D.D.S., M.D.

Patient-Controlled Analgesia and Postoperative Urinary Retention After Hysterectomy for Benign Disease

Petros JG, Alameddine F, Testa E, Rimm EB, Robillard RJ (St Elizabeth's Med Ctr of Boston, Mass; Tufts Univ, Boston; Cardinal Cushing Gen Hosp, Brockton, Mass; et al)

J Am Coll Surg 179:663–667, 1994 131-95-6–37

Purpose.—Postoperative urinary retention can result in increased morbidity resulting from catheterization, longer hospitalization, and infection. Increasing rates of postoperative urinary retention after uncomplicated hysterectomy led to a retrospective study of its causes.

Methods.—The charts for 366 consecutive women (mean age, 51 years; range, 29–85 years) who had undergone uncomplicated abdominal or vaginal hysterectomy because of benign disease were reviewed. Strict criteria excluded patients with previous urinary retention. The patient was considered to have had urinary retention if she required a subsequent catheterization after removal of the catheter placed at surgery and after 400 mL of urine was obtained.

Results.—Fifty-eight (16%) patients had postoperative urinary retention. The use of patient-controlled analgesia and vaginal hysterectomy was significantly related to postoperative urinary retention. Patients who used patient-controlled analgesia were almost 6 times more likely to have urinary retention than were patients given IM analgesia. Similarly, patients who underwent vaginal hysterectomy were almost 6 times more likely to have urinary retention than those who underwent abdominal hysterectomy. Older patients tended to have a higher risk of urinary retention. Other factors, such as operative time, amount of fluid given perioperatively, and type and amount of postoperative analgesia were not significantly related to urinary retention.

Conclusion.—Urinary retention after hysterectomy might be averted with IM administration of analgesic agents or by suprapubic insertion of a cystostomy catheter, particularly in patients who had undergone vaginal hysterectomy.

▶ I chose this article for review because it seems to make a well-considered argument against the use of postoperative patient-controlled analgesia after uncomplicated hysterectomy. Unfortunately, it is very difficult to evaluate that assertion, given that despite measuring the operative time, amount of perioperative fluid administered, and the amount of analgesics given, the authors did not measure pain or time for ambulations, which are 2 other factors that may significantly influence hospital stay and, therefore, costs. It is disconcerting that these factors were not considered. I am, therefore, unable to adequately interpret the findings of this article, which, if true, would be useful information and would controvert many other studies regarding efficacy of patient-controlled analgesia.—J.D. Haddox, D.D.S., M.D.

Balanced Postoperative Analgesia: Effect of Intravenous Clonidine on Blood Gases and Pharmacokinetics of Intravenous Fentanyl

Bernard JM, Lagarde D, Souron R (Hôtel-Dieu, Nantes, France)

Anesth Analg 79:1126–1132, 1994 131-95-6–38

Purpose.—Combining drugs to treat postoperative pain can produce additive or synergistic effects, reducing the need for individual constituents. This can decrease side effects. Although clonidine can reduce the requirement for opioids, it can cause marked sedation and associated respiratory problems. Therefore, using clonidine to reduce opioid dose remains questionable. A double-blind, randomized trial compared the effects of postsurgical IV infusions of fentanyl or of lower-dose fentanyl plus clonidine on pain, sedation, hemodynamics, and pharmacokinetics.

Methods.—Thirty-two patients (average age, 23 years; 13 men) who underwent surgery to correct scoliosis completed the study. They were randomly assigned to receive postsurgical IV infusions of fentanyl (75 μg/hr) or fentanyl (25 μg/hr) plus clonidine (0.3 μg/kg/hr).

Results.—In both groups, pain scores were low, and demands for supplemental ketoprofen were similar. Sedation was also similar. Arterial oxygen saturation of less than 90% for at least 20 seconds was noted at least once in 4 patients in the fentanyl group but never in the fentanyl-clonidine group. There were 106 episodes of arterial oxygen desaturation in the fentanyl group but none in the fentanyl-clonidine group. Respiratory rate and arterial blood gas concentrations were similar. Mean arterial blood pressure was significantly higher in the fentanyl group. Six patients in the fentanyl group required naloxone, and 2 required oxygen; none in the fentanyl-clonidine group required either. The mean arterial blood pressure was significantly lower in the combination group. There were no other significant hemodynamic differences. Concentrations of fentanyl remained stable in both groups during administration. However, plasma clearance and elimination rate constant of fentanyl were significantly lower in the combination group. The elimination half-life of fentanyl was not significantly different.

Conclusion.—Adding clonidine reduces the dose of fentanyl required for relieving postsurgical pain, but fentanyl doses should be greatly reduced when clonidine is used. Simultaneous infusion of clonidine might lead to accumulation of fentanyl in the body and can prolong the risk for opioid-related respiratory tract depression.

▶ This article was selected to highlight the potential usefulness of clonidine in reducing the use of opioids in the postoperative period. It is interesting to note the significant reduction in the fentanyl dosage that was required in the presence of clonidine to avoid perioperative problems.—J.D. Haddox, D.D.S., M.D.

Computer-Modulated Patient-Controlled Analgesia: Preliminary Evaluation of a Prototype

Mies RJM, van der Aa JJ, Dixon CL, Kaltenbach M, Derendorf H, Gravenstein N (Eindhoven Univ, The Netherlands; Univ of Florida, Gainesville)

Reg Anesth 19:270–276, 1994 131-95-6–39

Purpose.—It is believed that stable plasma concentrations of medication produce more stable pain relief. However, this is a difficult goal to reach with either traditional IM injection or patient-controlled analgesia. In theory, a pharmacokinetic model can be used to calculate infusion schemes that should allow the plasma drug concentrations to remain constant. Programmable infusion pumps, together with computer technology, should accomplish this goal. A prototype electronically controlled infusion pump that can monitor patient requests for a drug bolus and adapt the dosage accordingly, while weaning the infusion concentration over time, was developed and tested in an animal model.

Methods.—An open, 2-compartment pharmacokinetic model that calculates infusion needs in both the blood and well-perfused tissues and in less well perfused tissues was used to determine the morphine plasma concentration and elimination fluctuations. Bolus responses were used to compute the continuous infusion profile for each of 4 dogs. The predictive accuracy of this model was tested by using a computer-controlled infusion pump driven by the calculated model.

Results.—The pharmacokinetic model consistently underpredicted the actual plasma drug level. The error was greatest immediately after an in-

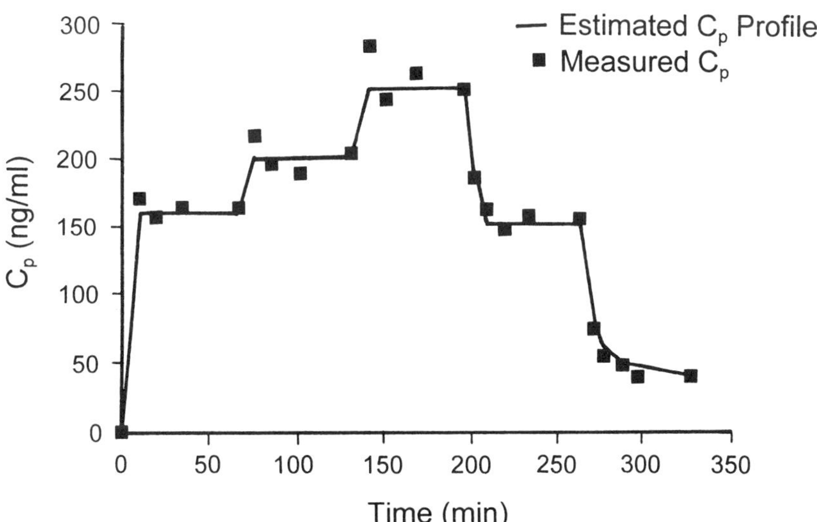

Fig 6–14.—Plasma concentration (C_p) profile (ng/mL) vs. time (minutes) after the first increase in C_p for dog C. (Courtesy of Mies RJM, van der Aa JJ, Dixon CL, et al: *Reg Anesth* 19:270–276, 1994.)

crease in the plasma drug concentration after a bolus and gradually became less marked (Fig 6–14). Nevertheless, use of the prototype pump achieved therapeutic concentrations of morphine in all 4 dogs.

Conclusion.—Although a computational error produced predicted drug levels different from the actual levels, the clinical significance was minimal because errors of this magnitude produced little or no change in pain intensity in patients in other studies. The ability of the prototype pump to maintain constant plasma drug levels suggests that this system may be useful for human pain control.

▶ This very interesting article explores the combination of patient-controlled analgesia with computer management of a pharmacokinetic model to achieve a relatively steady plasma level of morphine. As Figure 6–14 demonstrates, there was a slight error in calculation in the model; however, it predicted with an accuracy that is applicable clinically. This type of study is likely to become more frequent as our clinical experience and facility with computers increases. This may represent the cutting edge of a new marriage of technology.—J.D. Haddox, D.D.S., M.D.

A Double-Blind Placebo Controlled Study of a 5% Lidocaine/Prilocaine Cream (EMLA) for Topical Anesthesia During Thermolysis

Wagner RF Jr, Flores CA, Argo LF (Univ of Texas, Galveston)

J Dermatol Surg Oncol 20:148–150, 1994 131-95-6–40

Purpose.—Permanent hair removal with electrolysis or thermolysis can be painful, especially when sensitive areas such as the upper lip are involved. Most patients have refused injection of a local anesthetic with a fine needle. The efficacy of a eutectic mixture of local anesthetics (EMLA), a 5% lidocaine-prilocaine cream, applied as a local anesthetic during thermolysis on the upper lip, was evaluated in a double-blind study.

Methods.—The study subjects were 30 nonpregnant women with idiopathic hirsutism of the upper lip. Those who were eligible had skin types I, II, or III and were not currently taking any pain-relieving or mind-altering drug. Each received a 60-minute application of EMLA randomized to 1 side of the upper lip and placebo cream to the opposite side. After the creams were wiped away, thermolysis of the unwanted hair was performed with use of a sterile insulated probe. The patients used a visual analogue scale to evaluate the degree of pain they experienced during the procedure.

Results.—The scores on the pain-rating scale were significantly higher for the placebo-treated side than for the EMLA-treated side. There were more adverse events with EMLA than with placebo (12 vs. 2), but there were no lasting ill effects. Temporary problems associated with EMLA included redness, stinging, itching, and dermatitis.

Dermatologic Surgery Applications of EMLA

Procedure	*Comment*
Pulsed dye laser treatment	Vasoconstriction does not interfere with treatment efficacy
Argon laser treatment	
Carbon dioxide laser treatment of genital warts	
Split thickness skin grafting	
Thermocautery of genital warts	
Thermolysis	
Shave biopsy	More bleeding associated with EMLA than infiltration anesthesia with epinephrine
Punch biopsy	More bleeding associated with EMLA than infiltration anesthesia with epinephrine
Curettage of molluscum contagiosum	
Hyperhidrosis inhibition	
Dermabrasion of tattoo	
Leg ulcer dressing change	
Scraping herpetic leg ulcer	

Abbreviation: EMLA, eutectic mixture of local anesthetics (5% lidocaine-prilocaine cream).

(Courtesy of Wagner RF Jr, Flores CA, Argo LF: *J Dermatol Surg Oncol* 20:148–150, 1994.)

Conclusion.—When an oil-in-water emulsion with equal weights of lidocaine and prilocaine is applied to the skin or mucous membrane, the 2 agents diffuse from the emulsion into the skin. Patients have been discouraged from seeking permanent removal of unwanted hair growth on the upper lip and other areas because of the pain associated with multiple treatments. The use of EMLA should reduce pain and discomfort during thermolysis, electrolysis, and other dermatologic surgical procedures, such as those listed in the table.

▶ The versatility of EMLA cream has been repeatedly demonstrated for procedures requiring topical anesthesia. The 45- to 60-minute effective onset time must be considered in instructing and scheduling patient procedures.—D.A. Van Alstine, M.D.

Chronic Pain Treatment

A Comparative Study of the Effect of High-Intensity Transcutaneous Nerve Stimulation and Oral Naproxen on Intrauterine Pressure and Menstrual Pain in Patients With Primary Dysmenorrhea

Milsom I, Hedner N, Mannheimer C (Multidisciplinary Pain Ctr, Göteborg, Sweden; Univ of Göteborg, Sweden; East Hosp, Göteborg, Sweden)

Am J Obstet Gynecol 170:123–129, 1994 131-95-6–41

Introduction.—Women with dysmenorrhea experience pain that is associated with myometrial hypercontractility, which causes uterine ischemia. Both prostaglandin synthetase inhibitors and combined oral contraceptives have been shown to reduce pain but are not indicated in every patient. Transcutaneous electrical nerve stimulation (TENS) is a nonpharmacologic method for pain reduction. The effect of high-intensity TENS was compared with that of naproxen in women with dysmenorrhea to determine whether TENS could be used successfully to treat this condition.

Methods.—An open, randomized, crossover study was performed in 12 women with primary dysmenorrhea. Intrauterine pressure was recorded with a microtransducer catheter. Pain was assessed with a visual analog scale.

Results.—Before treatment, all the women in this study had high resting uterine pressure, high active uterine pressure, and a high frequency of pressure cycles. Orally administered naproxen significantly suppressed all uterine activity patterns. Transcutaneous electrical nerve stimulation induced prompt pain relief without any significant reduction in uterine activity. Pain scores were significantly reduced within 30–60 minutes of TENS treatment and within 19–120 minutes after naproxen treatment.

Conclusion.—High-intensity TENS is a safe and effective form of therapy for the reduction of pain in patients with primary dysmenorrhea. Although relief of pain after TENS was prompt, there were no indications of an accompanying reduction in uterine activity. It is possible that the pain relief experience after TENS treatment may be secondary to decreased myometrial ischemia.

▶ Although this study supports the efficacy of TENS in primary dysmenorrhea, the relative cost and availability of naproxen vs. TENS would be an issue for most patients. In patients who are intolerant to nonsteroidal anti-inflammatory drugs or those with contraindications to these agents, TENS might prove to be an important alternative therapy.—D.A. Van Alstine, M.D.

Effects of High-Frequency Transcutaneous Electrical Nerve Stimulation on Limb Blood Flow in Healthy Humans

Indergand HJ, Morgan BJ (Univ of Wisconsin, Madison)

Phys Ther 74:361–367, 1994 131-95-6–42

Introduction.—Although transcutaneous electrical nerve stimulation (TENS) has been used clinically for more than 2 decades, its hemodynamic effects have not been definitively established. The effects of high-frequency TENS on calf blood flow in healthy subjects were investigated.

Methods.—Seven women and 4 men, aged 20–44 years, comprised the study group. All were free of symptoms. Experimental protocols included TENS applications, cold pressor testing, and reactive hyperemia testing.

Results.—Calf blood flow was unaffected by sensory- or motor-level TENS. The mean arterial pressure and calf vascular resistance were also unaffected. During time-control experiments, calf blood flow, calf vascular resistance, and arterial pressure were unchanged. Dorsal foot skin temperature declined during sensory- and motor-level TENS. Immersing the hand in ice water for 90 seconds caused a rise in arterial pressure and a decrease in calf blood flow. After cessation of 5-minute vascular occlusion, calf blood flow increased substantially.

Conclusion.—Neither sensory-level nor low-intensity motor-level TENS delivered at high frequencies changes limb blood flow in healthy individuals with normal vascular resistance. Because the magnitude of hemodynamic response to many interventions depends on baseline values, caution must be exercised when applying these findings to other groups. These results may not be applicable to forms of TENS with different stimulation characteristics.

▶ Transcutaneous electrical nerve stimulation is a useful noninvasive, inexpensive method of controlling pain. An understanding of how TENS affects blood flow may further enhance our understanding of how TENS relieves pain. Additionally, changes in blood flow could be the result of changes in vascular sympathetic tone that could potentially be harmful in patients with vascular insufficiency.—E. Lang, M.D.

Clinical Evaluation of Pain Treatment With Electrostimulation: A Study on TENS in Patients With Different Pain Syndromes

Meyler WJ, de Jongste MJL, Rolf CAM (Univ Hosp of Groningen, The Netherlands)

Clin J Pain 10:22–27, 1994 131-95-6–43

Introduction.—Electrostimulation has a place as pain-modulation therapy, but observations on the efficacy of transcutaneous electrical nerve stimulation (TENS) have been inconclusive. Double-blind investi-

Success Rate of Transcutaneous Electrostimulation

IASP code, axis II	Number of patients	Success after 6 months	%
Nervous system			
Central	17	4	24
Peripheral	92	49	53
Autonomic	11	1	9
Psychological	11	1	9
Respiratory/ cardiovascular	17	13	76
Musculoskeletal	39	27	69
Gastrointestinal	2	0	0
Other/viscera	4	1	25

Abbreviation: IASP, International Association for the Study of Pain.
Note: Total number of patients = 193.
(Courtesy of Meyler WJ, de Jongste MJL, Rolf CAM: *Clin J Pain* 10:22–27, 1994.)

gations are difficult to perform because patients who receive TENS are aware of paresthesias. The clinical efficacy and side effects of TENS in a group of patients with intractable pain caused by various pain syndromes were evaluated.

Methods.—Various pain syndromes in 211 patients were treated with TENS. Because of insufficient follow-up data, 18 patients were removed from the study, leaving 193 patients. A multidisciplinary team categorized the patients according to the classification of chronic pain provided by the International Association for the Study of Pain. All patients used conventional TENS 3 times a day for 1 hour. This was the only additional treatment during the 6-month follow-up period. An independent investigator retrospectively reviewed the patient records after a 6-month treatment period and estimated the effect of TENS.

Results.—Most patients with pain caused by angina (75%), peripheral nerve damage (53%), and mechanical degenerative disease of the musculoskeletal system (69%) showed a favorable response to TENS (table). Only 10% to 25% of patients with pain caused by CNS or autonomic dysfunction or with prominent psychological or social distress responded favorably to TENS. Side effects (usually skin irritation or allergy) occurred in 35% of the patients but were generally minor and were resolved with supporting instructions.

Conclusion.—The beneficial effect of TENS in patients with chronic intractable pain appears to depend on the cause of the underlying pain. Most patients with an immediate favorable response will continue to have an effect from TENS for more than 6 months. Success requires thorough supporting instructions and supervision by skilled professionals.

▶ This is an interesting article, because it involves a large number of subjects and demonstrates that the beneficial response to TENS can last at least 6 months, which is something that I have also observed clinically. All too often, our referral base considers TENS to be an ineffective or placebo treatment. Previous placebo studies would suggest that those effects tend to wane over time in all but a few individuals. The 6-month period of this study would suggest that the effect of TENS in these patients is not the result of placebo effects alone.—J.D. Haddox, D.D.S., M.D.

Destruction of the Vesicoureteric Plexus for the Treatment of Hypersensitive Bladder Disorders

Gillespie L (The Pelvic Pain Treatment Ctr, The Women's Clinic for Interstitial Cystitis, Beverly Hills, Calif)

Br J Urol 74:40–43, 1994 131-95-6–44

Introduction.—Burning pelvic pain and frequency of urination characterize trigonitis, urethritis, and chronic cystitis. To eliminate the pelvic pain and hypersensitive bladder symptoms of interstitial cystitis, the vesicoureteric plexus was obliterated bilaterally in this study. All the women who participated in the surgery had abnormal nerve sensory latency and manifestations of petechial hemorrhaging.

Methods.—Neuroconductive studies, including bulbocavernosus reflex response, were performed to identify 175 women with increased pudendal sensory latency and intractable pelvic pain. The vesicoureteric plexus was dissected with either a transvaginal or laparoscopic approach. The plexus was isolated with endoclips; it was than incised and obliterated with a KTP laser. The procedure was performed bilaterally.

Results.—There was an association between the presence of occult gynecologic disease and a hypersensitive bladder; 55% of patients operated on had endometriosis that affected the pudendal nerve pathway. Pain relief and lessened symptoms were reported by 112 (64%) patients after surgery, 58 (33%) reported a moderate change in symptoms, and 5 (3%) reported no change after surgery. Postoperative determination of pudendal sensory latency yielded similar percentages; the results improved most in patients who reported significant relief, moderately in the middle group, and not at all in the group who reported no change after surgery. One complication—periureteric fibrosis—occurred, but there were no reports of postoperative hemorrhage or injury to the ureter.

Conclusion.—Excision of the bilateral vesicoureter ganglion offers some measure of pain relief from the hypersensitive bladder symptoms caused by interstitial cystitis. A good response is caused in part by patient selection, because pelvic pressure is not relieved by this procedure.

▶ This article presents a novel approach to the treatment of hypersensitive bladder disorders. The importance of correct patient selection is clear. The authors state that 45 patients were followed up for 2 years without symptom recurrence. I would like to know what happened to the other 75% of the patients. Nerve obliteration frequently has late complications, which were not evaluated in this report.—E. Lang, M.D.

Pain Insensitivity in Schizophrenia: A Neglected Phenomenon and Some Implications

Dworkin RH (Columbia-Presbyterian Med Ctr, New York)

Schizophr Bull 20:235–248, 1994 131-95-6–45

Background.—The insensitivity to pain of some individuals with schizophrenia has been recognized for a considerable time by surgeons and internists as well as psychiatrists. The validity of this phenomenon is supported by observations that such patients respond poorly to pin pricks, may be prone to gross self-mutilation, and frequently are initially seen for medical treatment of serious conditions such as acute perforating peptic ulcers, myocardial infarction, megacolon, and appendicitis, with no complaint of pain. Although reduced sensitivity to pain in individuals with schizophrenia has been studied in the laboratory, most relevant studies have significant methodological problems and fail to provide detailed descriptions of the nature of painful stimuli to which the subjects do and do not react, the type of patients who have reduced pain sensitivity, and the contribution of sensory and affective processes in pain insensitivity.

Implications of Reduced Pain Sensitivity.—Pain insensitivity in schizophrenia may predispose individuals to poor physical health because of delayed recognition of serious medical conditions and to serious or repeated injury. Furthermore, such individuals may be predisposed to self-mutilation (often severe), homelessness, premorbid development, and affective flattening.

Directions for Future Research.—Although a variety of techniques may be used to study pain in a clinical setting, the contributions of the sensory and affective aspects of pain may be distinguished by only 2 methods. The first involves psychophysical methods, such as cross-modality matching and magnitude estimation, and is complex and of questionable reliability. A second, more practical approach is based on signal detection theory (SDT) and distinguishes the sensory-discriminative aspects of the pain response of a subject from the extent to which an experience is reported as painful. The SDT approaches may produce an index of sensory discrimination, indicative of neurosensory system function, and a measure of response criterion, related to the affective response of a subject to the stimulus. In a recent study using SDT approaches to study pain insensitivity in individuals with schizophrenia, affected patients had less sensory discrimination of heat-induced pain than did control subjects, but they demonstrated normal response criterion for reporting pain. However, higher response criteria in patients with schizophrenia were associated with increased affective flattening and less complete affective experience. Therefore, pain insensitivity associated with schizophrenia may be indicative of affective as well as sensory abnormalities.

Conclusion.—Further research is necessary to more fully understand pain insensitivity in patients with schizophrenia. A more complete understanding of this phenomenon may enable amelioration of some of its negative consequences in affected patients and a better description of the relationship between different aspects of the psychopathologic features of schizophrenia.

▶ This fascinating review examines a neglected phenomenon. The relative insensitivity to pain found in the schizophrenic population has been recognized for more than 70 years. Further investigation into this finding might provide useful information regarding the provision of pain control to patients with chronic pain. Further research would be very important.—E. Lang, M.D.

Low-Back Pain of Pregnancy

Orvieto R, Achiron A, Ben-Rafael Z, Gelernter I, Achiron R (Tel Aviv Univ, Israel)

Acta Obstet Gynecol Scand 73:209–214, 1994 131-95-6–46

Purpose.—Low back pain is considered a normal consequence of pregnancy by many obstetricians, largely because of its high prevalence. The risk factors that lead to this widespread problem were evaluated, and the preventive steps that could eliminate or lessen the severity of low back pain were determined.

Methods.—A 30-item questionnaire was given to 449 healthy, pregnant women whose gestation had lasted at least 14 weeks. Patients were questioned about personal and demographic information, their obstetric history, and the occurrence and manifestations of low back pain during the present or previous pregnancies or between pregnancies. The definition of low back pain was any or all discomfort in the lower back region. Ultrasound was performed to determine gestational age, fetal weight, and placental location. Data were analyzed with analysis of variance and covariance and the Chi square and Student *t* tests.

Results.—Low back pain was reported in the present pregnancy by 246 women (54.8%), and 63 women (14%) reported the existence of low back pain before the pregnancy began. Most risk factors measured were not related to development of low back pain: maternal age, number of previous pregnancies, maternal height, weight, body mass index, and gestational age did not predispose to low back pain. There was a statistically significant risk for development of low back pain if the condition existed before the first pregnancy or if it was present during and between previous pregnancies. A higher prevalence of low back pain occurred in Sephardic women and women with a high body mass index. Its frequency increased with increasing gestational age. Ultrasound indicated a relationship between development of low back pain and posterior fundal location, but only among parous women. The finding that pain radiation corresponded to fetal weight was statistically significant. Women who were advised how to avoid low back pain reported a significant reduction in symptoms.

Conclusion.—Back care advice may significantly reduce or prevent the onset of low back pain during pregnancy.

▶ This is an interesting study that stresses the factors associated with back pain during pregnancy. Unfortunately, the investigators did not perform a physical examination of the patients who participated in the study. This provides information about factors associated with the back pain but no information as to the cause and types of back pain. Further research of this type is important, but an accurate definition and description of the cohort would provide more clinically applicable information.—E. Lang, M.D.

Tumor Necrosis Factor-α as a Biochemical Marker of Pain and Outcome in Temporomandibular Joints With Internal Derangements

Shafer DM, Assael L, White LB, Rossomando EF (Univ of Connecticut, Farmington)

J Oral Maxillofac Surg 52:786–791, 1994 131-95-6–47

Purpose.—Previous studies have stressed abnormal anatomical relationships and disk position as a cause of temporomandibular joint (TMJ) derangement. The relation between biochemical changes within the synovium and painful TMJ dysfunction has not received much attention. The relation between tumor necrosis factor-α (TNF) levels in synovial fluid and painful dysfunctional TMJs was examined.

Methods.—Synovial fluid was collected from 18 TMJs in 12 women, 16–35 years of age, who were undergoing either arthroscopy or arthrotomy because of internal derangements. Preoperative clinical findings and surgical outcome were compared with preoperative TNF levels in the synovial fluid samples. The mean follow-up was 6.6 months. Only data from patients with a postoperative follow-up of at least 3 months were included in the analysis. The outcome was rated poor in case of continued intracapsular pain, range of motion limited to less than 30 mm of maximal pain-free interincisal opening, or if further surgery was needed.

Results.—The data from 11 patients were evaluable. The mean preoperative TNF level was 14 ng/mL when pain on palpation was absent and

42 ng/mL when pain on palpation was present. The mean preoperative TNF level was 12 ng/mL when the surgical outcome was favorable and 26 ng/mL when the surgical outcome was poor. These differences were statistically significant. Furthermore, arthroscopic joint lavage reduced the mean TNF value from 48 ng/mL before the procedure to 7 ng/mL after.

Conclusion.—Preoperative TNF levels in synovial fluid from TMJs are correlated with preoperative pain and with surgical outcome. Levels of TNF in the synovial fluid of patients with TMJ derangements may be predictive of surgical outcome.

▶ This study highlights the complex nature of TMJ disease. There are some study shortcomings related to methods of collection of synovial fluid and the use of preoperative arthrograms. Conceptualization of TMJ disease as a purely mechanical phenomenon with a "mechanical" solution is clearly overly simplistic. The conclusion that preoperative TNF levels are significant predictors of surgical outcome is still not clearly proved and is of uncertain usefulness.—D.A. Van Alstine, M.D.

Valproate for Treatment of Chronic Central Pain After Spinal Cord Injury: A Double-Blind Cross-Over Study

Drewes AM, Andreasen A, Poulsen LH (Spinal Cord Injury Centre, Viborg County Hosp, Denmark)

Paraplegia 32:565–569, 1994 131-95-6–48

Purpose.—Patients with spinal cord injury frequently have chronic, intractable pain, particularly central or phantom body pain. Most recently, antiepileptic medications, particularly valproate, have been used with some success to control central pain in these patients. In a double-blind, placebo-controlled, crossover study, the efficacy of valproate in the treatment of chronic central pain in patients with spinal cord injuries was determined.

Methods.—Twenty adult patients with nonprogressive spinal cord injuries who complained of central pain for longer than 1 month were assigned to receive either valproate or placebo for 3 weeks. After a 2-week washout, the patients were given the other treatment for 3 weeks. The dose was adjusted with weekly monitoring of serum drug concentrations, liver function, pain intensity, and side effects. The effect of treatment was assessed in each treatment group.

Results.—Four patients experienced dizziness while taking valproate; no patients taking placebo experienced side effects. Pain improved in 6 patients taking valproate and 4 patients taking placebo and worsened in 2 patients taking valproate and 1 patient taking placebo. The median dose of valproate reached 1,800 mg, and the median serum drug concentration was 614 μmol/L.

Conclusion.—Valproate did not produce significant analgesic effects compared with placebo in patients with central pain after spinal cord injury, even though high doses were used and high serum concentrations were achieved. The available pharmacologic agents may be more effective in treating mild or moderate pain. Further study of pain control in this patient population is needed, because there is a paucity of research in this area, although pain is common in patients with spinal cord injuries.

▶ The treatment of chronic pain resulting from spinal cord injury continues to be a vexing problem. There are no consistently reliable treatment options.—D.A. Van Alstine, M.D.

Phantom Pain: Natural History and Association With Rehabilitation

Houghton AD, Nicholls G, Houghton AL, Saadah E, McColl L (Guy's Hosp, London, England; Royal Sussex County Hosp, London, England)

Ann R Coll Surg Engl 76:22–25, 1994 131-95-6–49

Purpose.—Phantom pain after amputation is common, but in most cases, the sensation of pain in the absent limb decreases over time. Few studies have dealt with the long-term prevalence of phantom pain, and almost no attention has been given to the effect of this phenomenon on rehabilitation. In a study of patients who had undergone lower limb amputation, the natural history of phantom pain and the relationship between phantom sensations and degree of rehabilitation were examined.

Methods.—A group of 338 patients with lower limb amputations who were referred to a disablement services center for prosthesis fitting were

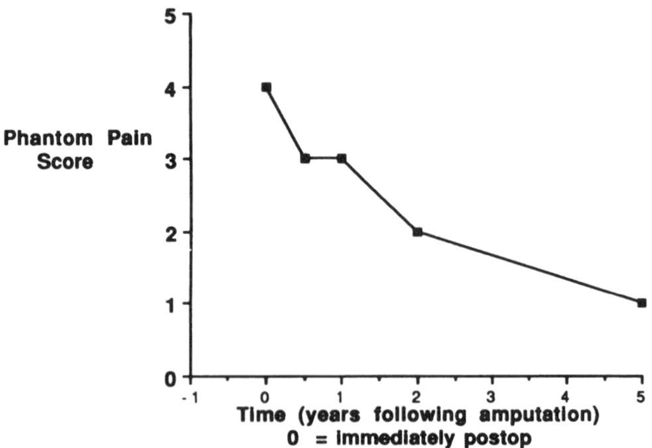

Fig 6–15.—The natural history of phantom pain with time in all amputees, both traumatic and vascular, under the care of one disablement services center. (Courtesy of Houghton AD, Nicholls G, Houghton AL, et al: *Ann R Coll Surg Engl* 76:22-25, 1994.)

asked to complete a questionnaire on the amount of pain they had in the limb before amputation, the degree of phantom pain at 6 months and at 1, 2, and 5 years after amputation, current extent of phantom pain, and current rehabilitation status.

Results.—The questionnaire yielded 212 (63%) responses, 176 of which were available for analysis. Ninety-eight amputations had been performed because of traumatic injuries and 78 because of vascular disease. Patients who had sustained traumatic injuries were younger than those with vascular disease. The 96 patients with below-knee amputation and the 74 with above-knee amputation did not differ in age, duration of amputation, or severity of preoperative or phantom pain. Those with below-knee amputation responded better to rehabilitation than did patients with above-knee amputation, and those with traumatic injuries responded better than did patients with vascular disease. Phantom pain was experienced by 78% of patients overall. The median phantom pain score decreased from a moderate level immediately after surgery to slight at 5 years after surgery (Fig 6–15). Phantom pain was equally present in both groups, but the relationship between preoperative and phantom pain was of greater duration in patients with vascular disease. No subgroup had a greater tendency than any other subgroup for phantom pain to impair rehabilitation.

Conclusion.—In agreement with other studies, phantom pain decreased over time for these amputees. There was a relationship between amount of preoperative pain and the development of phantom pain. Overall, 22% of patients believed that phantom pain had impaired their rehabilitation. Continuing efforts to control pain after amputation may help such patients during rehabilitation.

▶ This is a very interesting study with a large number of subjects. Unfortunately, the methodology relies on the memory of subject pain perception about 10 years, on average, after amputation. Despite that, it is the largest study to date on the natural history of phantom pain. It still would appear to provide some very useful information, especially for rehabilitation. It demonstrates a correlation between preoperative pain and phantom pain after amputation because of vascular disease as opposed to trauma. This correlation persisted until the patients were administered the questionnaire. This is consistent with previous studies that have suggested that preoperative pain control could possibly result in decreased prevalence or severity of phantom pain after amputation in vascular patients.—J.D. Haddox, D.D.S., M.D.

Thalamic Pain Syndrome: Anatomic and Metabolic Correlation

De Salles AAF, Bittar GT Jr (Pain Management Ctr, Univ of California, Los Angeles)

Surg Neurol 41:147–151, 1994 131-95-6–50

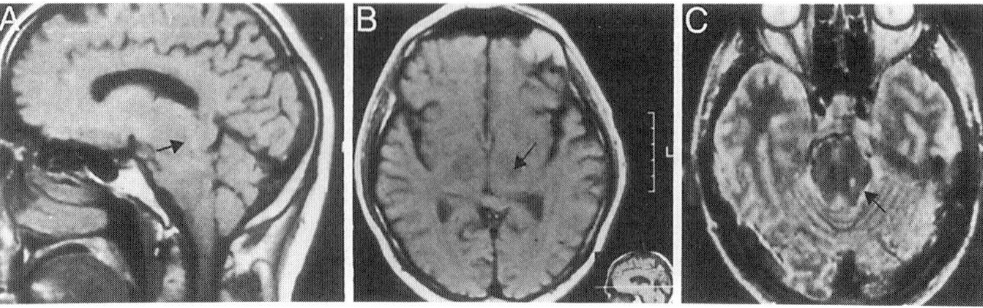

Fig 6–16.—Postoperative MRI. The T1-weighted sagittal image **(A)** shows the track of the needle crossing the ventroposterior median nucleus of the thalamus and the site of the biopsy in the mesencephalon, posterior to the left red nucleus and lateral to the aqueduct of Sylvius. The T1-weighted axial image **(B)** shows the defect of the needle track in the ventroposteromedial nucleus of the thalamus. The T2-weighted axial image **(C)** shows the site of biopsy in the mesencephalon. (Courtesy of De Salles AAF, Bittar GT Jr: *Surg Neurol* 41:147–151, 1994.)

Purpose.—The most common cause of thalamic pain syndrome is intracerebral hemorrhage, although any process that damages the thalamic nuclei can induce the syndrome. Thalamic pain syndrome was surgically induced in a patient undergoing brain-stem stereotactic biopsy.

Case Report.—Man, 54, had a progressive sleep disorder, dementia, and abnormal results of liver function tests. An abnormality in the midbrain was detected at MRI, and a stereotactic biopsy was performed to confirm the presumed diagnosis of an infiltrating brain-stem astrocytoma. Pathologic study of the specimen, however, failed to show tumor cells. In the following weeks, the patient experienced right-sided dysesthesia and a burning sensation on the right side of the face and right hand. Six months later, he underwent liver transplantation. His memory and behavior symptoms resolved and liver function improved. Postoperative MRI showed no progression of the brain-stem abnormality but disclosed the tract of the biopsy needle crossing the ventrobasal complex of the thalamus (Fig 6–16). A thalamic lesion was considered to be the cause of the pain experienced by the patient. The lesion may have involved the medial lemniscus immediately caudad to the ventroposteromedial nucleus. A positron emission tomography (PET) scan obtained a year after the biopsy showed persistence of thalamic hypometabolism. Secondary hypometabolism was also noted in the contralateral cerebellar hemisphere, but this subsequently resolved without parallel resolution of symptoms.

Conclusion.—The structure and metabolic alterations documented in this case add evidence to the theory that the pathophysiology of the thalamic pain syndrome involves disruption of modulatory sensations at the thalamic level. Observed changes in the PET scans of the thalamus were correlated to the patient's pain pattern.

▶ This is a very interesting case report regarding thalamic pain syndrome. Figure 6–16 demonstrates the needle tract, which correlated to an area of thalamic hypometabolism on the PET scan. This article was chosen to raise consciousness about this particular syndrome and to illustrate how newer imaging technologies may become clinically applicable.—J.D. Haddox, D.D.S., M.D.

Plasma, Brain, and Spinal Cord Concentrations of Thiopental Associated With Hyperalgesia in the Rat

Archer DP, Ewen A, Roth SH, Samanani N (Foothills Hosp, Univ of Calgary, Canada)

Anesthesiology 80:168–176, 1994 131-95-6–51

Purpose.—Low doses of barbiturates are widely believed to increase pain sensitivity. However, research on the electrophysiologic effects of these drugs on the neurons involved in nociception in the spinal cord have identified only depressant effects. The hyperalgesia resulting from low-dose thiopental infusions was quantified, and the associated levels of thiopental in the plasma, brain, and spinal cord were measured.

Methods.—In a rat model, nociception was measured using the threshold for motor response to pressure stimulation of the tail and tail flick latency. Thiopental was given IV to produce plasma levels that slowly increased or remained at steady state. Plasma and tissue thiopental levels were assessed by high-performance liquid chromatography.

Results.—Nociceptive threshold was reduced in association with the plasma thiopental concentration over a range of 2–20 $\mu g \cdot mL^{-1}$. This correlation was nonlinear. Nociceptive threshold was at a nadir at a mean plasma thiopental level of 13.7 $\mu g \cdot mL^{-1}$. The steady-state study revealed a similar decrease in nociceptive threshold, with an equilibrium plasma thiopental level of 7.6 $\mu g \cdot mL^{-1}$. Thiopental levels in brain and spinal cord samples were 1.7 and 3.5 $\mu g \cdot g^{-1}$, respectively.

Conclusion.—Consistent with previous studies, these findings indicate an association of hyperalgesia with small doses of thiopental. Decreases in nociceptive threshold and tail flick latency were associated with spinal cord levels of thiopental in a range reported by others to depress the electrophysiologic activity of neurons involved in nociception.

▶ This article was included because the animal model for studying hyperalgesia was interesting. It is believed that low doses of thiopental increase pain sensitivity. Quantification of this phenomenon will further advance our understanding of nociception.—E. Lang, M.D.

Joint Inflammation Is Reduced by Dorsal Rhizotomy and Not by Sympathectomy or Spinal Cord Transection

Sluka KA, Lawand NB, Westlund KN (Marine Biomedical Inst, Galveston, Tex; Univ of Texas, Galveston)

Ann Rheum Dis 53:309–314, 1994 131-95-6–52

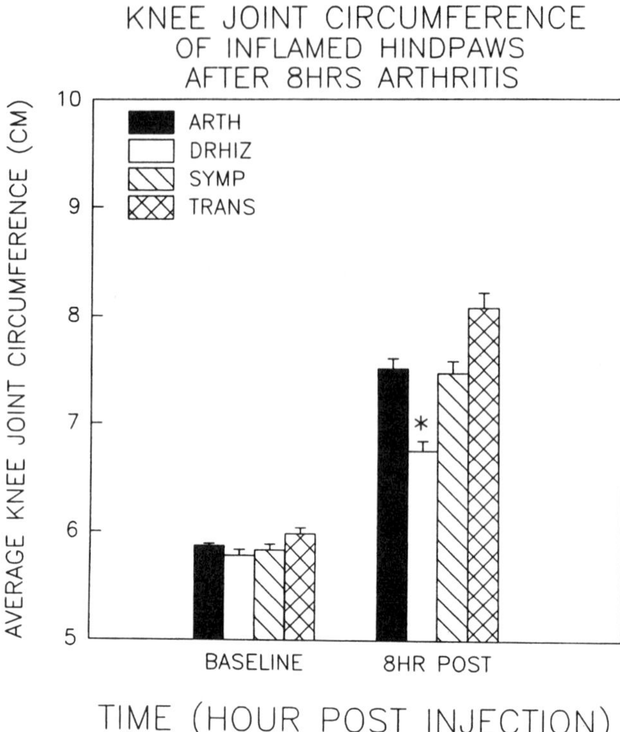

Fig 6–17.—The joint circumferences are represented as the average circumference of the inflamed knee joint measured before and 8 hours post induction of arthritis for all groups of animals: control arthritic, *ARTH*; dorsal rhizotomy, *DRHIZ*; sympathectomy, *SYMP*; and transection, *TRANS*. A significant decrease occurred for the arthritic animals with DRHIZ compared with all other groups. * $P < .05$. (Courtesy of Sluka KA, Lawand NB, Westlund KN: *Ann Rheum Dis* 53:309–314, 1994.)

Purpose.—Injection of kaolin and carrageenan into the knee of rats induces an acute arthritis that develops within 1–3 hours. This provides an excellent model for analyzing the involvement of the nervous system in inflammation. The roles of primary afferents, sympathetic postganglionic efferents, and supraspinal descending control in the development of pain and inflammation in acute arthritis were investigated.

Methods.—In a group of 32 Sprague-Dawley rats, rhizotomy of L2–S1 was performed in 6 rats, surgical and/or chemical sympathectomy of L2–S2 in 12 rats, and spinal cord transection of T8–10 in 10 rats. After an appropriate postsurgical recovery period, the knee joints of these rats and a control group of 10 rats were injected with 3% kaolin and 3% carrageenan. Joint circumference, thermographic readings, and behavioral changes were assessed.

Results.—Only the rats who underwent dorsal rhizotomy had a significant reduction in knee joint circumference and temperature that was not seen in the control rats or the rats who underwent sympathectomy or

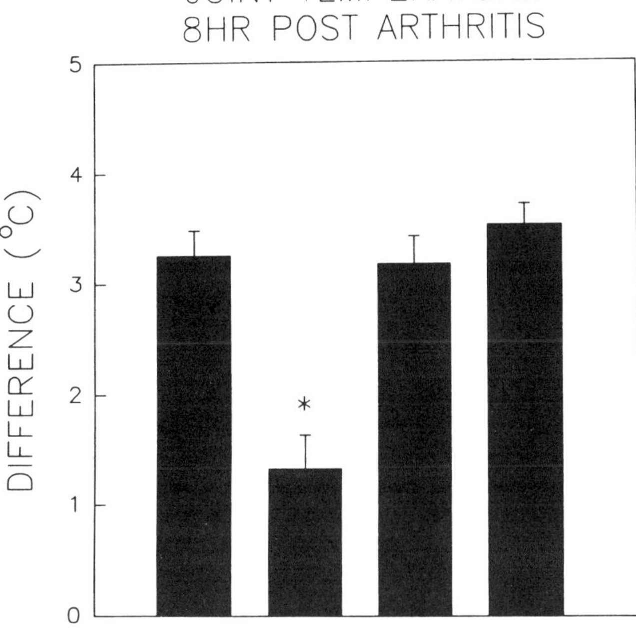

Fig 6–18.—The joint temperature for each group taken 8 hours post arthritis. The data are represented as the difference in temperature between the ipsilateral inflamed and contralateral untreated knees. A significant difference was observed between the dorsal rhizotomy (*DRHIZ*) group and all other arthritic groups. **P* < .05. (Courtesy of Sluka KA, Lawand NB, Westlund KN: *Ann Rheum Dis* 53:309–314, 1994.)

spinal cord transection (Fig 6–17). Thermographic readings of affected knee joints were significantly increased in all except the dorsal rhizotomy group (Fig 6–18). No significant differences were observed in pain-related behavior ratings between the sympathectomy group and the control group with arthritis.

Conclusion.—The central terminals of primary afferent fibers are instrumental in the inflammatory response of rats with acute arthritis. Peripheral joint inflammation is influenced by the central terminals of sensory afferents. The sympathetic nervous system is not involved in acute inflammation in the arthritic rat model.

▶ This article was also included because the animal model for studying hyperalgesia was interesting. Through the use of animal models like these, it is possible to understand the role of the nervous system in maintaining joint inflammation.—E. Lang, M.D.

Electrophysiological Characteristics of Localized Twitch Responses in Responsive Taut Bands of Rabbit Skeletal Muscle Fibers

Hong C-Z, Torigoe Y (Univ of California, Irvine)

J Musculoskel Pain 2:17–43, 1994 131-95-6–53

Purpose.—In humans, the local twitch response (LTR) is a useful objective sign of the myofascial pain syndrome caused by trigger points. However, the study of basic LTR and trigger point mechanisms in humans has been limited because of ethical reasons. Rabbit skeletal muscle was used to investigate localized twitch responses by electromyography.

Methods.—Rabbit localized twitch responses (R-LTRs) were studied in 9 rabbits. The animals were anesthetized with a method that preserved most peripheral reflexes mediated by the CNS. Manual-probe stimulus, mechanical-tap stimulus, and needle insertion using a solenoid-driven needle were used to elicit R-LTRs.

Results.—The best recording of the R-LTRs from the responsive band was achieved when the trigger spot was stimulated mechanically. Responses to snapping stimulation had a longer duration than those to mechanical tap stimulation. These in turn were longer than R-LTRs produced by needle stimulation (Figs 6–19 and 6–20).

Conclusion.—These findings support the impression that one trigger spot of the rabbit may contain multiple loci of hypersensitivity. The near-complete loss of R-LTRs after lidocaine block or transection of the motor nerve shows that propagation of the R-LTR occurs mainly through a CNS reflex instead of solely through direct muscle fiber transmission. Because R-LTRs are comparable to human LTRs in many ways, this animal model is promising for the study of LTRs and possibly of taut bands and trigger points characteristic of myofascial pain syndrome.

▶ The current lack of a reasonable animal model for myofascial pain has made research into the pathophysiology of this disorder difficult. Our understanding of the effect of tricyclic antidepressants and nonsteroidal anti-inflammatory drugs on myofascial pain would also be enhanced. The possibility that this represents a model for use in future studies makes this article an important contribution.—D.A. Van Alstine, M.D.

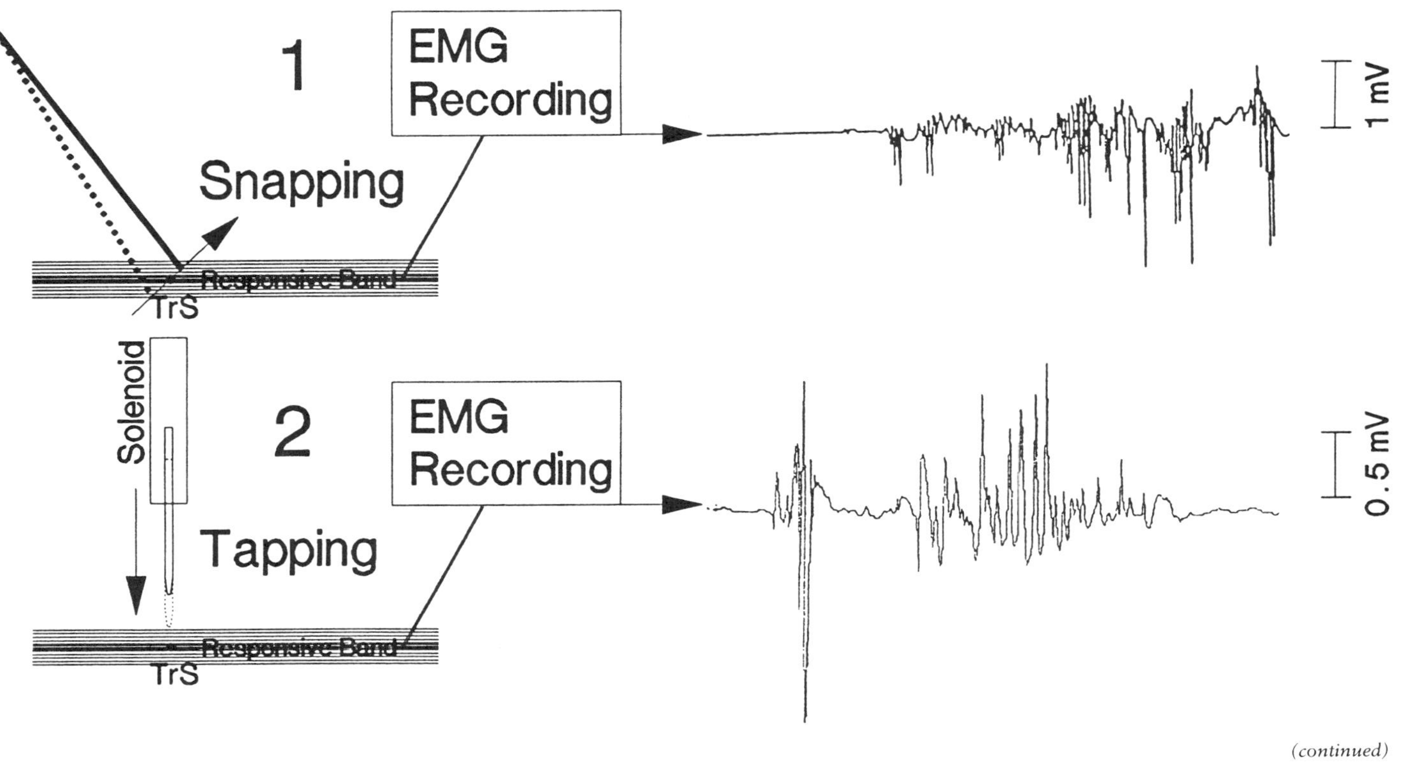
1
EMG
Recording
Snapping
Responsive Band
TrS
1 mV
Solenoid
2
EMG
Recording
Tapping
Responsive Band
TrS
0.5 mV

(continued)

Fig 6–19 (cont).

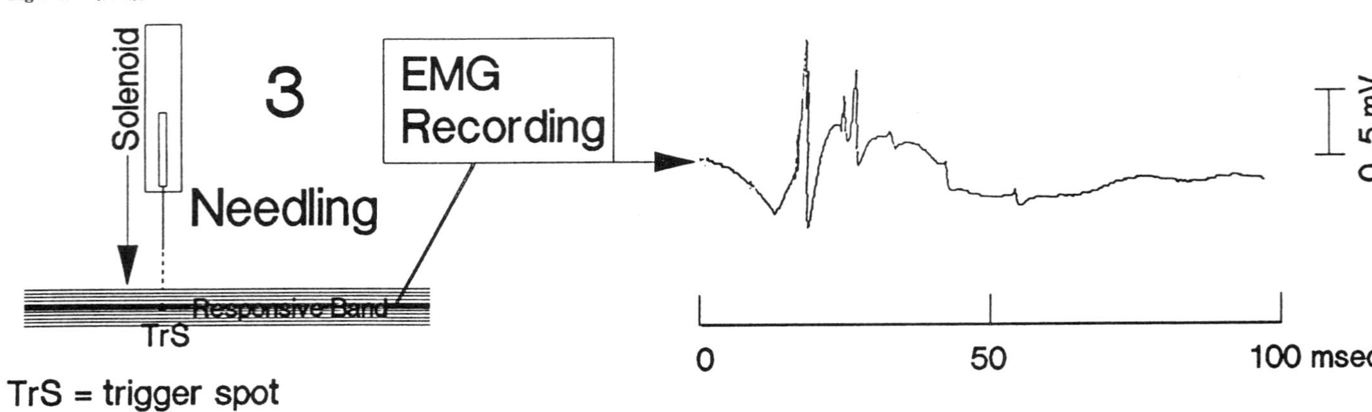

Fig 6–19.—Electromyographic (*EMG*) recordings (with monopolar needles) of rabbit localized twitch responses elicited by mechanical stimulation: Trace 1, by snapping; Trace 2, by tapping; and Trace 3, by needling. (Courtesy of Hong C-Z, Torigoe Y: *J Musculoskel Pain* 2:17–43, 1994.)

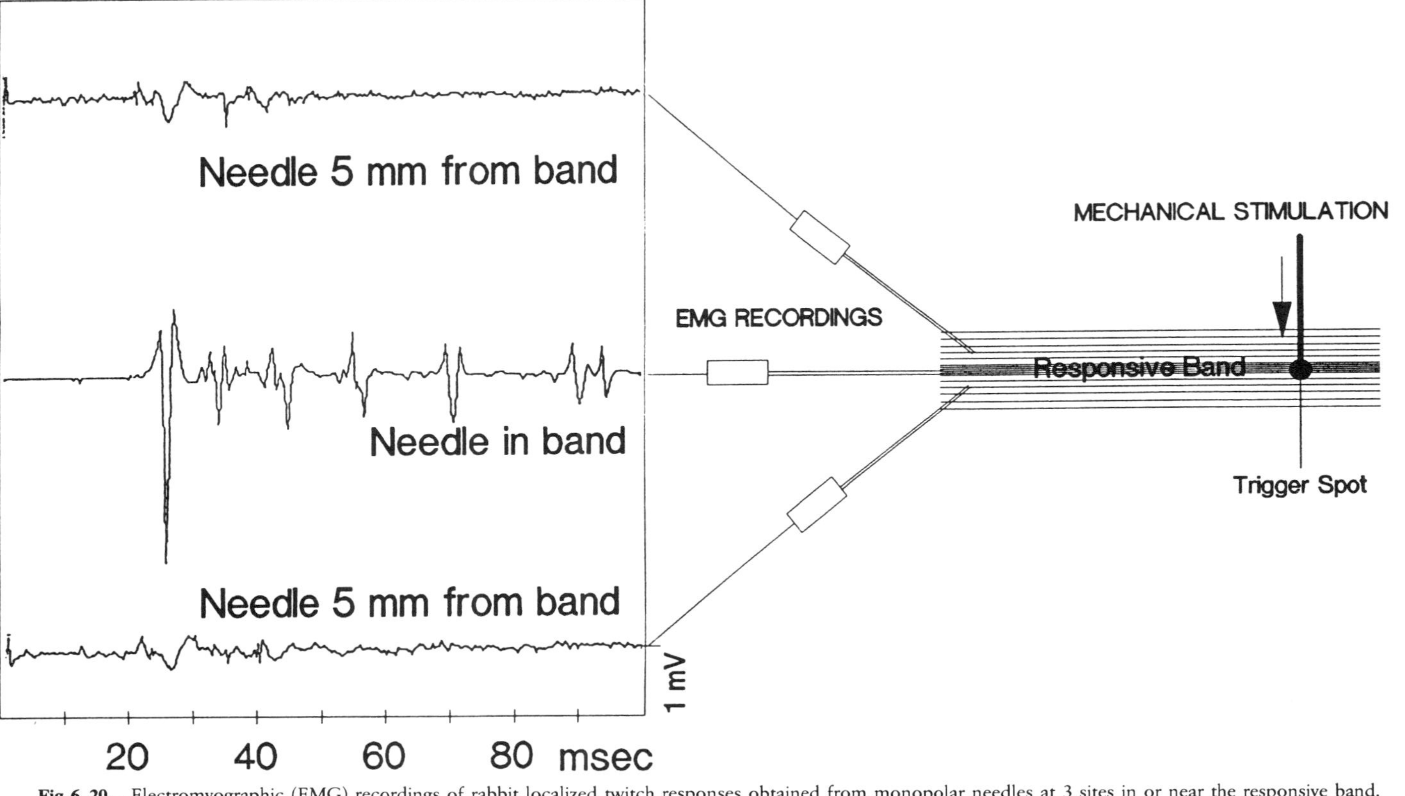

Fig 6–20.—Electromyographic (EMG) recordings of rabbit localized twitch responses obtained from monopolar needles at 3 sites in or near the responsive band. Tracings observed 5 mm to each side of the responsive band showed only distant EMG waveforms, indicating that the twitch response was restricted to the muscle fibers within the responsive band. The responses were elicited by a solenoid-driven tap at the trigger spot. (Courtesy of Hong C-Z, Torigoe Y: *J Musculoskel Pain* 2:17–43, 1994.)

Single Cell Morphology and High-Energy Phosphate Levels in Quadriceps Muscles From Patients With Fibromyalgia

Nørregaard J, Harreby M, Amris K, Bangsbo J, Bartels EM, Danneskiold-Samøe B (Frederiksberg Hosp, Copenhagen; Glostrup County Hosp, Denmark; Univ of Copenhagen; et al)

J Musculoskel Pain 2:45–51, 1994 131-95-6–54

Purpose.—Authorities continue to debate whether pain in patients with fibromyalgia is of central or peripheral origin. Whether previous findings of changes in single-cell morphology and adenosine triphosphate (ATP) levels in fibromyalgic muscles could be reproduced was tested. Whether rubberband morphology and reduced energy content of fibromyalgia quadriceps muscle could be found under completely blinded conditions in a control group was studied.

Methods.—Muscle fiber bundles of 2–5 cells from needle biopsies were obtained from the vastus lateralis muscle of 20 patients with fibromyalgia and 20 age- and sex-matched control subjects. The bundles were scored for waviness and constrictions, and ATP and adenosine diphosphate (ADP) levels were determined with high-performance liquid chromatography.

Results.—Scores for histologic constructions and waviness specimens did not differ between groups (table). Score was significantly correlated with age and constriction. After correcting for age differences, a regression analysis of scores showed no trend toward higher scores in patients with fibromyalgia than in the control group. The ATP and ADP contents of the muscles were also comparable in the 2 groups.

Conclusion.—There were no significant differences in morphology between fibromyalgic and normal muscle in this series. Future research should be done to determine whether reported reduced energy content of the trapezius muscle in fibromyalgia results from a disturbance in microcirculation.

"Rubberband Scoring" and High-Energy Content in the Two Groups

	Fibromyalgia		Controls	
"Rubberband scoring"				
Constrictions	0.43	[0.2-0.55]	0.45	[0.30-1.0]
Waviness	0.50	[0.30-0.70]	0.78	[0.35-1.06]
High-energy phosphates				
ATP [mmol/kg dry weight]	21.4	[20.5-22.8]	22.0	[21.1-23.1]
ADP [mmol/kg dry weight]	2.4	[2.2-2.5]	2.3	[2.2-2.5]

Median and interquartile range.
Abbreviations: *ADP*, adenosine diphosphate; *ATP*, adenosine triphosphate.
(Courtesy of Nørregaard J, Harreby M, Amris K, et al: *J Musculoskel Pain* 2:45-51, 1994.)

► This type of study is important in elucidating the pathophysiology of pain syndromes of muscular origin. A control study with nonfibromyalgia myofascial pain would be instructive.—D.A. Van Alstine, M.D.

Systemic Lidocaine Blocks Nerve Injury-Induced Hyperalgesia and Nociceptor-Driven Spinal Sensitization in the Rat

Abram SE, Yaksh TL (Med College of Wisconsin, Milwaukee; Univ of California, San Diego)

Anesthesiology 80:383–391, 1994 131-95-6–55

Purpose.—Systemic lidocaine can produce analgesia in a variety of neuropathic pain states, but its site of action is unclear. Research has shown that repetitive C-fiber stimulation leads to facilitated processing of sensory information in the dorsal horn. Chronic nerve compression induces hyperalgesia with spontaneous neuronal activity generated by voltage-sensitive sodium channels, in addition to spinal facilitation. The effects of systemic local anesthetic on thermal hyperalgesia induced by chronic nerve compression and on behavioral pain responses to subcutaneous formalin were evaluated in rats.

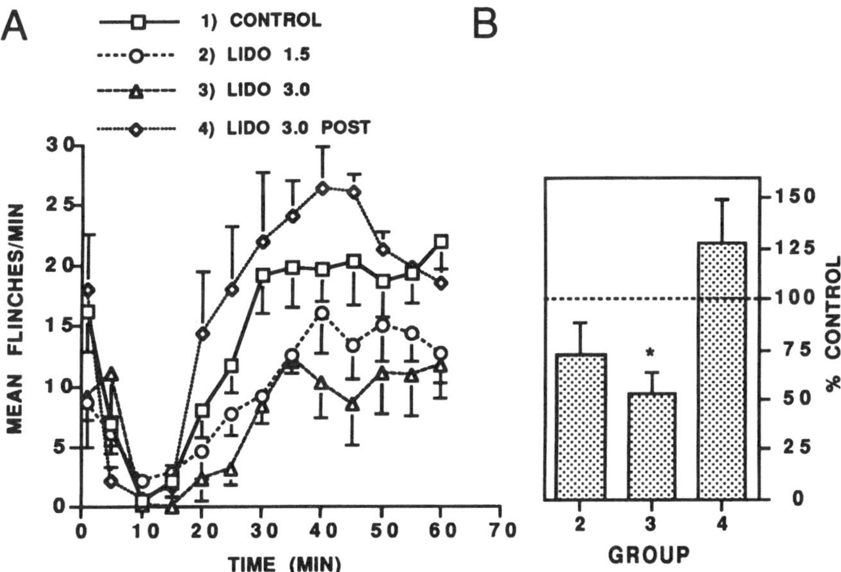

Fig 6–21.—A, mean number of flinches per minute (± SEM), plotted as a function of time after injection of formalin. The treatment groups were the following: (1) control (IV saline); (2) low-dose lidocaine (1.5-mg bolus); (3) high-dose lidocaine (3-mg bolus); (4) high-dose lidocaine, 2 minutes after formalin administration (3-mg bolus). **B,** mean values for phase 2 activity for groups 2, 3, and 4 expressed as a percent of control values. (From Tallarida RJ, Murray RB: *Manual of Pharmacologic Calculations with Computer Programs*, ed 2, 1987, pp 137–139). *Asterisk* represents significantly different from control (one-way analysis of variance, $P < .05$). (Courtesy of Abram SE, Yaksh TL: *Anesthesiology* 80:383–391, 1994.)

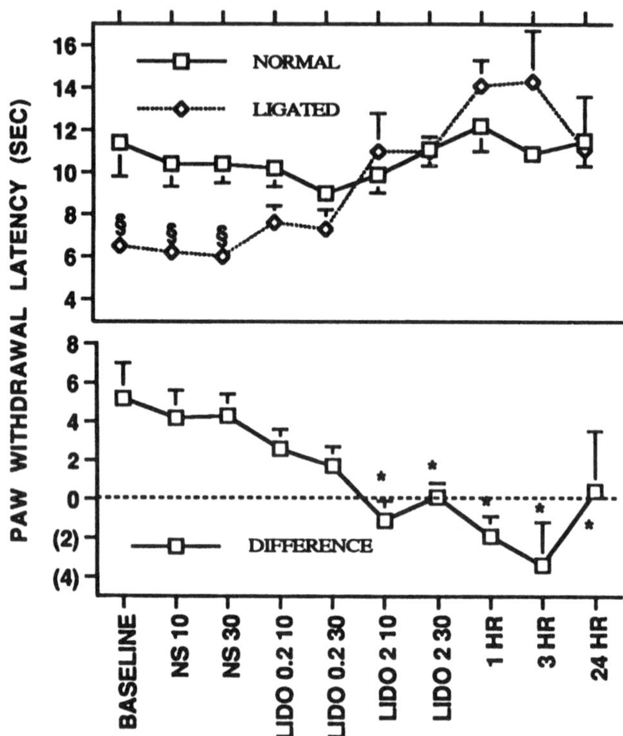

Fig 6–22.—Mean paw withdrawal latencies (± SEM) for normal and ligated limbs 10 and 30 minutes after a bolus injection of 3 mL of normal saline (NS 10, NS 30), 10 and 30 minutes after a bolus injection of 3 mL of lidocaine, .2 mg/mL (Lido .2 10, Lido .2 30), 10 and 30 minutes after a bolus injection of 3 mL of lidocaine, 2mg/mL (Lido 2 10, Lido 2 30), and 1, 3, and 24 hours after the lidocaine infusion, 2 mg/mL, was discontinued. *Section mark* indicates significantly different from nonligated paw (one-way analysis of variance, $P < .05$); the *asterisk* represents significantly different from baseline (repeated-measures analysis or variance, $P < .05$). (Courtesy of Abram SE, Yaksh TL: *Anesthesiology* 80:383-391, 1994.)

Methods.—The formalin test was used as a model of acute pain and centrally mediated delayed sensory sensitization. Starting 5 minutes before subcutaneous formalin injection in the left hind paw, rats were given lidocaine IV at doses of 3 mg plus 25 μg/min by infusion or 1.5 mg plus 12.5 μg/min. These doses produced mean serum levels of 6.3 and 3.6 μg/mL, respectively. In another set of experiments, the Bennett model of chronic sciatic nerve compression was used to create neurogenic thermal hyperalgesia in one hindlimb. Three to 5 days later, these animals received IV lidocaine at a dose of 0.6 mg plus 5 μg/min by infusion, which produced a mean serum level of 1.0 μg/mL.

Results.—Lidocaine did not significantly affect the first phase of the formalin test or the thermal response latencies in normal limbs. However, high-dose lidocaine significantly decreased phase 2 flinching behavior (Fig 6–21). Low-dose lidocaine reversed the thermal hyperalgesia induced by sciatic nerve ligation during the 30-minute infusion period and for 3 hours thereafter (Fig 6–22).

Conclusion.—These animal models show that systemic local anesthetic can alter behavioral responses to noxious stimulation via 2 distinct mechanisms. It decreases the hyperesthetic state resulting from peripheral nerve injury and reduces the degree of spinal sensitization caused by C-afferent fiber activation. The main effect of systemic lidocaine on neuropathic pain, therefore, seems to occur through suppression of spontaneous impulse generation from injured nerve segments or associated dorsal root ganglia.

▶ This study expands our understanding of the effect of lidocaine on acute and neuropathic pain. The evidence for multiple sites of action of lidocaine has been suggested in other articles in the literature. Repeating this study using mexiletine as a comparative agent would be interesting.—D.A. Van Alstine, M.D.

Relationship Between Increased Blood Pressure and Hypoalgesia: Additional Evidence for the Existence of an Abnormality of Pain Perception in Arterial Hypertension in Humans

Rosa C, Vignocchi G, Panattoni E, Rossi B, Ghione S (CNR Inst of Clinical Physiology, Pisa, Italy; Univ of Pisa, Italy)

J Hum Hypertens 8:119–126, 1994 131-95-6–56

Purpose.—Both animal and human studies show an association between hypertension and decreased perception of pain (hypoalgesia). Thus, unrecognized myocardial infarction, which is more common in patients with hypertension, may be related to a diminished response to pain. Studies of hypoalgesia in humans have used electrical tooth pulp stimulation. Two other techniques were used here to confirm the association between hypertension and hypoalgesia.

Methods.—Study participants were 77 outpatients with untreated essential hypertension and 37 outpatients and 27 healthy volunteers with normal blood pressure. An electrical constant current stimulator was used for quantitative assessment of cutaneous sensitivity. Measurements were repeated after 1 month. In a second test, 8 volunteers with normal blood pressure and 8 patients with essential hypertension were examined for thresholds of the polysynaptic components R2 and R3 of the blink reflex to electrical stimulation of the supraorbitalis nerve. Tooth pulp was stimulated in 85 participants in the cutaneous sensitivity test and in all participants in the blink reflex study. All measurements were obtained without knowledge of the subjects' blood pressure status.

Results.—Compared with both normotensive groups, the patients with hypertension had significantly higher cutaneous perception, pain, and tolerance thresholds. Differences between the 2 normotensive groups were not significant. Stepwise multiple regression analysis showed that in all instances blood pressure accounted for most of the variability. Patients with hypertension were significantly older than members of the 2 normotensive groups, but age did not contribute to the correlations. Tests of tooth pulp pain thresholds yielded similar findings, and thresholds of R2 and R3 were also significantly higher in patients with hypertension.

Conclusion.—A previously reported association between hypertension and hypoalgesia was confirmed in cutaneous sensitivity and blink reflex tests. The endogenous opioid system and the baroreceptor system have been implicated in reduced perception of pain in patients with hypertension.

▶ The connection between hypertension and pain threshold is interesting. The postulated higher activation of the intrinsic opioid system as a cause is, as yet, unsupported. Would a prospective study on the prevalence of untreated essential hypertension in patients with chronic pain be revealing?—D.A. Van Alstine, M.D.

Morphine Does Not Affect Laser Induced Warmth and Pin Prick Pain Thresholds

van der Burght M, Rasmussen SE, Arendt-Nielsen L, Bjerring P (Univ of Aarhus, Denmark; Univ of Aalborg, Denmark)

Acta Anaesthesiol Scand 38:161–164, 1994 131-95-6–57

Purpose.—The degree of analgesia provided by opiates varies. Clinical evidence suggests that continuous, deep visceral pain is generally opioid responsive, whereas cutaneous and neurogenic pain respond only occasionally. The effect of morphine on cutaneous warmth and pin-prick pain thresholds was evaluated with an argon laser as the source of pain.

Methods.—Fifteen healthy adult volunteers received IV morphine, .15 mg/kg, and an additional 15 volunteers received a placebo injection. An argon laser beam was directed to the skin of the right hand at increasing power. The warmth threshold was defined as the power at which a definite feeling of warmth occurred. The pin-prick pain threshold was the power at which a distinct pin-prick sensation was noted. This procedure was performed before medication and at 10, 20, 30, and 40 minutes afterward.

Results.—The warmth threshold increased maximally to 20.7% above baseline at 30 minutes after injection in the group given morphine. The corresponding increase in the placebo group was 14.3%, which is not significantly different from that of the medicated group. Similarly, the pin-prick pain threshold increased maximally to 9.4% above baseline at 30 minutes after injection in the group given morphine, with a corresponding increase of 4.6% in the placebo group. Again, these responses were not statistically distinguishable.

Conclusion.—The clinical impression that morphine has little effect on intermittent cutaneous pain was supported.

▶ This study has several ramifications. By using a laser, the authors were able to somewhat selectively supply an adequate stimulus to selective fiber types. The lack of effect on warmth sensation (probably C-fiber–mediated) and pin-prick pain (A-delta fiber) in this model, using intermittent stimuli, has implications for acute postoperative and labor pain. This clinical pain tends to have both incident (intermittent) and rest (continuous) components. This study is consistent with clinical experience that would suggest that opioids are much more effective in relieving rest than incident pain, thereby lending credence to the use of weak local anesthetic-opioid mixtures, as opposed to opioids alone, for central neuraxial blockade in the postoperative setting. Having said that, there are clearly instances in which opioids alone appear to be adequate. This model should be investigated further, as should others that allow selected fiber types to be stimulated, to further elucidate our understanding of pain mechanisms.—J.D. Haddox, D.D.S., M.D.

Effects of Extracorporeal Shock-Wave Lithotripsy on Referred Hyperalgesia From Renal/Ureteral Calculosis

Giamberardino MA, de Bigontina P, Martegiani C, Vecchiet L (G D'Annunzio Univ of Chieti, Italy; La Sapienza Univ, Rome)

Pain 56:77–83, 1994 131-95-6–58

Purpose.—Patients with unilateral renal-ureteral colic from calculosis of the upper urinary tract often experience referred hyperalgesia in the lumbar region of the affected side after the stone fragment has been eliminated with extracorporeal shock-wave lithotripsy (ESWL). The evolution of referred hyperalgesia was examined with clinical and instrumental means in 9 patients and 12 healthy volunteers.

Methods.—Fifteen patients met eligibility criteria and underwent sensory evaluation of the cutaneous, subcutaneous, and muscular tissues of the lumbar region of the affected side. After ESWL, patients were reevaluated at 1 month to determine whether at least 50% of the stone fragments had been eliminated and at 8 months to confirm complete elimination. Those criteria were met by 9 patients (4 men and 5 women; mean age, 42 years). Sensory evaluation of parietal tissue was again performed, and the patients were asked to keep a diary of their symptoms. Control subjects underwent pain threshold measurement to electrical stimulation at the L1 level.

Results.—All patients had muscle pain on percussion and were hypersensitive to digital pressure and pinch palpation before ESWL; 5 demon-

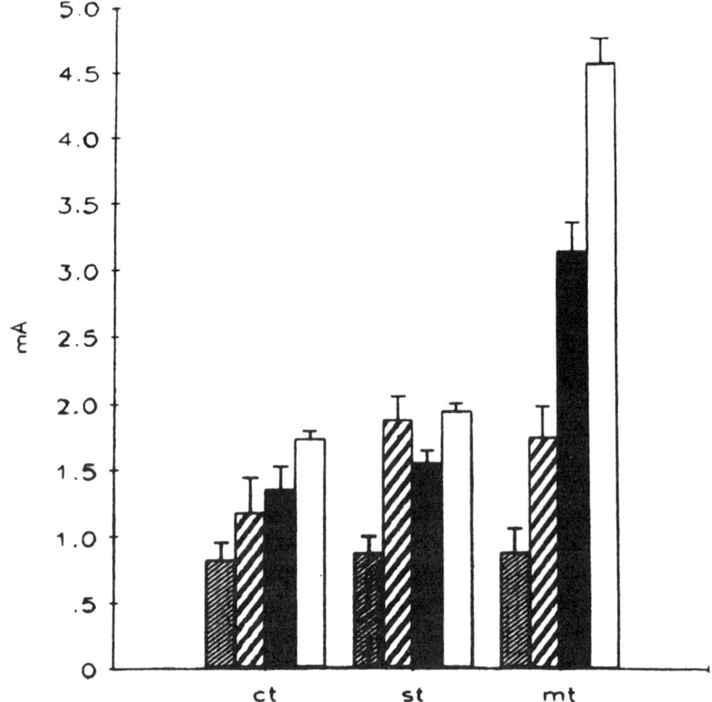

Fig 6–23.—Pain thresholds to electric stimulation of cutaneous (*ct*), subcutaneous (*st*), and muscular tissue (*mt*) at the lumbar level (metamere L1) of 1 side in 12 normal subjects (*open bars*) and in 9 patients affected with unilateral ureteral calculosis examined before extracorporeal shock-wave lithotripsy (ESWL) (*hatched bars*) and 1 month (*striped bars*) and 8 months (*filled bars*) afterward. Values are means ± SEM. (Courtesy of Giamberardino MA, de Bigontina P, Martegiani C, et al: *Pain* 56:77–83, 1994.)

strated a positive dermatographic reaction as well. Cutaneous, subcutaneous, and muscular pain thresholds to electrical stimulation were significantly lower than the values obtained in healthy volunteers. One month after ESWL, pinch palpation, the dermatographic procedure, and pin scratch-induced hyperalgesia test yielded negative results; muscle percussion and digital pressure, however, produced positive results. Thresholds of the 3 tissues were higher than before treatment but still significantly lower than normal in muscle. At 8 months, no patients had clinical signs of hyperalgesia. Thresholds of the 3 tissues remained lower than normal and were significantly different for subcutaneous tissue and muscle (Fig 6–23).

Conclusion.—The persistence of parietal tissue hyperalgesia in the area of referred pain from renal-ureteral calculosis depends only in part on the continuing presence of the stone after ESWL. Therefore, a certain amount of hyperalgesia, especially in the deep tissues, appears to be independent of the primary focus. The mechanism of this phenomenon remains uncertain.

► This paper was selected as an excellent contemporary description of referred hyperalgesia. The authors used a collection of readily accessible methods to quantify and characterize the hyperalgesic zone. These methods may be of use in other studies investigating similar phenomenon. The relevance of these findings is in the diagnosis of pain states and, perhaps, a better understanding of central sensitization.—J.D. Haddox, D.D.S., M.D.

Success Rates in Producing Sympathetic Blockade by Paratracheal Injection

Hogan QH, Taylor ML, Goldstein M, Stevens R, Kettler R (Med College of Wisconsin, Milwaukee; St Joseph's Hosp, Milwaukee, Wis)

Clin J Pain 10:139–145, 1994 131-95-6–59

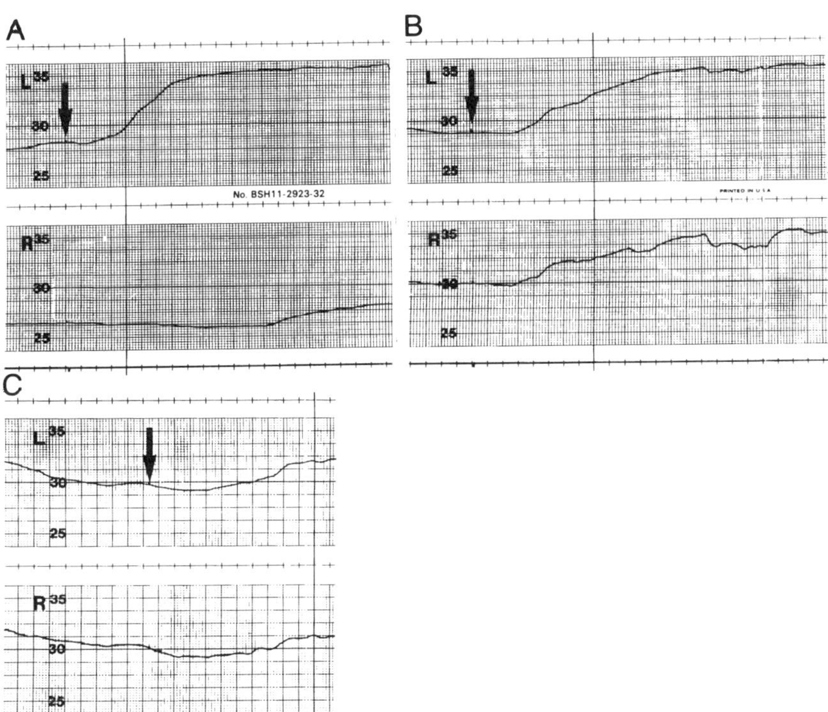

Fig 6–24.—Examples of the hand temperature responses to cervical paratracheal sympathetic blocks (*at arrow*). Large box (5 mm) = 1 min. **A,** unilateral temperature increase (7.2°C) after a block of the left side, probably indicating a selective unilateral sympathetic blockade. **B,** bilateral temperature increase (**left,** 6.5°C; **right,** 5.2°C) after a block of the left side, probably indicating bilateral sympathetic blockade or systemic effects of the local anesthetic. **C,** modest bilateral temperature increase (**left,** 2.2° C; **right,** 1.2°C) after a block of the left side, the most common pattern; also apparent is a gradual temperature decrease during and preceding the performance of the injection. (Courtesy of Hogan QH, Taylor ML, Goldstein M, et al: *Clin J Pain* 10:139–145, 1994.)

TABLE 1.—Success of Horner's Syndrome and Unilateral Warming

	$\Delta Ti \geq 1.5°C$	
	Yes	No
+ Horner's	57	27
– Horner's	3	13

(Courtesy of Hogan QH, Taylor ML, Goldstein M, et al: *Clin J Pain* 10:139–145, 1994.)

Purpose.—There are no standards for judging the effectiveness of a sympathetic block. A retrospective study was performed to review 100 anterior paratracheal injections and evaluate eye changes and hand temperatures to determine the physiologic effectiveness of the block.

Methods.—A total of 40 patients received 100 blocks because of a variety of indications. Fingertip temperature was taken. A lidocaine block was administered into the anterior tubercle of C-6.

Results.—Horner's syndrome occurred after 84 blocks. With hand warming as the standard, in 60 blocks, the hand on the injection side warmed by at least 1.5°C (Fig 6–24), and in 31 blocks, the opposite hand also warmed by at least 1.5°C. Therefore, only 27 of the blocks, all of which produced Horner's syndrome, were considered successful (Table 1). With an ipsilateral temperature of at least 34°C as the standard, 28 of 70 blocks were considered successful, including 1 without Horner's syndrome (Table 2).

Conclusion.—The presence of Horner's syndrome plus a temperature increase higher on the injection side suggests a successful block, but pathophysiologic inferences on the basis of a block should be made with caution.

▶ This article, which summarizes the results of 100 paratracheal sympathetic blocks, should be in the reference file of anyone who does these pro-

TABLE 2.—Success of Horner's Syndrome and Warming of the Ipsilateral Hand by 1.5°C More Than the Contralateral Hand

	$\Delta Ti\text{-}\Delta Te \geq 1.5°C$	
	Yes	No
+ Horner's	27	57
– Horner's	0	16

(Courtesy of Hogan QH, Taylor ML, Goldstein M, et al: *Clin J Pain* 10:139–145, 1994.)

cedures. All too often, inferences regarding pain mechanisms are made according to the results of these interventions, many of which are inadequately documented. This can lead to inappropriate measures and excessive expense and morbidity. This is a very thoughtful paper, the results of which should not be taken lightly.—J.D. Haddox, D.D.S., M.D.

Complications

Cerebrospinal Fluid Cutaneous Fistula

Howes J, Lenz R (Royal Cornwall Hosp, Truro, England)

Anaesthesia 49:221–222, 1994 131-95-6–60

Purpose.—Certain rare side effects of epidural analgesia administered because of acute or chronic pain are only now coming to light. Although previous reports have described CSF-cutaneous fistula, contributing factors have been present in all cases. Two patients with CSF-cutaneous fistula occurring after epidural anesthesia for postoperative pain relief are reported.

Patients.—The patients were a 59-year-old woman who underwent elective proctocolectomy and a 65-year-old man who underwent elective repair of an abdominal aortic aneurysm. Epidural catheters were placed after induction of anesthesia at the L2–3 and T9–10 interspaces, respectively. In both patients, loss of resistance to air was used to identify the epidural space. The day after the epidural catheters were removed, clear fluid was seen dripping from the puncture site in both cases.

Patient 1 complained of a typical postdural headache that began on the fourth postoperative day. This headache and the fluid leak failed to respond to 3 days of conservative management, so on the seventh day a blood patch was performed at the involved interspace with 10 mL of autologous blood. The symptoms resolved, and the patient was mobilized with no further headache or fluid leakage. There were no spinal or neurologic sequelae.

In patient 2, a typical spinal headache developed the day after the catheter was removed. The leaking fluid was confirmed to be CSF, and a blood patch was performed with 20 mL of autologous blood. Mobilization was uneventful, but 2 weeks later increasingly severe pain developed in the right buttock. In the pain clinic, a tender, well-localized area in the distribution of the right S5 nerve root was identified. Steroid and local anesthetic infiltration of this area yielded a good result. Another such treatment was given 2 weeks later. The pain was almost completely gone by 4 months.

Discussion.—In 2 patients, CSF-cutaneous fistula, a rare complication of epidural analgesia, developed. Patient 1 was receiving high-dose steroids to treat ulcerative colitis, which may have delayed healing. In patient 2, dural puncture was the only factor that predisposed to fistula development. If an epidural catheter close to the dural puncture site is a predisposing factor for fistula development, this complication may become more common as combined spinal-epidural techniques come into wider use. Back pain may have occurred as a side effect of the epidural blood patch in patient 2.

▶ This article was chosen to demonstrate an unusual complication associated with epidural catheter placement. The authors postulate that placing an epidural catheter in proximity to the site of a dural puncture may predispose to formation of a CSF-cutaneous fistula. Although rare, it is important to be aware of potential complications of this nature.—E. Lang, M.D.

Postblock Epidural Hematoma Causing Paraplegia

Ganjoo P, Singh AK, Mishra VK, Singh PK, Bannerjee D (Sanjay Gandhi Postgraduate Inst of Med Sciences, Lucknow, India)

Reg Anesth 19:62–65, 1994 131-95-6–61

Purpose.—Although it is a safe procedure, epidural block is occasionally associated with permanent neurologic deficit and other serious complications. Epidural hematoma that compresses the spinal cord has been reported as a cause of postblock paraplegia; however, large hematomas have been noted only in patients with coagulation or bleeding disorders. The occurrence of a large epidural hematoma that caused cord compression after epidural hematoma in a patient with no apparent bleeding or clotting abnormality was reported.

Case Report.—Man, 72, received continuous epidural anesthesia during transurethral prostatectomy. The patient had no obvious preexisting bleeding or clotting disorder, and he remained hemodynamically stable throughout the operation. When the epidural catheter was removed at 12 hours, the patient appeared to have recovered from the effects of the anesthetic: Sensation in his lower extremities had returned and the patient was moving his legs, although he did not get out of bed. However, on the third postoperative day, numbness and weakness occurred in both legs and progressed to complete paraplegia and bowel incontinence over the next few hours. At CT myelography, a complete extradural block from L1 upward was seen that compressed and displaced the dura anteriorly. Urgent laminectomy was performed about 20 hours after the onset of symptoms, at which time a large extradural clot that extended from D8 to L3 was evacuated. The hematoma was not explained by any bleeding site or vascular abnormality. The operation yielded no significant improvement in the patient's motor or sensory deficit.

Conclusion.—Spinal cord compression caused by epidural hematoma is a rare but possible complication of epidural block in patients with apparently normal hemodynamics. This possibility must be kept in mind when evaluating patients with postblock neurologic deficits. In the reported case, valuable time was lost because epidural hematoma was not considered in a patient with normal coagulation parameters.

► This article was chosen to demonstrate another unusual complication associated with epidural catheter placement. The exact incidence of epidural hematoma is unknown, but it is paramount to keep it in mind when evaluating patients with postblock neurologic defects.—E. Lang, M.D.

Delayed Diagnosis of the Cause of Facial Pain in Patients With Neoplastic Disease: A Report of Eight Cases

Huntley TA, Wiesenfeld D (Royal Melbourne Hosp, Australia)

J Oral Maxillofac Surg 52:81–85, 1994 131-95-6–62

Purpose.—Facial pain is a common initial complaint of many patients with temporomandibular dysfunction (TMD). In the current series of 8 patients with facial pain, 5 in whom TMD was initially diagnosed, were later found to have a tumor.

Patients.—The patients were 5 women, 2 men, and 1 boy (age range, 17–69 years). Swelling was a common feature (Fig 6–25). The patients had sought medical care from several physicians, as many as 11 in 1 case. Diagnostic delays ranged from 3 to 48 months. Final diagnoses included schwannoma, carcinoma in 2, osteoblastoma, ameloblastoma, lymphoma, angiosarcoma, and neurofibroma. The use of CT was important to the diagnosis in 6 of the 8 patients (Figs 6–26 and 6–27). In 1 patient, there was no evidence of tumor on the initial scan, but a subsequent scan demonstrated tumor in the left infratemporal fossa. Although the tumor was evident on initial CT scans in another patient, it was misdiagnosed as masseteric and medial pterygoid hypertrophy. Three patients eventually died, 2 are alive with disease, and 2 are alive with no signs of disease; 1 patient was lost to follow-up.

Conclusion.—All patients with massive neoplastic disease in this series had a surprising lack of accompanying signs and relatively innocuous symptoms. Failure to determine the correct diagnosis resulted in substantial treatment delays. Several features should alert clinicians to diagnoses other than TMD in patients with facial pain: constant pain that is not influenced by jaw movement; increasing severity of symptoms or symptoms that remain unchanged; the presence of swelling; neurologic signs such as unexplained sensory changes in the distribution of the trigeminal nerve or hearing loss; and marked trismus, especially of rapid onset during treatment.

► A high suspicion for alternative diagnoses for the cause of pain cannot be overstressed. Unusual signs and symptoms or failure to respond as expected to a specific treatment should trigger a reevaluation of the diagnosis. Unfortunately, in an era of rigid cost-containment strategies, delays in further workups for unresponsive patients will doubtless continue.—D.A. Van Alstine, M.D.

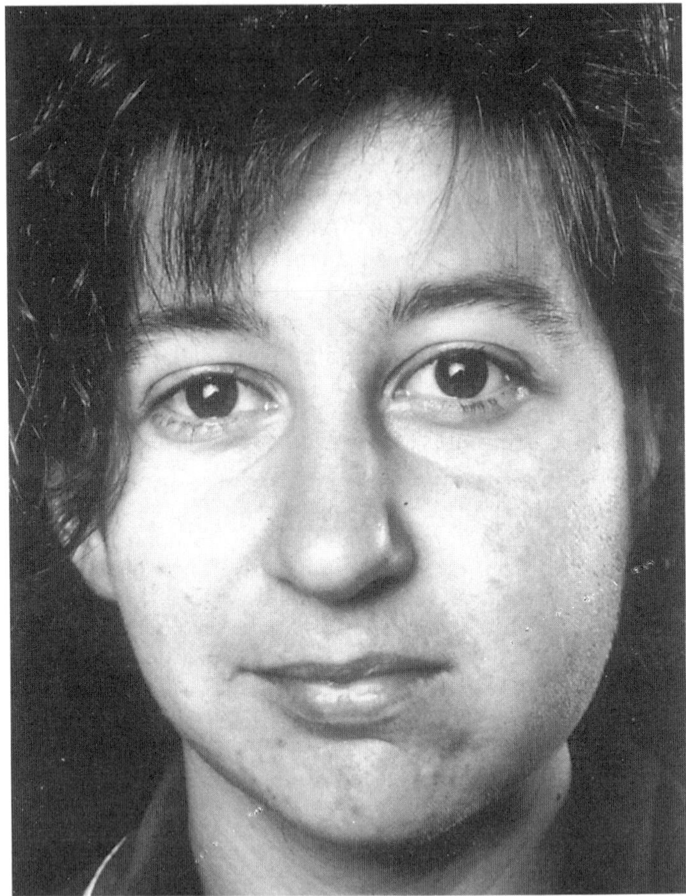

Fig 6–25.—Clinical photograph demonstrating facial swelling. (Courtesy of Huntley TA, Wiesenfeld D: *J Oral Maxillofac Surg* 52:81-85, 1994.)

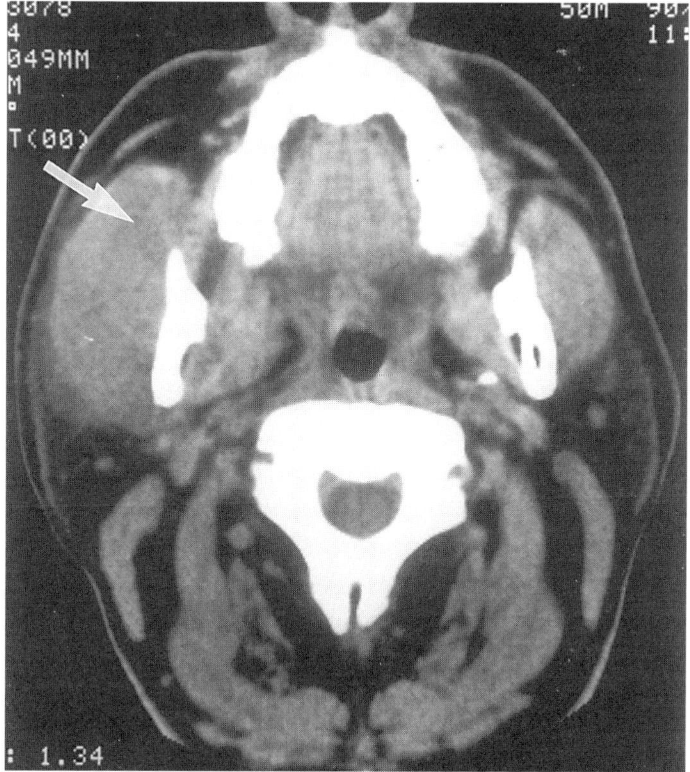

Fig 6–26.—Computed tomography scan demonstrating a right perimandibular mass extending into the infratemporal fossa (*arrow*). (Courtesy of Huntley TA, Wiesenfeld D: *J Oral Maxillofac Surg* 52:81-85, 1994.)

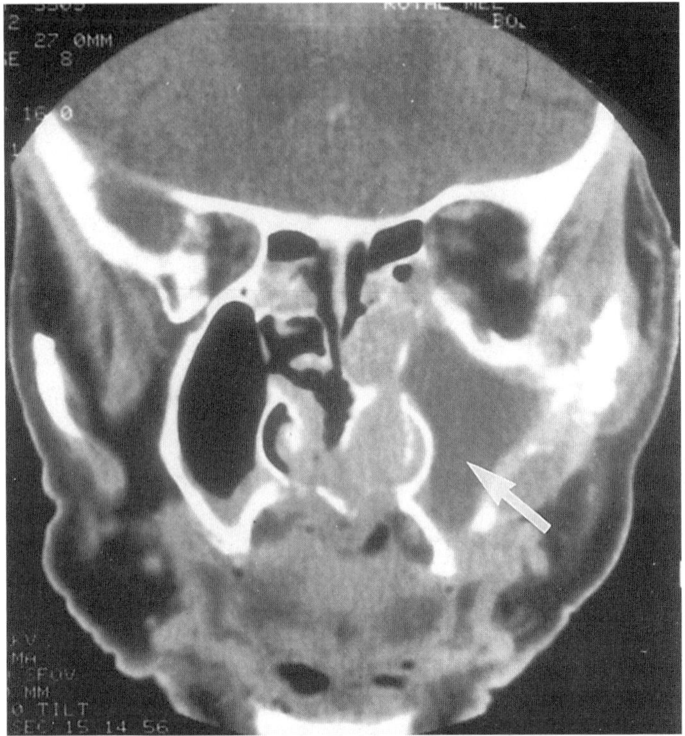

Fig 6–27.—Computed tomography scan demonstrating obliteration of the left maxillary and ethmoidal sinuses and nasal cavity (*arrow*). (Courtesy of Huntley TA, Wiesenfeld D: *J Oral Maxillofac Surg* 52:81-85, 1994.)

Does the Design of the Sprotte Spinal Needle Reduce the Force Needed to Deform the Tip?

Lipov EG, Sosis MB, McCarthy RJ, Ivankovich AD (Rush-Presbyterian-St Luke's Med Ctr, Chicago)

J Clin Anesth 6:411–413, 1994 131-95-6–63

Purpose.—The use of pencil-point spinal needles has become popular for decreasing postspinal headaches caused by CSF leakage after dural puncture. Recently, during subarachnoid insertion with a 24-gauge Sprotte needle in 2 patients, the needle tip bent when resistance was encountered. Although there was no CSF when the stylet was removed to check positioning, there was bending in the window area of the needle. In both cases, removing the needle was difficult. These occurrences prompted a study of the force needed to deform the tip of various spinal needles when axial and perpendicular forces were applied.

Methods.—An independent testing laboratory performed the independent-measure, multigroup study. An Instron gauge was used to determine the force necessary to bend 22- and 24-gauge Sprotte, 22- and 25-gauge Whitacre, and 22- and 25-gauge Quincke needles after microscopic verification of needle uniformity.

Results.—The force required to bend the Sprotte needles was less than that needed to bend Whitacre and Quincke needles of comparable gauge when lateral or axial pressure was applied. Microscopic inspection of the needles demonstrated a wide variability in the window area placement in a single lot of Sprotte needles. Needle tip assessment showed that the Sprotte needles were most likely to bend at the needle window, whereas the Quincke and Whitacre needles deformed at the point of clamping.

Conclusion.—Sprotte needles are inherently weak to lateral and axial pressure. This may result in a higher number of needle tip deformations on needle insertion. The nature of this deformation may make it difficult to withdraw the needle and may result in needle tip fracture.

▶ Reductions in the frequency of dural puncture headache are well documented with the pencil-point spinal needle designs. It is important, however, that we do not sacrifice safety and reliability to achieve that goal. In this series, Whitacre needles did not have a tendency to fail at the injection window. Newer versions of the Sprotte-style needle have the exit hole placed closer to the needle tip; the strength characteristics of this design have not been tested. Other needle designs are in development.—D.A. Van Alstine, M.D.

Epidural Catheter-Induced Traumatic Radiculopathy in Obstetrics: One Center's Experience

Yoshii WY, Rottman RL, Rosenblatt RM, Kotelko DM, Rasmus KT, Rosen PJ, Wright WC, Stone JJ (Cedars-Sinai Med Ctr, Los Angeles)

Reg Anesth 19:132–135, 1994 131-95-6–64

Purpose.—Continuous epidural anesthesia is widely used in obstetric practice. Few reports have described prolonged neurologic dysfunction directly related to trauma from the epidural catheter. Seven cases of prolonged neurologic dysfunction occurring after continuous lumbar epidural anesthesia in obstetric patients over a 1-year period were reported.

Methods and Results.—The epidural blocks were used for labor analgesia in 5 patients, all of whom had spontaneous vaginal deliveries. In the other 2 patients, the blocks were placed for elective, repeat cesarean delivery. Six different anesthesiologists delivered the blocks. There was no unusual resistance to any of the epidural catheters, but all resulted in unilateral paresthesias. All of the patients experienced varying degrees of hyperesthesia to touch. These symptoms were limited to 1 or 2 adjacent dermatomes and were unilaterally distributed to the same side as the initial paresthesia. The symptoms were severe and painful in 4 patients. In the other 3, they were similar but significantly milder and were not noticed until routine anesthesiologic follow-up the next day. Three patients were given carbamazepine, and 1 of these was given epidural methylprednisolone as well. The symptoms resolved completely within 1 day to 1 month in 5 patients; in the other 2 patients, some symptoms were still present at 2–9 months of follow-up.

Discussion.—The probable mechanism of neurologic dysfunction in these patients is epidural catheter-induced traumatic radiculopathy. The most critical features in causing this form of neurotrauma may be epidural catheter stiffness and tip construction. Paresthesias as a result of epidural catheter insertion may be more significant than previously thought; the milder symptoms in this series might not have been recognized if the authors' experience had not alerted them to this syndrome.

▶ This article was chosen to demonstrate another unusual complication associated with epidural catheter placement. Patients often ask about nerve damage after epidural or spinal anesthesia. This report suggests that parasthesias occurring during placement of epidural catheters should not be ignored and that the catheter should probably be repositioned. Reports like these can help make us aware of complications and avoid morbidity.—E. Lang, M.D.

Subdural Anesthesia as a Complication of an Interscalene Brachial Plexus Block: Case Report

Tetzlaff JE, Yoon HJ, Dilger J, Brems J (The Cleveland Clinic Found, Ohio)
Reg Anesth 19:357–359, 1994 131-95-6–65

Purpose.—Although interscalene brachial plexus block offers an alternative to general anesthesia for shoulder surgery, the procedure is not without complications. Serious complications of interscalene brachial plexus block include misdirection of local anesthetic into the epidural, subdural, or subarachnoid space. A high central block was produced after a local anesthetic was injected during an attempted interscalene plexus block.

Case Report.—Man, 43, was given IV midazolam before capsular repair of chronic shoulder instability. An interscalene brachial plexus block was placed with a 25-gauge ¾-inch needle. During a 3-minute period, .25 mL of a combination of 1.4% mepivacaine, 1:200,000 epinephrine, and 4 mL of sodium bicarbonate was injected. This was followed by injection of 3 mL of the solution during a 2-minute period and slow injection of the remaining volume. A complete sensory and motor nerve block was obtained. Before the start of the procedure, the patient's pulse rate was 68 and blood pressure was 110/60 mm Hg.

About 20 minutes after injection was completed, the patient became short of breath, apneic, and reported tingling in his right arm. Within minutes, he was unable to move his arm and displayed slurred speech, but he did not lose consciousness. His pulse rate was 86 and blood pressure was 100/55 mm Hg. Administration of 100% oxygen was begun, along with 5 mg of ephedrine, and general anesthesia was induced with 100 mg sodium thiopental. Surgery proceeded without further difficulty, and the patient experienced an uneventful postoperative course.

Discussion.—Complications of interscalene anesthesia include stellate ganglion block, recurrent laryngeal nerve block, phrenic nerve block, and intravascular injection. Injection into the subdural, epidural, or subarachnoid space resulting from misdirection of the needle occurs less commonly. Unintentional epidural block is rare. If a high central block occurs, the patient's symptoms are a clue to the type of central block produced. In this case, the slow onset of symptoms eliminated the possibility of subarachnoid injection, and the apnea precluded epidural injection. The scalene block that was achieved indicated that injection was correctly placed in the sheath of the brachial plexus, but partial injection into the subdural space must have occurred. Equipment for monitoring and resuscitation should be available whenever interscalene anesthesia is attempted.

▶ This article stresses an unusual complication of interscalene brachial plexus block. When performing these blocks, it is important to have monitoring and resuscitation equipment available. The article also describes how to differentiate between subarachnoid, epidural, and subdural injections.—E. Lang, M.D.

Staphylococcal Meningitis Following Synchromed Intrathecal Pump Implant: A Case Report

Bennett MI, Tai YMA, Symonds JM (St James Univ Hosp, Leeds, England; Guest Hosp, Dudley, England; Russells Hall Hosp, Dudley, England)

Pain 56:243–244, 1994 131-95-6–66

Purpose.—Staphylococcal meningitis can occur as a complication of intraventricular shunts in neurosurgical patients. The infection is usually treated with shunt removal and intrathecal or intraventricular vancomycin. A patient in whom staphylococcal meningitis was successfully treated without the need for intrathecal drug pump removal is reported.

Case Report.—Man, 18, with cerebral palsy received an implanted intrathecal drug pump for the treatment of painful adductor muscle spasms caused by spastic paraplegia. The pump delivered continuous intrathecal baclofen at a rate of 450 μg/day. Ceftazidime and vancomycin were given as routine prophylaxis. On day 39, the patient was readmitted with pyrexia, vomiting, and headache. A pyogenic infection was detected at lumbar puncture, and culture grew *Staphylococcus epidermidis*. The symptoms did not respond to rifampicin and flucloxacillin, which were active in vivo against the pathogen.

Because the intrathecal pump had a bacterial filter between the reservoir and outport, catheter contamination was assumed to be the source of continuing infection. The baclofen in the reservoir was replaced on day 60 with vancomycin, 50 mg/mL, which was continuously infused at 5 mg/day. Two days later the pyrexia resolved, and a third lumbar puncture on day 70 showed that the infection was resolving. The CSF vancomycin concentration was 55 mg/L, so the infusion rate was reduced to 2.5 mg/day. The patient continued to take oral rifampicin and flucloxacillin at home for 2 weeks, after which baclofen was added to the vancomycin in the pump. There was no evidence of infection in the CSF on day 116. Vancomycin infusion was continued until day 186, when the CSF was again clear. The CSF was still normal 34 days later, and the patient has remained well.

Discussion.—In this case, staphylococcal meningitis associated with intrathecal pump implantation responded to intrathecal vancomycin without the need for removal of the pump and catheter system. This is the first such case reported. Although further experience is needed, the experience suggests that intrathecal vancomycin, 2.5–5 mg/day, is sufficient as long as the clinical and laboratory findings are satisfactory.

▶ This article was chosen to demonstrate a serious complication of placement of an intrathecal pump. It is imperative that before placement of these devices, the cost-benefit risk ratio be clear to the clinician and patient. It is surprising that the infection did not necessitate removal of the pump.—E. Lang, M.D.

Reversible Urinary Retention Secondary to Excessive Morphine Delivered by an Intrathecal Morphine Pump

Uppal GS, Haider TT, Dwyer A, Uppal JA (Inland Empire Spine Inst, Riverside, Calif; Univ of Southern California, Los Angeles; Univ of Colorado, Denver)

Spine 19:719–720, 1994 131-95-6–67

Purpose.—Intractable pain caused by cancer is often treated with intrathecal morphine infusion through an implanted pump, and some orthopedic surgeons are using this approach for patients with refractory pain in the back or leg.

Case Report.—Man, 70, required opioid treatment of back pain after undergoing a number of unsuccessful operations over 2 decades. Computed tomographic scans demonstrated arachnoiditis in the lumbar spine but no bony compression, and an MRI study showed scar tissue in the area of surgery. Back pain had persisted despite conservative measures but was almost totally relieved by an intrathecal dose of 0.5 mg of morphine. A pump then was implanted subcutaneously in the abdominal wall and connected with an intrathecal catheter. Treatment with morphine, 2 mg/24 hr, controlled pain well for 3 weeks; abdominal pain and difficulty in urination developed, however, and a cystometrogram revealed a flaccid neurogenic bladder. Spinal CT scans failed to demonstrate compression of the cord or dura. Normal bladder function returned after the dose of morphine was reduced to 0.5 mg/24 hours. Postvoid residual urine at the time of discharge was less than 30 mL.

Conclusion.—If urinary retention develops in a patient receiving opioids via intrathecal pump and cord compression is ruled out, the dose should be reduced until the condition is reversed.

▶ Having seen this complication in a young male in whom an intrathecal pump was implanted by one of our neurosurgeons, I thought this paper should be highlighted. At the first sign of urinary difficulty, a trial of naloxone or nalbuphine would be helpful in determining cause, without the need for imaging. Certainly, if these drugs did not correct the problem, imaging would be prudent. The paper highlights yet another potential problem with the use of intrathecal opioids, and it should generate considerable respect for this procedure and its potential complications before it is undertaken.—J.D. Haddox, D.D.S., M.D.

7 Nursing

Introduction

The 46 articles selected for inclusion in Chapter 7 represent the wide scope of knowledge needed by nurses in the management of patient pain. Many of the studies reported were conducted by nurses, but they have usefulness for other clinicians. Other studies, conducted by clinicians and investigators from other disciplines, have clear relevance for nursing practice. The overlap in research reflects the multidisciplinary nature of most pain management. It is likely this disciplinary overlap will increase as more institutions adopt critical pathways and protocols for care that incorporate the work of more than one type of care provider.

Articles included in this chapter indicate the kinds of pain management knowledge needed by nurses. Many of the other chapters in this book elaborate on topics mentioned in this section. Thus, nurse readers may want to begin with the nursing chapter, but they certainly should not stop there.

Articles on measurement show an increasing tendency to test the appropriateness of established measurement instruments for different populations. This approach is much preferable to each investigator or group of clinicians developing an instrument for their own use. Also included in the section on measurement is a discussion of quality-of-life measures, which are becoming increasingly important in the study of pain.

The cornerstone of pain management is the use of drugs, and nurses usually are the individuals who administer them. The development of new drugs and routes of administration is occurring rapidly and affects what nurses need to know to practice safely and effectively. Again, the selections in this chapter represent a small subset of what is available in other chapters. The focus is less on individual drugs and more on the routes of administration and the complications and side effects that occur with various drugs and routes of administration.

At an earlier time in nursing research, there was considerable discussion of the psychological characteristics related to patients' experience of pain. The literature reviewed during this past year produced only one such study by a nurse, which may be somewhat indicative of a move away from describing factors that influence pain and toward giving attention to how to manage it.

Increased attention by clinicians, case managers, payers, and others to the development and use of guidelines for clinical practice is reflected in the literature with an increase in guideline-oriented publications. Many of these relate to the United States Agency for Health Care Policy and Research guidelines on the management of acute postoperative pain and management of cancer pain (1, 2). There are indications that the development of research-based practice guidelines will be accelerated.

Although much has been written about nurses' use of nondrug interventions, empirical research on this is sparse. Only one study of cognitively based interventions was found in the nursing literature of the past year. In addition, the article that reviews the poor quality of research on the use of ice to relieve pain illustrates another major research gap that could be appropriately addressed by nurses.

Also at an earlier time, the pain literature was primarily focused on young or middle-aged adults undergoing abdominal surgery, with some attention given to patients with pain caused by cancer. It is encouraging to see the increased attention given to pain in younger and older populations and in various clinical populations. Pain is a complex phenomenon, and we are only beginning to understand how the nature of the condition associated with the pain and various patient characteristics influence the pain experience.

The last section of this chapter is focused on organizational and policy issues related to pain management. It underscores the fact that although effective pain management is the individual clinician's responsibility, it also is an institutional responsibility.

As nurses, we commonly express the view that we are patient advocates. It seems peculiar to me, therefore, that our literature is so devoid of any attention to patient preference in pain management. This is true not only of the nursing literature but of the pain literature in general. One purpose of this YEAR BOOK OF PAIN is to identify gaps in the research on pain. The gap between what we say about patient advocacy and the lack of research on patient preferences is particularly wide.

Ada K. Jacox, R.N., Ph.D.

References

1. Carr DB, Jacox A, et al: *Acute Pain Management: Operative or Medical Procedures and Trauma. Clinical Practice Guideline.* Rockville, Md, Agency for Health Care Policy and Research, 1992. PHS, USDHHS, AHCPR Publication 92-0032.
2. Jacox A, Carr DB, Payne R, et al: *Cancer Pain Guideline Panel. Management of Cancer Pain. Clinical Practice Guideline.* Rockville, Md, Agency for Health Care Policy and Research, 1994. PHS, USDHHS, AHCPR Publication 94-0592.

Measurement and Methodological Issues

Alternate Oucher Form Testing: Gender, Ethnicity, and Age Variations

Jordan-Marsh M, Yoder L, Hall D, Watson R (Univ of California Los Angeles

Med Ctr, Torrance)
Res Nurs Health 17:111–118, 1994 131-95-7–1

Purpose.—Although many tools for assessing pain in children have been reported, few studies have examined their systematic clinical use. Such use will require wide applicability across age groups and the absence of sex- and ethnicity-related effects. The few studies that have assessed ethnically diverse samples of children have found ethnicity-related differences. The Oucher form, modified to reduce its size and shorten the screening technique, was evaluated to determine sex, ethnicity, and age variations in the assessment of pain in children.

Methods.—A convenience sample of 79 acute care or clinic pediatric patients were studied. Age range was 3–12 years. Most of the original sample scored 0 on the Oucher so only 19 children were included in the final comparison. The children used 2 versions of the Oucher in random order: the original, poster-sized format and a reduced, 8½- × 11-inch form. The Oucher, which includes both a 0–100 numerical scale and 5 photographs of a young, male, white child reflecting various levels of discomfort, was selected on the basis of its visual appeal to the clinical team. The screening process was shortened by asking the children to count to 100 by 10s rather than 1s.

Results.—Scores on the Oucher scales were highly correlated, regardless of the size or presentation order of the 2 formats. No differences were noted by age, gender, or black, white, or Hispanic ethnicity.

Conclusion.—Preliminary research supports the use of the smaller Oucher form and the shortened screening process for the assessment of pain in children. The numerical Oucher can be used for children aged 5–12 years, regardless of sex or ethnicity. Because of the small sample size, the lack of ethnic differences on the photographic Oucher should be interpreted cautiously. If further studies reveal ethnic differences, alternative photographic versions that represent different ethnic groups might be created.

▶ This comparison of the usefulness of two measurement instruments in a population of pediatric patients with cancer is a good example of the kinds of study that need to be done on the multiple instruments available for measuring pain. Measurement instruments do not work the same in different clinical groups and different ages. Comparing already developed tools in various populations is far preferable to the practice in some institutions of developing new measures with unknown psychometric properties. We need to know a great deal more about which of the available instruments work better with different groups so that our knowledge in this and other areas is cumulative.—A.K. Jacox, R.N., Ph.D.

Measuring Pain in Pediatric Oncology ICU Patients

West N, Oakes L, Hinds PS, Sanders L, Holden R, Williams S, Fairclough D, Bozeman P (St Jude Children's Research Hosp, Memphis, Tenn)
J Pediatr Oncol Nurs 11:64–68, 1994 131-95-7–2

Purpose.—Most pediatric patients with cancer will experience significant pain during the course of their illness, whether from the disease or from diagnostic, monitoring, or treatment procedures. Research suggests that pain is commonly undertreated in children with cancer, in part because of their limited ability to communicate their pain and the methods used by care givers to assess the presence of pain. Such assessment is particularly difficult in the ICU. Various pain measurement tools were assessed for feasibility and accuracy in pediatric oncology ICU patients.

Methods.—Thirty 5- to 13-year-old patients in a pediatric oncology ICU were included. The patients rated the presence and severity of their pain on 2 measurement tools, the Faces Pain Scale (FPS) and the Poker Chip Tool (PCT). The children's parents used the same scales to rate their child's pain independently. In addition, the children's nurses rated their patients' pain using the Objective Pain Scale (OPS).

Findings.—Patients' and parents' pain ratings were significantly correlated on the FPS but not the PCT. A moderate correlation was noted between nurses' ratings on the OPS and patients' ratings on the FPS. The nurses' ratings were only weakly correlated with the children's PCT ratings. Most participants, including patients, parents, and nurses, preferred the FPS to the PCT.

Conclusion.—For children who can cooperate with a self-report measurement, the FPS appears to be an accurate and clinically useful tool for measuring pain in the pediatric oncology ICU. The low interrater agreement suggests that patients, parents, and nurses rate intensity of pain in different ways. Continued research is needed to develop an accurate behavioral observational pain scale that incorporates physiologic indicators.

▶ The comment after Abstract 131-95-7–1 is relevant for this study, which compared use of measurement instruments with patients who were ethnically diverse and had various clinical conditions.—A.K. Jacox, R.N., Ph.D.

Development and Evaluation of the Family Pain Questionnaire

Ferrell B, Rhiner M, Rivera LM (City of Hope Natl Med Ctr, Duarte, Calif)
J Psychosoc Oncol 10:21–35, 1993 131-95-7–3

Purpose.—Pain has a major impact on the quality of life of patients with cancer. The family is important to cancer patients; home care of cancer patients is increasing, and family members provide the vast majority of this care. Overall patient care might be enhanced by an understanding of the family's knowledge of and attitudes toward pain. The development and testing of an instrument to measure family caregivers' experience with and knowledge of cancer pain were reported.

Methods.—The instrument, called the Family Pain Questionnaire (FPQ), was developed with the use of data from a larger study of cancer pain as seen from the perspective of caregivers. The study sample comprised the primary family caregivers of 85 patients with cancer who were receiving analgesics. Seventy-two percent of these caregivers were women. Almost 66% were the patient's spouse; 26% were the patient's child. Eighty-five percent of all caregivers lived with the patient. The FPQ was developed with data obtained through interviews with the caregivers and refined through expert opinion and additional psychometric testing. The 21-item FPQ was modeled after tools used to measure health care professionals' knowledge and attitudes about pain. It assessed the caregivers' knowledge of basic pain principles such as addiction, pain relief, and routine analgesia. It also assessed caregivers' personal experiences with pain and included the caregivers' perceptions of the patient's pain and their own distress regarding the pain.

Results.—Mean scores on the FPQ indicated that the caregivers' weakest area of knowledge was related to their tendency to give low medication doses for fear of not having enough for later. The scores reflected significant fear of respiratory depression and addiction. Knowledge was highest for items regarding the need to give medication before the pain becomes severe and belief in the usefulness of nondrug approaches to pain management. Scores were high for all 4 items in the experience scale: patient's current pain, patient's current pain relief, distressfulness of pain to the patient, and distressfulness of pain to the caregiver. The caregivers rated the patients' pain as much more severe than the patients did.

Conclusion.—Cancer pain has an important impact on family caregivers; it appears to be an overwhelming and all-consuming experience for the caregivers. The FPQ identifies areas of pain management in which caregivers need education. The FPQ will be useful in research and clinical practice to evaluate the caregiver's role and experiences in pain management.

▶ Understanding the impact of cancer and cancer pain management on patients' families has been a neglected area. This instrument for measuring the knowledge of and attitudes toward pain among family caregivers of patients with cancer should be a helpful adjunct to clinicians in evaluating the educational needs of the families of patients.—A.K. Jacox, R.N., Ph.D.

The Accuracy of Memory for Pain: Not So Bad Most of the Time

Salovey P, Smith AF, Turk DC, Jobe JB, Willis GB (Yale Univ, New Haven, Conn; State Univ of New York, Binghamton; Univ of Pittsburgh, Pa; et al)

APS J 2:184–191, 1993 131-95-7-4

Purpose.—The clinical treatment of chronic pain syndromes requires systematic assessment of pain based to some degree on patients' self-reports. The accuracy of autobiographic and retrospective accounts of pain severity is often questioned, however. The accuracy of memory for pain was investigated.

Methods.—A multiyear research program was conducted to explore accuracy in the reporting of chronic pain episodes. Six experiments were done to investigate sources of error in the retrospective reporting of pain episodes. The experiments focused on complexities in the language used to describe pain, the relative accuracy of retrospective accounts of pain intensity vs. pain-related behavior, and the effects of current mood and levels of pain on memory of previous painful experiences.

Results.—Pain and pain behaviors documented over 1 month were accurately recalled later. Diary-keeping had little impact on memory for pain and was not systematically affected by transient mood. Pain reports appeared to be robust against the influence of transient moods. Pain experienced at the time of recall systematically influenced its recall. Thus, with the exception of the biasing effect of present pain on the reporting of past pain, the accuracy of pain recall was high.

Conclusion.—In general, self-reports of pain can be trusted. Pain seems to be recalled with reasonable accuracy, and pain-related behaviors are recalled with equal accuracy. Although much maligned, retrospective self-reports of pain obtained systematically with measures of proven reliability appear to be relatively trustworthy.

▶ This interesting set of studies in patients with chronic pain challenges the assumption that retrospective accounts of pain severity in these patients may be inaccurate. Of the several variables that the author studied, only pain at the time of recall affected the reliability of the previously experienced pain. Much more needs to be understood regarding the factors that influence the accuracy of pain recall in various populations, as indicated by the numerous inconsistencies in the literature cited by the researchers. The condition with which the pain is associated may be one factor that influences pain recall.—A.K. Jacox, R.N., Ph.D.

Nurses' Assessment of Postoperative Patients' Pain

Zalon ML (Univ of Scranton, Pa)

Pain 54:329–334, 1993 131-95-7-5

Purpose.—Nurses are directly responsible for providing measures to relieve pain. Their assessment of pain is essential to providing pain-relieving measures. However, research indicates that incomplete pain relief is an acceptable goal among nurses. Nurses' pain assessments were compared with patients' pain assessments.

Methods.—One hundred nineteen nurses and 119 patients (66 women) who had undergone abdominal surgery were surveyed at 2 community and 2 university hospitals. Their average age was 51 years (range, 19–83 years). Patients completed a 10-cm visual analogue scale (VAS) ranging from "no pain" to "pain as bad as it could be." Within 10 minutes, nurses also marked a VAS. Just before assessment, about 40% of nurses spent less than 5 minutes with their patients and about 50% spent 5–15 minutes. Neither nurse nor patient saw the other's assessment.

Results.—Nurses' assessments of patients' pain significantly correlated with patients' assessments. However, nurses overestimated the severity of mild pain and underestimated the severity of severe pain. Patient age, sex, acuity of illness, number of days after surgery, and the amount of time the nurses spent with patients did not significantly affect the nurses' assessments. The patients' pain was unrelated to age. There were no differences in accuracy of assessment among the different hospital units. It was observed that nurses did not consistently use a standardized method to assess pain that has been recommended by experts.

Conclusion.—Underestimating pain is a serious clinical problem. Research on systematic assessment methods would be valuable for the management of postoperative pain. Also, research linking the accurate pain assessment with adequate pain relief is suggested.

▶ This well-designed study documents the continuing difficulty in clinicians' ability to accurately assess patients' pain. The thoughtful discussion of the findings is useful, because it goes beyond describing discrepancies between patients' and nurses' assessments to try to identify factors contributing to the discrepancy. These included nurse behaviors such as variability in how—or even whether—pain was assessed by nurses, as well as variations in how patients marks a VAS or report pain to nurses. It is well known that there are frequent differences between clinicians' and patients' assessments of pain. This study suggests some reasons for this.—A.K. Jacox, R.N., Ph.D.

Multidimensional Pain Assessment in Premature Neonates: A Pilot Study

Stevens BJ, Johnston CC, Horton L (Univ of Toronto, Ont, Canada)
J Obstet Gynecol Neonatal Nurs 22:531–541, 1993 131-95-7-6

Purpose.—Repeat painful procedures in premature infants may have significant, permanent consequences. Less is known about the specific responses of premature infants than those of healthy, full-term infants.

The physiologic and behavioral responses of premature neonates to a painful stimulus were investigated.

Methods.—Forty neonates aged 32–34 weeks' post conception and younger than 5 days postnatal age were examined. Physiologic and behavioral responses were observed during a routine heel-stick and squeeze procedure.

Results.—During the most invasive phase of the procedure, mean heart rate increased and mean oxygen saturation decreased. The variance of the changes in intracranial pressure was great. Behavioral parameters observed were, in order of frequency, brow bulge, eye squeeze, nasolabial furrow, and open lips. Significant differences occurred between cries in the stick and squeeze phases. Changes in intracranial pressure scores were significant only between the baseline and stick phases. Most facial actions differed significantly between the baseline and stick and baseline and squeeze phases. The peak fundamental frequency and minimal fundamental frequency of crying were significantly greater during the stick phase than during the squeeze phase. Illness severity did not affect the physiologic parameters, and facial expression did not significantly affect the peak spectral energy of the cry during the squeeze phase.

Conclusion.—Premature infants can express their pain in ways similar to those of healthy, full-term neonates. Behavioral responses were more promising indicators than physiologic responses, which were significant but nonspecific for pain.

▶ Understanding of premature infants' responses to noxious, painful stimuli has progressed from initially denying that infants were capable of feeling the stimulus to acknowledgment that they may feel it but that it is difficult to measure. This well-designed study has identified behavioral responses such as brow bulge, eye squeeze, nasal labial furrow, and open lips, all of which can be observed by clinicians and all of which are very similar to facial expressions observed in healthy full-term neonates. This significant study should contribute greatly to the measurement of pain and the assessment of pain in premature infants.—A.K. Jacox, R.N., Ph.D.

Assessment of Patient Satisfaction Utilizing the American Pain Society's Quality Assurance Standards on Acute and Cancer-Related Pain

Miaskowski C, Nichols R, Brody R, Synold T (Univ of California, San Francisco)

J Pain Symptom Manage 9:5–11, 1994 131-95-7-7

Purpose.—An important aspect of a quality assurance program that deals with pain management, as recommended by the American Pain Society (APS), is to determine how well satisfied patients are with how their pain is treated. Accordingly, a survey was undertaken at a 411-bed, acute-care, municipal hospital in San Francisco to estimate patient satis-

TABLE 1.—Patient Satisfaction Survey

1. At any time during this hospital stay have you needed treatment for pain?
2. How long have you been in pain?
3. Have you experienced pain in the last 24 hours?
4. Did you tell the doctors or nurses you were having pain?
5. On a scale of 0 to 10 with 0 representing "no pain" and 10 representing the "worst pain you can imagine," what was the worst pain you had in the past 24 hours?
6. On a scale of 0 to 10 with 0 representing "no pain" and 10 representing the "worst pain you can imagine," how much pain do you have right now?
7. On a scale of 0 to 10 with 0 representing "no pain" and 10 representing the "worst pain you can imagine," where did the pain go to after you got pain medication?
8. How satisfied are you with the amount of pain relief you received?
9. How satisfied are you with how the staff responded to your reports of pain?
10. Who do you believe is responsible for your pain relief while you are in the hospital?
11. Of the following health team members (i.e., doctor, nurse, social worker, physical therapist, pharmacist, other), who has been helpful to you when you were in pain?
12. When you asked for pain medication what was the longest time you had to wait to get it?
13. Was there a time when the medication you were given for pain didn't help and you asked for something more or different to relieve the pain?
14. If your answer is yes, how long did it take before your doctor or nurse changed your treatment to a stronger or different medication and you got it?
15. If longer than one hour, why do you think it took so long?
16. Did your doctors or nurses ask you to be sure to tell them when you have pain?
17. Did your doctors or nurses tell you we consider treatment of pain very important?

(Courtesy of Miaskowski C, Nichols R, Brody R, et al: *J Pain Symptom Manage* 9:5–11, 1994.)

faction with various aspects of their pain management. An unrandomized group of 72 medical or surgical patients from 9 nursing units participated in the study. The APS patient questionnaire (Table 1) was used.

Results.—All patients reported requiring treatment of pain at some point, and approximately half had been in pain for 8 days or longer. The mean pain intensity score was 4.25 at the time of the interview, and the highest score in the previous 24 hours was 7.6. More than one fourth of

TABLE 2.—Recommendations for Patient Satisfaction Surveys

1. Use a surveyor who is not directly involved in the patients' care, or conduct the survey after the patient has been discharged from the facility.
2. Evaluate analgesic prescriptive practices (i.e., number of analgesics ordered, types of analgesics ordered, frequency, route of administration, and dose).
3. Evaluate patient satisfaction with pain management practices and satisfaction with care providers using a descriptive, numeric rating scale.
4. Explore with the patient, in a nonthreatening manner, the incongruity between their pain intensity ratings and the level of satisfaction with pain relief or the staff's response to reports of pain.
5. Use additional survey responses (e.g., rating of pain relief, waiting time for pain medications, and requests for changes in pain management plan) to determine patient satisfaction with pain management practices.
6. Ask patients to rate how much pain they expect to have following surgery or as a result of a procedure and how much pain relief they expect to be provided to them.
7. Ask patients direct questions about what they would change about pain management in the institution.

(Courtesy of Miaskowski C, Nichols R, Brody R, et al: *J Pain Symptom Manage* 9:5–11, 1994.)

the patients had pain intensity scores of 5 or higher after receiving medication for pain. The average number of pain medications ordered was 2.34, but only 16% of patients received medication around the clock. About half of the patients had to wait longer than 15 minutes to receive their medication. Most patients believed that the physician was responsible for treating their pain while they were hospitalized. Nevertheless, they perceived nurses as being the most helpful of those who participated in their care. More than 70% of patients were at least somewhat satisfied with their pain relief. Those with the highest pain intensity scores were the least satisfied.

Conclusion.—Certain changes in the survey instrument (Table 2) would provide stronger data and help in developing improved pain management practices. Large enough samples would allow the study of varying practices in different specialty areas or on individual nursing units.

▶ One of the difficulties in knowing whether pain practices are changing is the lack of baseline data on present practices and patient satisfaction with them. This report of the use of a modified version of the APS questionnaire for measuring patient satisfaction with their pain management provides a useful model for others to use. The authors make useful suggestions about the need to explore with patients their reasons for rating their satisfaction with pain management as high even when they experienced inadequate pain relief.—A.K. Jacox, R.N., Ph.D.

▶ This study evaluates the treatment of and response to pain among inpatients. About half of the patients studied did not have relief of their pain with the prescribed therapies. Although the study was performed in patients who required acute care, the findings can be generalized. Patients with cancer also frequently need analgesic therapy and undergo acute care. The significance of this report is the documented failure to adequately treat pain that is often moderate to severe in intensity. This is especially important when considering the treatment of cancer-related pain, because patients with cancer, who often need higher doses of analgesics, are most frequently treated in general medical centers. It is unlikely that the documented inadequacy in treating pain would be any different for patients with cancer in the same medical facility.

Response to the analgesic needs of patients with cancer may be even more significantly compromised if the experience in the treatment of nonmalignant pain is extrapolated. Health care professionals need to be made aware of the inadequacies of pain management as part of quality assurance in meeting the therapeutic needs of the patient. Failure to adequately treat pain in general medical practice becomes even more profound in the patient with cancer, who often has severe, unremitting pain.—N.A. Janjan, M.D.

Quality of Life Issues in Pain Management Research

Wells N (Vanderbilt Univ Med Ctr, Nashville, Tenn)

APS Bul July/Aug:6–10, 1994 131-95-7–8

Purpose.—Quality-of-life (QOL) measures can help investigators determine whether intervention outcomes represent benefits to the patient. Measurements of QOL help determine new risk-to-benefit ratios of pain management.

Definition.—In 1958, The World Health Organization defined QOL as a "state of complete physical, mental and social well-being and not just the absence of disease and infirmity." More current definitions incorporate the psychological, social, and physical responses to illness and treatment and indicate that QOL, like pain, is multidimensional in its ef-

Selected Quality-of-Life Instruments

Instrument	Generality	Dimensions	# Items (# Pain)	Items weighted	Sensitivity	References
Sickness Impact Profile	Generic	fx, psy, soc	136 (0)	Fixed	Moderate	Bergner et al., 1981 **Bergner, 1993**
Nottingham Health Profile, Part 1	Generic	fx, phy, psy, soc	38 (8)	Fixed	Moderate	Hunt et al., 1981 McEwen, 1993
Medical Outcome Survey-Short Form	Generic	fx, phy, psy, soc	20 (1)	No	?	Stewart et al., 1988
Profile of Mood States-Bipolar	Generic	psy	72 (0)	No	High	McNair et al., 1971 Lorr & McNair, 1988
Psychosocial Adustment to Illness	Generic	fx, psy, soc	46 (0)	No	?	Derogotis, 1986
Functional Living Index-Cancer	Disease-cancer	fx, phy, psy, soc	22 (2)	No	?	Schipper et al., 1984
Quality of Life Index (QL Index)	Disease-cancer	fx, phy, psy	14 (1)	No	High	Padilla et al., 1983 Padilla & Grant, 1985
Linear Analogue Self-Assessment (LASA)	Disease-cancer	fx, phy	4-6 (1)	No	High	Coates et al., 1983

(continued)

Table *(continued)*

Functional Assessment Cancer Therapy-General	Disease-cancer	fx, phy, psy, soc	33 (1)	No	High	Cella et al., 1993
EORTC-QL30Q	Disease-cancer	fx, phy, psy, soc	30 (2)	No	Moderate	Aaronson et al., 1993
Quality of Life Index-Cancer	Disease-cancer	fx, phy, psy	70 (1)	Variable	Moderate	Ferrans, 1990 Ferrans & Powers, 1985
Symptom Distress Scale	Disease-cancer	fx, phy, psy	10 (1)	No	High	McCorkle & Young, 1978 McCorkle, 1987
Brief Pain Inventory	Symptom-pain	fx, phy, psy, soc	23 (6)	No	High	Daut et al., 1983 Cleeland, 1989
Brief Pain Inventory-Short Form	Symptom-pain	fx, phy, psy, soc	8 (6)	No	High	Cleeland, 1989

This list is not meant to be comprehensive. The reader is referred to Cella and Tulsky, 1990; Donovan et al., 1989; Moinour et al., 1989; and Moinour and Chapman, 1991 for a review of quality-of-life instruments.

Abbreviations: fx, functional status; *phy*, physical symptoms; *psy*, psychological well-being; *soc*, social relations.

(Courtesy of Wells N: *APS Bulletin* July/Aug:6–10, 1994.)

fect on life experience. Four core dimensions of QOL are functional status, physical symptoms, psychological well-being, and social relations.

Measurement.—In general, self-report instruments are most appropriate for QOL measurement. In guiding instrument selection, the degree of sensitivity, clinical relevance, length of instrument, and ease of understanding are considered. In a comparative study of several QOL instruments, it was recommended that instruments be combined to overcome their individual shortfalls (table). Some generic instruments use referent groups to determine the importance of QOL; however, with this type of fixed value, patients can adjust the value of various QOL dimensions as physical status changes. In another approach, individual ratings of importance are obtained by making adjustments related to change over time. However, this type of scoring increases the length and complexity of the instrument. Measures of QOL can describe responses to illness and treatment, provide patients with more information about expected treatment effects, and help patients select treatment options.

Clinical Relevance.—When evaluating QOL instruments, emphasis on aspects particularly affected by illness or treatment may be warranted. Patients receiving active cancer therapies need brief instruments. Some instruments are easier to understand than others. Sensitivy of the instruments to change in QOL dimensions must also be considered. One clincial trial on immediate-release and controlled-release opioids included a QOL measure that showed that controlled-release opioids reduced pain intensity and produced better QOL. Investigators should perhaps begin to consult with QOL researchers to enhance study design, much in the same way that they routinely consult with statisticians.

▶ The impact of pain on QOL is receiving increased attention. This review of QOL measures and the problems in using them should be helpful to clinicians and researchers.—A.K. Jacox, R.N., Ph.D.

Pain and Cognitive Characteristics of Patients

Perceived Control Over Pain: Relation to Distress and Disability

Wells N (Vanderbilt Univ Med Ctr, Nashville, Tenn)

Res Nurs Health 17:295–302, 1994 131-95-7–9

Purpose.—Pain control depends on a patient's belief about his/her ability to control pain, ability to cope, and expectation of relief. In theory, patients who believe they control their outcomes are confident that they can learn coping behaviors and expect a good outcome have better pain relief than do patients who believe that someone or something else controls their outcomes, who do not have confidence that they can learn behaviors that will mediate their pain, or who expect the worst. This study was done to determine whether control beliefs are related to levels of distress or disability in patients with chronic pain unrelated to malignancy.

Methods.—A group of 71 patients (age range, 18–70 years) was evaluated at a pain treatment center. Most patients had low back, cervical, upper shoulder or arm, or lower limb pain or pain at multiple sites. There were almost twice as many women as men. Patients had been in pain for an average of 3.8 years. Thirty-one patients were receiving Worker's Compensation benefits, and 32 were unemployed because of pain. Beliefs about pain control were measured using the Pain-Related Control Scale and the Pain-Related Self-Statements scale. Pain intensity was measured weekly using the Visual Analogue Scale. Stress and disability were measured using the Profile of Mood States and the Sickness Impact Profile.

Results.—Pain, feelings of helplessness and catastrophizing, and inability to cope were significantly related to distress and disability levels. Negative control beliefs significantly increased disability levels.

Conclusion.—The finding that pain control beliefs and distress and disability are interrelated may help to identify those patients for whom intervention may be helpful in controlling their pain.

► The relationship between personality variables and how patients experience various pain is typical of much of the research done in the 1960s and 1970s. In choosing a population different from that previously studied, the author has extended the study of the relationship between control beliefs and the outcomes of distress and disability to patients with nonmalignant pain originating from multiple sites. The importance of this kind of knowledge will be apparent as it is incorporated into programs of research that test interventions for pain and describe how these characteristics relate to the effectiveness of the interventions.—A.K. Jacox, R.N., Ph.D.

Guidelines for Pain Management

Management of Cancer Pain: Adults

Cancer Pain Guideline Panel (Rockville, Md)
Am Fam Physician 49:1853–1868, 1994 135-95-7-10

Background.—Cancer pain can be effectively treated in up to 90% of patients by relatively simple means. The key to effective pain management in such patients is flexibility, because diagnosis, stage of disease, response to pain and interventions, and personal preferences vary among patients. The management of cancer pain in adults was reviewed.

Cancer Pain Management.—A team approach that involves the patient, family, and health care providers is best for effective cancer pain management. Pain and its management are discussed with the patients and their families. Patients are encouraged to actively participate in management, and patients who are reluctant to report pain are reassured that there are many safe, effective ways to relieve pain. The cost of proposed drug treatment is considered. Clinicians should also share documented pain assessment and management strategies with others providing health care to the patient, and they should know state and local regulations for controlled substances.

Assessment.—Pain should be assessed at regular intervals, at each new report of pain, and at appropriate times after interventions. The cornerstone of pain assessment is the patient self-report.

Pharmacologic Treatment Options.—Drug therapy is effective, involves relatively little risk, is inexpensive, and generally works rapidly. Initially, the simplest dosage schedules and least invasive pain management methods should be used. Patients with mild to moderate pain and without contraindications should be given aspirin, acetaminophen, or a nonsteroidal anti-inflammatory drug. An opioid should be added if pain persists or increases. The opioid potency or dose is increased if pain becomes moderate to severe. Doses should be given on a regular schedule. Long-term cancer pain requires around-the-clock medication, with additional doses as needed. Various drugs and administration routes are not recommended for cancer pain treatment. Adverse effects of opioids can include constipation, nausea and vomiting, sedation and mental clouding, respiratory depression, and subacute overdose.

Physical and Psychosocial Interventions.—Physical methods for alleviating pain include cutaneous stimulation, exercise, repositioning, immobilization, and counterstimulation. Cognitive-behavioral interventions include relaxation and imagery, cognitive distraction and reframing, patient education, psychotherapy and structured support, and support groups and pastoral counseling.

Invasive Interventions.—Less invasive analgesic management precedes invasive palliative approaches with rare exceptions. Surgery, nerve blocks, neurosurgery, and some forms of radiation therapy are invasive options.

Conclusion.—Although cancer pain and its associated symptoms cannot always be completely eliminated, the appropriate use of available treatment methods can relieve pain in most patients. Pain management improves a patient's quality of life and enhances his or her ability to work productively, enjoy recreational activities, and function normally.

▶ In March 1994, the U.S. Agency for Health Care Policy and Research released the *Clinical Practice Guideline: Management of Cancer Pain,* in several forms: the full 257-page guideline; the *Quick Reference Guide Management of Cancer Pain: Adults* (1); a consumer version of the guideline. The version used in this article and in many other journals was the quick reference guideline. Approximately 1 year after the release of the guideline, more than 2.5 million copies have been disseminated to health care providers and consumers. In addition, the *Quick Reference Guide* and the consumer guideline have been reprinted in numerous journal articles, such as this one. This is an excellent way to increase clinician awareness of the guidelines.—A.K. Jacox, R.N., Ph.D.

Reference

1. Jacox A, Carr DB, Payne R, et al: *The Quick Reference Guide Management of Cancer Pain: Adults.* Rockville, Md; Agency for Health Care Policy and Research 1994. PHS, USDHHS AHCPR Publication 94-0593.

▶ This publication informs family physicians about the Agency for Health Care Policy and Research cancer pain management *Guidelines* and the principles of cancer pain management. Providing notification to family physicians about the publication of the *Guidelines* is important, because many patients receive supportive care from their primary care physicians, and because family physicians often serve as medical directors for nursing homes and hospices. The multidisciplinary focus of the *Guidelines* also helps the family physician to instruct other health care professionals and to incorporate the principles of cancer pain management into practice. Now available, the *Guidelines* legitimize and help optimize the control of cancer-related pain through the information provided about accepted therapies. This review article fulfills the intent of the *Guidelines* by informing health care professionals who may be unfamiliar with either the principles or available therapeutic options for the treatment of cancer-related pain.—N.A. Janjan, M.D.

How to Use the New AHCPR Cancer Pain Guidelines

McCaffery M, Ferrell BR (City of Hope Med Ctr, Duarte, Calif)

Am J Nurs 94:42–46, 1994 131-95-7–11

Introduction.—The subject of relief from cancer-related pain has become a clinical specialty, although professional education about pain is sometimes meager and inaccurate. Misconceptions about pain can be a barrier for health care providers. The Agency for Health Care Policy and Research (AHCPR) has found that cancer pain is often undertreated.

New Guidelines.—To improve this situation, the AHCPR has released cancer pain guidelines to offer the best available information to health care providers about how to assess and relieve cancer-related pain. These guidelines provide a concise and thorough review of current knowledge and research about cancer pain.

Research.—The cancer pain guidelines are based on research. Nineteen databases were searched, 9,600 citations were screened, and 625 research studies were reviewed. During a 2-year period, the multidisciplinary team of authors met 6 times, wrote 17 drafts, and field-tested the guidelines at clinical sites. The project involved 468 consultants, peer reviewers, and site testers.

Results.—The results of this process are a series of 4 publications that cover various aspects of managing cancer-related pain: the *Clinical Practice Guideline*; 2 patient *Guidelines*, regarding pain in adults and children; and 2 *Quick Reference Guides* for clinicians, concerning pain in adults and in infants, children, and adolescents.

Examples.—This article offers 11 common clinical situations, which include a patient example, quotations from the *Guidelines* to support recommendations and actions, and nursing interventions to resolve the problem. *Guidelines* ordering information is also included.

▶ This description of the AHCPR cancer pain *Guidelines,* which was written by a member of the panel and a consultant to the panel that developed the *Guidelines,* is a useful reference for clinicians. The 18 examples present common clinical scenarios that nurses who treat patients with cancer are likely to encounter. The article illustrates a good way to introduce clinicians to the *Guidelines* and how to use them.—A.K. Jacox, R.N., Ph.D.

▶ The cancer pain *Guidelines* that were developed and published by the AHCPR provide information about the causes and management of cancer-related pain. In addition, the *Guidelines* represent an extremely important policy statement by the National Institutes of Health, indicating that the control of pain is a priority in cancer therapy. Pain is recognized as the most frequent consequence of cancer and its therapy. Adequate control of cancer-related pain is important to improve tolerance to aggressive antineoplastic therapy and relieve symptoms associated with the disease in order to improve the quality of life. The *Guidelines* emphasize that the management of cancer-related pain is not restricted to hospice care and identifies the need to treat pain in patients with cancer at any stage of the disease.—N.A. Janjan, M.D.

Clinical Practice Guideline Development: A Historical Perspective and Nursing Implications

Miaskowski C, Jacox A, Ferrell BR, Hester NO, Paice JA (US Dept of Health and Human Services, Rockville, Md)

Oncol Nurs Forum 21:1067–1085, 1994 131-95-7–12

Introduction.—Pain management is a priority in oncology nursing. Undertreatment of cancer-related pain affects a patient's mood, daily living, and quality of life. In 1994, the Agency for Health Care Policy and Research (AHCPR) released its ninth *Clinical Practice Guidelines: Management of Cancer Pain.* It contains 66 recommendations for assessing and managing cancer pain. The major recommendations are summarized in the *Quick Reference Guide* for clinicians on pain in adults. Topics covered include pain assessment; pharmacologic management, including a chart that lists drugs and routes of administration that are not recommended for treating cancer pain (Table 1); physical and psychosocial interventions; nonpharmacologic management; treatment in elderly patients; and assessment and management tools. A flowchart is included that shows the sequence of management of cancer pain (Table 2), as is a sample of 3 pain intensity scales (Fig 7–1). Information is provided

TABLE 1.—Drugs and Routes of Administration Not Recommended for Treatment of Cancer Pain

Class	Drug	Rationale for not recommending
Opioids	Meperidine	Short (2-3 hour) duration. Repeated administration may lead to CNS toxicity (tremor, confusion, or seizures). High oral doses required to relieve severe pain, and these increase the risk of CNS toxicity.
Miscellaneous	Cannabinoids	Side effects of dysphoria, drowsiness, hypotension, and bradycardia preclude its routine use as an analgesic.
	Cocaine	Has demonstrated no efficacy as an analgesic or coanalgesic in combination with opioids.
Opioid agonist-antagonists	Pentazocine Butorphanol Nalbuphine	Risk of precipitating withdrawal in opioid-dependent patients. Analgesic ceiling. Possible production of unpleasant psychomimetic effects (e.g., dysphoria, hallucinations).
Partial agonist	Buprenorphine	Analgesic ceiling. Can precipitate withdrawal.
Antagonist	Naloxone Naltrexone	May precipitate withdrawal. Limit use to treatment of life-threatening respiratory depression.
Combination preparations	Brompton's cocktail	No evidence of analgesic benefit to using Brompton's cocktail over single opioid analgesics.
	DPT (Meperidine, Promethazine, and Chlorpromazine)	Efficacy is poor compared with that of other analgesics. High incidence of adverse effects.
Anxiolytics alone	Benzodiazepine (e.g., alprazolam)	Analgesic properties not demonstrated except for some instances of neuropathic pain. Added sedation from anxiolytics may limit opioid dosing.
Sedative/ hypnotic drugs alone	Barbiturates Benzodiazepine	Analgesic properties not demonstrated. Added sedation from sedative/hypnotic drugs limits opioid dosing.
Routes of administration		**Rationale for not recommending**
Intramuscular (IM)		Painful. Absorption unreliable. Should not be used for children or patients prone to develop dependent edema or in patients with thrombocytopenia.
Transnasal		The only drug approved by the FDA for transnasal administration at this time is butorphanol, an agonist-antagonist drug, which generally is not recommended. (See opioid agonist-antagonists above.)

(Courtesy of Miaskowski C, Jacox A, Ferrell BR, et al: *Oncol Nurs Forum* 21:1067–1085, 1994.)

about the AHCPR, the process of development of the *Clinical Practice Guidelines*, and the implications of the *Guideline* development process for oncology nurses.

Process of Development.—The AHCPR was established to enhance the quality and effectiveness of health care services. It accomplishes this by funding research grants, assessing health care technologies, and providing support for the development of the *Clinical Practice Guidelines*. It facilitates the development of the *Guidelines* by convening a multidisciplinary panel of experts and health care consumers. The panel defines

TABLE 2.—Agency for Health Care Policy and Research (AHCPR) Clinical Practice Guidelines

Published AHCPR-Sponsored Clinical Practice Guidelines	**Date of Release**
Acute Pain Management: Operative or Medical Procedures and Trauma	2/92
Urinary Incontinence in Adults	3/92
Pressure Ulcers in Adults: Prediction, Prevention, and Early Intervention	5/92
Management of Functional Impairment Due to Cataract in the Adult	2/93
Depression in Primary Care	4/93
Volume 1: Detection and Diagnosis	
Volume 2: Treatment of Major Depression	
Sickle Cell Disease: Screening, Diagnosis, Management, and Counseling in Newborns and Infants	4/93
Evaluation and Management of Early HIV Infection	1/94
Diagnosis and Treatment of Benign Prostatic Hyperplasia	2/94
Management of Cancer Pain	3/94
*Diagnosis and Management of Unstable Angina**	3/94
AHCPR-Sponsored Clinical Practice Guidelines Under Development	**Expected Date of Release**
*Heart Failure: Evaluation and Care of Patients With Left Ventricular Systolic Dysfunction**	Summer/94
Treatment of Pressure Ulcers in Adults	Summer/94
Acute Low Back Problems in Adults	Summer/94
*Otitis Media With Effusion in Children**	Summer/94
Quality Determinants of Mammography	Fall/94
*Poststroke Rehabilitation**	Fall/94
Recognition and Initial Assessment of Alzheimer's and Related Dementias	1995
*Cardiac Rehabilitation**	1995
Smoking Prevention and Cessation	1996
Diagnosis and Treatment of Anxiety and Panic Disorders	1996

*Developed or being developed under contract.
(Courtesy of Miaskowski C, Jacox A, Ferrell BR, et al: *Oncol Nurs Forum* 21:1067–1085, 1994.)

the major questions regarding the clinical condition to be addressed and reviews and analyzes the scientific evidence, the benefits and harms of each intervention, and health care costs associated with the entire *Guideline*. The panel invites comments from other organizations, re-

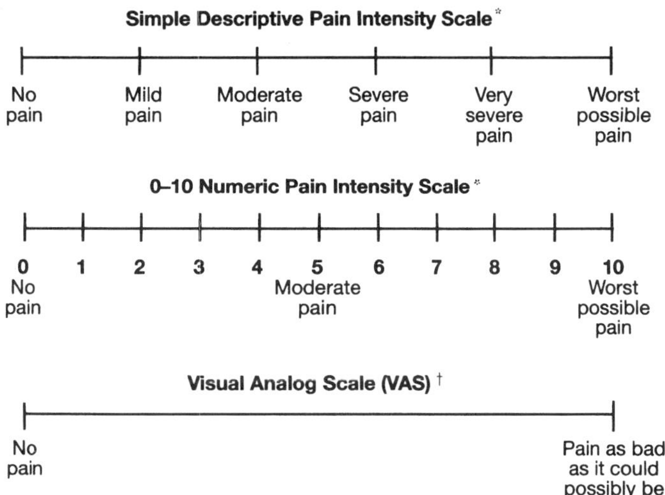

Fig 7–1.—Pain intensity scales. *If used as a graphic rating scale, a 10-cm baseline is recommended. †A 10-cm baseline is recommended for visual analogue scales (VAS). (Courtesy of Miaskowski C, Jacox A, Ferrell BR, et al: *Oncol Nurs Forum* 21:1067–1085, 1994.)

searchers, manufacturers, and individuals. Drafts are subject to peer review. Finally, each *Guideline* is subject to a pilot test with clinicians and others, such as hospital administrators.

Implications.—Ten *Clinical Practice Guidelines* have been published, and others are in development. All need to be reviewed by oncology nurses, and the recommendations need to be implemented in their practice settings. Oncology nurses must determine the scope of their responsibilities in implementing recommendations from the *Guidelines* and must disseminate the *Guidelines* to other nurses, health care providers, and patients.

▶ The development and dissemination of clinical practice guidelines has a long history in health care. Guidelines have included anything from documents based on one or a few individuals' clinical opinions to the AHCPR-sponsored *Guidelines* that are based on research and are widely tested among peers for their validity. This article describing the development of the AHCPR cancer pain *Guidelines* is another example of the numerous articles about the *Guidelines* that increase their dissemination to the clinicians for whom they were written. Like many other articles, this one includes a complete reprint of the *Quick Reference Guide Management of Cancer Pain: Adults.* The tables and figures provided give clinicians information practical to use.—A.K. Jacox, R.N., Ph.D.

Postanesthesia Nursing Care for Ambulatory Surgery Patients Post-Spinal Anesthesia

Kang SB, Rudrud L, Nelson W, Baier D (Gundersen Clinic-Lutheran Hosp, La Crosse, Wis; Univ of Wisconsin, Madison)
J Post Anesth Nurs 9:101–106, 1994 131-95-7–13

Purpose.—Despite the resurgent interest in spinal anesthesia, it is better accepted for hospitalized surgical patients than for ambulatory patients. Reasons for this include the high prevalence of postdural puncture headache (PDPH) and the uncertainty of patient recovery time before discharge. The indications, benefits, and complications of spinal anesthesia for ambulatory surgical patients were reviewed, including recommended nursing care in the postanesthesia care unit (PACU).

Spinal Anesthesia for Ambulatory Surgery.—Recent studies have found a direct association between the incidence of PDPH and the size of the needle used for dural puncture. Use of a 27-gauge needle or a needle with a pencil-point–like tip, such as a Whitacre or Sprotte needle, can reduce the frequency of PDPH to acceptable levels. Furthermore, use of the short- or intermediate-acting local anesthetics xylocaine or bupivacaine, rather than the long-acting anesthetic tetracaine, can allow safe discharge from the hospital within 4–6 hours after induction. With these techniques, spinal anesthesia is a valid and desirable option for anesthesia in ambulatory surgical patients. Its use requires a knowledgeable PACU staff, because nursing care, along with surgical and anesthesia management, is an essential component of successful ambulatory surgery.

Indications and Contraindications.—Spinal anesthesia can be used for ambulatory procedures such as orthopedic surgery of the lower extremity, including knee arthroscopy and podiatric procedures; various obstetric and gynecologic procedures, including dilation and curettage and laparoscopy; general surgical procedures such as inguinal hernia repair and hemorrhoidectomy; and urologic procedures such as cystoscopy and varicocele repair. The patient must be cooperative and willing to undergo this form of anesthesia. Good candidates include those who do not wish to receive general anesthesia, such as those with a previous unfavorable outcome. Other indications include a history of airway problems, difficult intubation, asthma, chronic obstructive pulmonary disease, spontaneous pneumothorax, and pseudocholinesterase deficiency. Some arthroscopy patients may wish to be awake to watch the procedure. Contraindications include refusal of spinal anesthesia, mental retardation, emotional instability, hypovolemia, aortic stenosis, coagulation abnormalities, severe back problems, and infection in the needle puncture site.

Benefits and Complications.—The main benefit of spinal anesthesia is that it averts the complications of general anesthesia such as grogginess, drowsiness, and nausea and vomiting. Spinal anesthesia also averts intubation, allowing the patient to watch the operation or converse with the surgeon. Potential complications in addition to PDPH include hypotension, bradycardia, respiratory depression, postoperative back pain, and urinary complications.

PACU Nursing Care.—Guidelines for nursing care in the PACU are presented, including monitoring and management for hypotension, bradycardia, hypoventilation, and respiratory arrest; criteria to resume ambulation; and home discharge instructions. Discharge criteria include normal and stable vital signs for at least 1 hour, full recovery of lower extremity motor function with no instability during standing or walking, recovery of lower extremity and perineal sensory function, spontaneous urination, a dry surgical site, control of pain, and reliable transportation home.

Conclusion.—Spinal anesthesia is a useful option for selected ambulatory surgery patients. It provides excellent anesthesia while averting the common complications of general anesthesia. With current techniques, the frequency of PDPH is minimized, and the patient can go home in a reasonable amount of time.

▶ This article provides useful information about how to care for ambulatory surgical patients after receiving spinal anesthesia. Written by a physician and 3 nurses, the article provides references for its statements and outlines practical measures to use with this patient population.—A.K. Jacox, R.N., Ph.D.

Drug-Related Interventions

MODES OF ADMINISTRATION

Interpleural Analgesia: A New Technique
Martin B, Meherg D (St Joseph's Hosp, Tampa, Fla)
Crit Care Nurse 14:31–35, 1994 131-95-7–14

Purpose.—Interpleural analgesia is an effective pain management technique for patients with multiple rib fractures or those who have undergone renal surgery, cholecystectomy, thoracotomy, or unilateral breast surgery. Benefits include rapid, prolonged analgesia and the avoidance of hemodynamic instability. In a new technique for interpleural analgesia in patients who have had thoracotomy, a special chest drainage catheter was used.

Methods.—The catheter was placed within a chest tube that incorporates an injection lumen for anesthetic administration. The chest tube catheter was inserted during surgery at the apex of the affected side (Fig 7–2), thus averting the complications associated with percutaneous insertion. Bupivacaine was instilled into the interpleural space through the injection lumen. The bolus dosage ranged from 10 to 30 mL of bupivacaine 0.25% or 0.5% with 1:200,000 epinephrine. The procedure for injection (table) includes positioning the patient supine with the head of

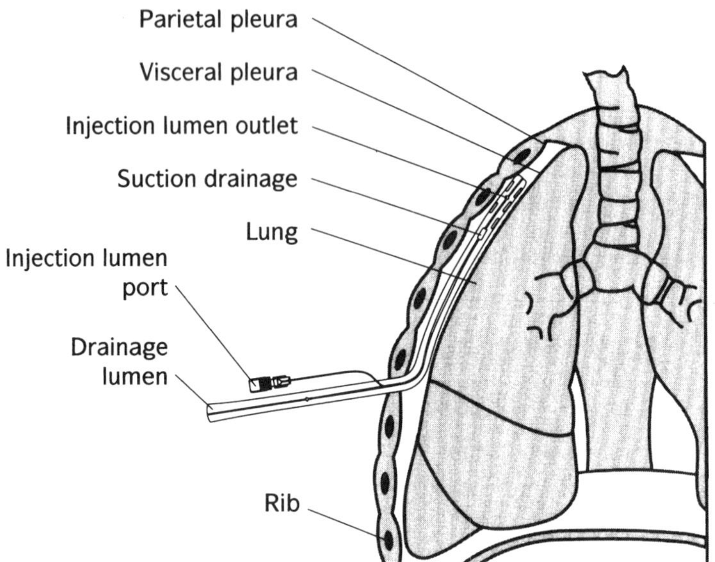

Fig 7–2.—Interpleural chest drainage catheter in place. (Courtesy of Martin B, Meherg D: *Crit Care Nurse* 14:31–35, 1994.)

the bed elevated 30 degrees and monitoring for signs and symptoms of toxicity.

Case Report.—Woman, 71, with a history of smoking had a noncalcified left lower lobe nodule. Left thoracotomy and left lower lobectomy were performed. During surgery, a chest tube with an interpleural injection lumen was inserted. A second dose of bupivacaine was administered during recovery after anesthesia. Her pain score before the third dose was 6 on a scale of 1–10, and incentive spirometry volume was 250 mL. One hour after the injection, her pain score was 0 and her incentive spirometry volume was 500 mL. On the fifth day after surgery, the chest tube was removed, interpleural analgesia therapy was discontinued, and meperidine therapy was continued for pain management.

Conclusion.—Nursing management of interpleural analgesia includes astute assessment of pain scores and functional measures and ongoing evaluation of the effectiveness of the pain management.

▶ This is another good description of a relatively new analgesic technique. There are many useful suggestions for the nursing care of patients that involve using the techniques.—A.K. Jacox, R.N., Ph.D.

Procedure for Interpleural Injection

Purpose: To introduce analgesic dose of a local anesthetic agent into pleural space for pain management
Skill Level: RN
Supportive data: Bupivacaine is injected in analgesic dosage into interpleural space via chest tube that has an injection lumen.

Equipment: Bupivacaine (Marcaine); Sterile normal saline for injection; Iodophor swab; 1 22-g 1″ needle; 1 30-mL syringe

Steps	Key points
1. Explain procedure and rationale to patient.	
2. Prepare prescribed analgesic dose.	Maximum dose: 225 mg bupivacaine with epinephrine or 175 mg bupivacaine. Dilute with normal saline to achieve desired concentration if necessary. Bupivacaine 0.25% = 2.5 mg/mL Bupivacaine 0.5% = 5.0 mg/mL
3. Position patient supine with head of bed elevated 30°.	Facilitates dissemination throughout pleural space.
4. Obtain patient's pain score and incentive spirometry volume.	Used to evaluate effectiveness of analgesic.
5. If chest tube connected to suction, turn suction off.	Prevents loss of analgesic through drainage lumen.
6. Clean injection lumen port with iodophor.	
7. Inject prescribed dose through injection lumen.	Expect resistance to injection due to small gauge of injection lumen.

(continued)

Table (*continued*)

8. Maintain head of bed at 30° for 20-30 minutes.	
9. Keep chest tube suction off for 15 minutes	
10. Monitor for signs and symptoms of toxicity.	Includes: tinnitus, metallic taste, light-headedness, somnolence, visual or auditory disturbance, unusual anxiety, restlessness, delirium, slurred speech, nystagmus, muscle tremors, seizures, respiratory arrest, dysrhythmias, cardiovascular collapse.
11. Document the following:	
■ Administration time	
■ Pain score before and 1 hour after procedure	
■ Heart rate, blood pressure, respiratory rate every 4 hours	Hypertension and tachycardia may occur from intravascular injection or absorption of epinephrine.
■ Incentive spirometry volume before and 1 hour after procedure	

(Courtesy of Martin B, Meherg D: *Crit Care Nurse* 14:31–35, 1994.)

Patient-Controlled Analgesia: A Comparison With Nurse-Controlled Intravenous Opioid Infusions

Murphy DF, Graziotti P, Chalkiadis G, McKenna M (Sir Charles Gairdner Hosp, Perth, Western Australia)

Anaesth Intensive Care 22:589–592, 1994 131-95-7–15

Purpose.—Most clinical trials of patient-controlled anesthesia (PCA) using IV opioids have compared this method with IM opioids and found PCA to be significantly better. However, it would be more reasonable to compare PCA with nurse-administered IV opioids. Nurse-controlled analgesia (NCA) with IV opioids has provided good pain relief. In a recent study, PCA and NCA were compared with IV opioids in patients who had undergone major surgery.

Methods.—The study sample included 200 patients who had undergone major abdominal or thoracic surgery. All were given IV pethidine, as needed, in the recovery room. As they left the recovery room, PCA or NCA pethidine was started, as assigned randomly. The PCA group received pethidine in 20-mg doses with a 5-minute lockout period and no background infusion. The NCA group received 500 mg of pethidine in 500 mL of physiologic saline solution given by infusion at a rate titrated to achieve adequate analgesia, as judged by the patient. This group also received 20- to 40-mL bolus injections as required. The 2 groups were compared for pain scores, level of sedation, nausea and other adverse effects, and cumulative pethidine requirement during the first 24 hours after surgery.

Results.—The 2 groups were comparable in terms of age, weight, and type of surgery. The NCA group had consistently but not significantly lower pain scores than the PCA group did; overall mean pain scores on a scale of 0–10 were 1.7 and 2.1, respectively. Hourly cumulative opioid dose was 587 mg in the NCA group and 531 mg in the PCA group; the difference was not significant. Neither were there any significant differences in the frequency or severity of nausea or sedation.

Conclusion.—Nurse-controlled infusion of pethidine appears to be as effective as PCA for the management of postoperative pain. Therefore, NCA with IV opioids may be a useful alternative when PCA is either unavailable or unsuitable. The study could identify no patient characteristics that identified those who are unlikely to use PCA effectively. Many patients for whom difficulties with PCA might have been anticipated accepted it surprisingly well.

▶ This demonstration that PCA and NCA are equally effective in managing pain suggests an alternative other than administration of IM opioids for those patients who are unable to use PCA. It is interesting that the authors noted that neither PCA nor NCA IV opioid techniques used alone should be thought of as the gold standard for postoperative pain relief, because there is a large body of evidence to show that a combination of analgesics provides better pain relief than use of opioids alone.—A.K. Jacox, R.N., Ph.D.

Psychosocial and Pharmacologic Predictors of Satisfaction With Intravenous Patient-Controlled Analgesia

Jamison RN, Taft K, O'Hara JP, Ferrante FM (Brigham and Women's Hosp, Boston; Harvard Med School, Boston)

Anesth Analg 77:121–125, 1993 131-95-7–16

Purpose.—Although its use has become widespread, the factors underlying patient satisfaction with IV patient-controlled analgesia (PCA) for the management of postoperative pain are not well understood. Satisfaction levels are high despite the finding that patients do not use IV PCA uniformly to obtain complete analgesia. The influence of various patient- and nurse-assessed factors on patient satisfaction with IV PCA was examined.

Methods.—The study sample comprised 68 women scheduled to undergo abdominal hysterectomy. Before surgery, each patient completed a battery of tests to assess emotional distress, locus of control, perceived support, and optimism. After surgery, the patients rated the intensity of their pain, emotional distress, expected recovery time, nightmares, and satisfaction with IV PCA. Nurse ratings of anxiety, estimated recovery, and satisfaction with IV PCA were also obtained, and data on cumulative and hourly IV PCA use and dose-demand ratio were collected.

Results.—Most (77%) of the patients found IV PCA helpful in pain management. A number of factors were significantly related to degree of patient dissatisfaction with IV PCA: pain intensity, nightmares, patients' perceived support, expected time of recovery, optimism, preoperative anxiety, and postoperative depression. Ratings of dissatisfaction were not related to locus of control or duration of IV PCA use. Emotional distress both before and after surgery was significantly related to dose-demand ratio and hourly analgesic use.

Conclusion.—Patient dissatisfaction with IV PCA appears to be related to pain intensity, perceived support, anticipated recovery, and anxiety. Pharmacologic and nonpharmacologic interventions to address each of these factors may be useful in optimizing patient satisfaction with this popular method of postoperative pain management. Cause-and-effect mechanisms should be sought in future studies.

▶ Although locus of control is believed by some to influence patient response to IV PCA, this study did not support that assumption but found that other psychological factors, such as mood, expectations of recovery, and anxiety, were related to satisfaction with PCA. Patients with higher ratings of emotional distress received more analgesic and made more unsuccessful demands, which suggests there is much to learn with regard to factors influencing the use of IV PAC.—A.K. Jacox, R.N., Ph.D.

How Safe Are Intramuscular Injections?

Beecroft PC, Kongelbeck SR (Children's Hosp, Los Angeles)

Clin Issues Crit Care Nurs 5:207–215, 1994 131-95-7–17

Introduction.—Adverse effects can occur from IM injections. These include fibrosis and contractures after multiple injections or large injection volumes; nerve injury in young, comatose, anesthetized, or chronically ill thin children; abscesses caused by short needles or increased muscle tension; gangrene in patients with circulatory compromise or insulin-dependent diabetes; local and systemic reactions caused by adverse drug reactions or immune responses; and inadequate drug absorption because of route of administration.

Factors That Contribute to Adverse Effects.—These factors include injection site except for the ventrogluteal area; injectate, with specific drugs or high concentrations; needle length, particularly the use of longer needles in infants, shorter needles in adults, or injections in obese patients; injection frequency, particularly at the same site; and patient, particularly those with underlying disease or low body weight.

General Practice Recommendations.—The ventrogluteal site is preferred. Injectates with solubility problems, chemical reactivity, or poor absorption characteristics should not be used. Medical personnel should be familiar with injection landmarks and appropriate needle length for individual patients. Patients who require multiple injections should be evaluated periodically.

Critical Care Recommendations.—Medical personnel should be aware that muscle mass may have deteriorated in critically ill patients, and unless small volumes of injectate can be used, IM injections should be avoided.

Conclusion.—Guidelines for IM injections to prevent or limit complications were presented. These injections should be avoided in critically ill patients in most cases.

► After reviewing the extensive research documenting the negative effects of IM injections, one would have expected the authors to argue strongly against the use of IM injections unless no other route is available. They do suggest that the use of IM injections in critically ill patients should be reevaluated and in most cases avoided. They also, however, give guidelines for the administration of IM injections. It would be interesting to see this well-documented paper used as the basis for a strong argument for more vigorous rejection of the IM as a route of injection.—A.K. Jacox, R.N., Ph.D.

A Prospective Comparison Study Between a Butterfly Needle and a Teflon Cannula for Subcutaneous Narcotic Administration

Macmillan K, Bruera E, Kuehn N, Selmser P, Macmillan A (Edmonton Gen Hosp, Alta, Canada)

J Pain Symptom Manage 9:82–84, 1994 131-95-7–18

Purpose.—In some patients local site problems develop when narcotics are administered subcutaneously (SC). It has been proposed that the SC sites initiated with the Teflon cannula would last longer and be more comfortable for the patient than sites initiated with the butterfly needle.

Methods.—In this prospective randomized crossover trial, the 25-gauge butterfly needle was compared with the combination of a 26-gauge introducer needle and a 24-gauge Teflon cannula designed for SC use in 8 women and 12 men with a primary tumor. Patients were randomly assigned to receive medication through either the Teflon cannula or the butterfly needle. The needle remained in place until signs or symptoms of toxicity, such as redness, swelling, tenderness, bruising, or leaking were observed. At the end of the study, patients were asked to verbally indicate which needle was more comfortable.

Results.—The duration of the SC site was significantly longer (11.9 days) with the Teflon cannula compared with the butterfly needle (5.3 days). Nurses and patients preferred the Teflon cannula because it did not need to be changed so frequently.

Conclusion.—On the basis of site duration and preferences, the Teflon cannula appears to be the better choice than the butterfly needle. Cost should be considered: The Teflon cannula costs about $7 (Canadian) per needle, whereas the butterfly needle costs about $.84 (Canadian). The Teflon cannula could not accommodate large infusion volumes; when the clysis was initiated, solution leaked out of the SC site or the pump alarm occluded. The Teflon cannula managed 30–50 mL of fluid per hour.

▶ This is another example of a clinical group doing a practically oriented study to use as a basis for deciding which type of needle should be used to administer SC infusions. Although a formal cost analysis was not completed, the authors appropriately used the data they collected to define the circumstances under which they would use the more expensive needle.—A.K. Jacox, R.N., Ph.D.

Use of the Edmonton Injector for Parenteral Opioid Management of Cancer Pain: A Study of 100 Consecutive Patients

Bruera E, Velasco-Leiva A, Spachynski K, Fainsinger R, Miller MJ, MacEachern T (Edmonton Gen Hosp, Alta, Canada)

J Pain Symptom Manage 8:525–528, 1993 131-95-7–19

Purpose.—In most patients with advanced cancer, parenteral opioids are needed to treat pain before death. Although portable infusion devices are safe and effective, some are very expensive and complex to use. An experience with the Edmonton Injector was described.

Methods and Findings.—Patterns of Edmonton Injector use were studied in 100 consecutive patients with cancer. Seventy-eight patients used the injector for a mean of 23 days. Thirty-seven patients began using the injector because of nausea and 31 because of severe pain. The median opioid dose equivalent to parenteral morphine was 264 mg/day, and the mean duration of the subcutaneous injection site was 6.5 days. The most common reasons for change were accidental needle pulling in 59% of patients and erythema in 12%. Local infection developed in only 1% of the 196 sites. The mean treatment cost was $1.65 (Canadian) per patient per day. There were no mechanical problems, and none of the patients refused to start or continue the treatment.

Conclusion.—The Edmonton Injector is a safe, easy-to-use device that permits cost-effective parenteral administration of opioids in most patients with pain from cancer. Confusional syndromes and a history of severe alcoholism or drug addiction are contraindications to use of this device.

▶ This likely is the kind of report that we will see increasingly in the literature. It is a study showing that a simply designed, low-cost device can be used to successfully manage pain in patients with cancer. Its value would have been increased if there had been comparison with a group of patients whose pain was managed with another method.—A.K. Jacox, R.N., Ph.D.

▶ Alternative methods for administering parenteral analgesics and antiemetics are particularly important in patients with advanced cancer. Increasingly important are issues related to cost-effectiveness and morbidity of therapy. These factors must be related to clinical status and prognosis. The Edmonton Injector was shown to be an effective means of delivering parenteral opioids with low associated morbidity. Increasing the cost-effectiveness and ease of analgesic administration is imperative to overcome recognized socioeconomic barriers in the treatment of cancer-related pain.—N.A., Janjan, M.D.

The Use of Multiple Routes of Opioid Drug Administration in an Advanced Cancer Patient

Coyle N, Foley KM (Mem Sloan-Kettering Cancer Ctr, New York)

J Pain Symptom Manage 8:234–241, 1993 131-95-7–20

Purpose.—Sophisticated infusion devices are now available for the management of cancer pain, leading to controversy about the role of such "high-tech" approaches. There are no comparative data from randomized trials, so decisions about the use of these approaches must be considered on a case-by-case basis. A stepwise approach, in which simpler approaches are tried first and followed by more sophisticated techniques if necessary, is appropriate for many patients. A case history that illustrates this stepwise approach was reported.

Case Report.—Woman, 57, had recurrent rectal adenocarcinoma 2 years after abdominoperineal resection, for which she received chemotherapy. Pain developed in her left buttock and right lumbar paraspinal area as a result of metastasis to the lumbosacral spine. The pain resolved with radiation therapy, but pain recurred as a result of cauda equina compression and lumbosacral plexopathy. The patient was given escalating doses of controlled-release morphine. She was admitted to the hospital the next month with severe pain and distress, which prompted a switch from oral to IV morphine. Because of difficulties in obtaining venous access, the route was switched again to subcutaneous (SC) administration with an ambulatory infusion pump. However, paroxysmal pain was not controlled with increasing SC doses, so a trial of epidural opioids plus local anesthetics was planned. The patient still had intermittent episode of severe pain, so epidural infusion was gradually increased. Subcutaneous infusion was decreased with the goal of using this route for self-administered "rescue" doses only. The patient was still having 1 or 2 paroxysms of pain per day.

Bilateral hydronephrosis and renal failure developed, which necessitated removal of the temporary epidural catheter and increased SC infusions. An epidural catheter was implanted; SC infusions were discontinued, then started again for minor left thigh pain. The patient was discharged home with both epidural and SC infusion pumps, as well as 2 nephrostomy bags. This required a 24-hour home health aide and an advanced-technology home care system. The patient did well at home for 1 month, with close cooperation between the home care agency and a nurse clinician from the pain service. The patient was readmitted for family respite and treatment of infection, and her pain worsened. She requested increased sedation and stated that she wanted to remain in the hospital and under sedation. She was given IV lorazepam and increased doses of epidural lidocaine to control severe abdominal pain and paroxysmal leg pain. The patient slept much of the time, but had severe abdominal pain when aroused. This pain responded to IV hydromorphone and increased doses of epidural hydromorphone and lidocaine. Severe myoclonus developed; IV hydromorphone was switched to methadone, and IV lorazepam was gradually increased. The patient was heavily sedated and responded only to noxious stimuli for 3 days until she died.

Conclusion.—In well-selected patients with cancer, advanced technology for pain relief can be important in supportive care. Continuous evaluation of the costs and benefits of this form of therapy is essential. Although the cost of home care was high in this complex case, the care was justified by the nature and severity of the patient's pain. Successful pain management can enhance patients' quality of life and allow them to remain at home for a meaningful period.

▶ Although up to 90% of cancer pain can be controlled with relatively simple approaches, there is a subset of patients for whom pain management is much more difficult. This detailed description of a patient for whom simple solutions progressed to more complex approaches as the pain progressed from a simple to a complex type is particularly impressive in that much of the pain management occurred in the patient's home. This article is a fine illustration of what a knowledgeable, experienced clinician can do in managing a complex problem.—A.K. Jacox, R.N., Ph.D.

▶ This article presents some of the issues related to the clinical management of severe cancer-related pain. These issues, which will require prospective cost-benefit analysis, include clinical status, prognosis, cause and level of symptoms, efficacy and morbidity of the therapeutic intervention, durability of response and need for retreatment, and functional outcome. The easiest, permanent, and most cost-effective therapeutic option is the best solution to any clinical presentation.

The inability to exactly predict the rate, extent, or site of symptomatic disease progression and survival, however, is the most significant factor that confounds the effectiveness of a clinical intervention. As illustrated, techniques that adequately manage pain at one point in the clinical course are ineffective with progression of the disease. Comparative analysis will be needed to determine whether an earlier, more aggressive intervention, such as placement of an epidural catheter, that obviates the need for a number of intervening types of therapy before the epidural catheter is ultimately placed is more cost-effective and reduces suffering. However, use of an invasive therapy is tempered by the level of difficulty in performing the procedure and the possible risks involved, and the inability to predict which patients will survive long enough to benefit from the more aggressive approach. Also, a more invasive therapy that is used initially may not prove to be adequate, and other approaches may still be needed later in the clinical course. Determining the indications for specific therapeutic approaches in the management of cancer-related pain will be imperative to optimize outcome and cost-effectiveness.—N.A. Janjan, M.D.

Intercostal Nerve Block

Litwack K (Univ of New Mexico, Albuquerque)

J Post Anesth Nurs 9:301–302, 1994 131-95-7–21

Introduction.—The intercostal nerve block is commonly used to provide pain relief to patients after upper abdominal and thoracic surgery. A summary of the technique, indications, and complications of intercostal nerve block was provided for postanesthetic care unit personnel.

Indications.—The technique is useful to decrease the need for opiates, to improve postoperative pulmonary function, and as an alternative to local anesthetic to treat cancer pain.

Drugs and Technique.—With the patient in the lateral or supine position, either short or long duration of nerve block is achievable by injecting 3-5 mL of 0.5% bupivacaine or 1% etidocaine per intercostal nerve, or 6% to 8% phenol in Renografin for a neurolytic block. Three intercostal nerves are injected for each intercostal nerve to be blocked.

Complications and Contraindications.—Risks include pneumothorax and intravascular injection. Contraindications include possible pneumothorax, infection at the injection site, shock, anticoagulation, and local anesthetic allergy.

Advantages and Disadvantages.—The advantages of intercostal block over epidural block are ease of administration and avoidance of urinary retention, hypotension, and motor weakness. Disadvantages include pneumothorax and repeated injections for continued pain relief.

Nursing Implications.—Patients should be monitored for systemic toxicity and pain relief. Resuscitation equipment should be available.

Conclusion.—Intercostal nerve block is effective for control of postoperative pain control and is relatively safe if the proper technique is used and the patient is carefully monitored.

▶ This brief description of the use of intercostal nerve blocks is packed with useful information for nurses providing care to patients receiving the blocks.—A.K. Jacox, R.N., Ph.D.

Subarachnoid Opioid Analgesia Reduces Long-Term Postsurgical Pain After Nephrectomy

Gwirtz KH, Beckes KA, Maddock RP, Gettelfinger GL, Li W (Indiana Univ, Indianapolis)

Reg Anesth 19:98–103, 1994 131-95-7–22

Purpose.—In postoperative patients, prevention of pain is critical to optimizing analgesia. Preemptive management of acute postoperative pain not only improves perioperative analgesia, but it may also provide lasting relief from postoperative pain. The effects of subarachnoid analgesia administered at the end of major surgery on long-term residual pain were assessed retrospectively.

Methods.—The study included 27 postdonor nephrectomy patients. At the time of surgery, patients chose their preferred method of postoperative analgesia: 19 received subarachnoid analgesia and 8 received patient-controlled analgesia. Within the subarachnoid analgesia group, patients were given morphine alone or in combination with fentanyl or bupivacaine, or both: 13 received morphine at a mean dose of 0.59 mg plus fentanyl, 25 μg, and bupivacaine, 3.75 mg. The patients participated in a telephone interview 2–12 months after surgery and were asked to rate their current pain in terms of severity, frequency, limitation of function, and need for oral analgesics.

Results.—The subarachnoid analgesia group had significantly lower average scores for intensity and frequency of pain and limitation of function up to 1 year after donor nephrectomy. Need for oral analgesics was low in both groups. There was no difference in the average doses of systemic opioids as a supplement to volatile anesthetic.

Conclusion.—Subarachnoid analgesia for the management of acute postoperative pain appears to decrease residual pain for up to 1 year after surgery, compared with patient-controlled analgesia. This benefit is presumed to occur through interference with the process of central sensitization. Further study of the social and cost effects of intraspinal analgesia in reducing prolonged postoperative discomfort and debility is encouraged.

▶ This article is another important contribution to the growing body of literature showing that preemptive management of acute postoperative pain improves both perioperative analgesia and pain management postoperatively. This and other studies illustrate that it is both possible and desirable to reduce postoperative pain by using preventive measures. It is an approach that merits much greater attention and use in the clinical setting.—A.K. Jacox, R.N., Ph.D.

Epidural Analgesia for Effective Pain Control

Naber L, Jones G, Halm M (Univ of Iowa Hosp and Clinics, Iowa City)

Crit Care Nurse 14(5):69–72, 77–83, 1994 131-95-7–23

Introduction.—Pain control management includes hospital acute pain services and intrathecal and epidural techniques for regional control. Epidural pain management by critical care nurses was reviewed.

Patient Selection.—Patients undergoing treatment for postoperative conditions, trauma, cancer, and chronic pain can benefit from epidural administration of narcotics. Epidural analgesia is contraindicated in patients who have injection site infection, generalized systemic infection, those receiving anticoagulant therapy; increased intracranial pressure, or allergy to narcotics; those who have undergone laminectomy; patients who refuse epidural anesthesia; and when there is lack of nursing personnel to monitor the patient.

Research and Benefits.—Epidural narcotics block spinal cord opioid receptors but leave sensation and motor and sympathetic performance intact. The route of administration provides longer pain relief with fewer and smaller doses, which leaves the patient more alert, facilitates early improvement of pulmonary function, and may relieve stress and contribute to earlier ambulation.

Catheter Placement.—Proper catheter placement and verification of placement are important to avert complications (Table 1).

TABLE 1.—Potential Complications and Side Effects of Epidural Analgesia

Complication	Cause/Risk factors	Clinical Manifestations	Prevention/Treatment
CATHETER-RELATED:			
Catheter migration	Rare: Catheter migrates to subarachnoid or subdural location, causing larger fraction of injected drug to enter CSF	Increased analgesia, seizures, respiratory depression, cardiovascular collapse, death	Check catheter dressing/site routinely; notify physician if migration suspected (eg, wet dressing).
Catheter occlusion	Secondary to blood or fatty clot or catheter against vein wall	Signs/symptoms of lack of analgesia (eg, increased pain rating)	Notify physician if occlusion suspected.
Catheter shearing	Improper technique (insertion or removal)	Signs/symptoms of lack of analgesia (eg, increased pain rating)	Stabilize and avoid bending catheter; notify physician if dressing is wet or leaking fluid; test fluid for glucose.
Hematoma	Bleeding into epidural space from venule or arteriole as a result of catheter placement or erosion; patients with abnormal PT or PTT at increased risk	Enlarged, hardened area at site, numbness/tingling of extremities	Avoid administration of anticoagulants.
Neurologic injury/paresthesia	Epidural abscess or hematoma compresses sensory and/or motor nerves	Numbness/tingling of areas below affected spinal level (lower extremities with lumbar epidural catheter)	Assess epidural site for enlarged or hardened area and signs/symptoms of infection; assess motor strength and sensory level every 4 hours; notify physician of increased loss of sensation and/or decreased motor strength.

Postdural puncture headache	CSF leaks from intrathecal space through puncture hole in dura; increased stretch and tension on pain-sensitive intracranial nerves and tentorium when assuming upright position	Severe headache, diplopia, photophobia, tinnitus	Conservative treatment: Bedrest, hydration, analgesics, abdominal binder, IV caffeine If headache continues: autologous blood patch: injection of 10 mL of patient's blood into epidural catheter; clot seals dural puncture, preventing CSF leak; success rate 89%-95% in first hour; few complications reported.
NARCOTIC-RELATED: Respiratory depression (most serious)	Early respiratory depression occurs within 2 hours as result of narcotic absorbed by epidural veins into systemic circulation; rapid achievement of narcotic concentrations in brain via internal vertebral system	Respiratory distress/arrest	Assess LOC and respirations every hour for 24 hours, then every 4 hours. Use respiratory monitoring. (ie, pulse oximetry and/or apnea monitor) whenever possible; support respirations; notify anesthesiologist/physician if respirations decrease from baseline. Administer oxygen and/or naloxone as ordered.
	Late respiratory depression develops 2-16 hours after injection due to cephalic diffusion of narcotic in CSF in fourth ventricle of brain. Incidence 0.3%-5%. Narcotic combines with	Decreased LOC, decreased depth of respirations and tidal volume, followed by decreased respiratory rate	Obtain ABGs; administer naloxone per orders for respiratory rate less than eight/minute. Teversal with naloxone known to cause cardiac instability; administer in small doses (0.08-0.12 mg) and repeat every 2-3 minutes until adverse side effect is reversed. Monitor patient using

(continued)

Table 1 *(continued)*

	opioid receptors of central respiratory centers. Risk factors: Elderly and in poor medical condition, large narcotic doses, residual opioids/sedatives and water-soluble narcotics (morphine). Increased risk with use of intrathecal technique and thoracic epidural catheters		pulse oximetry and/or apnea monitor; support patient with oxygen.
Hypotension	Epidural narcotics do not produce sympathetic nerve blockage; little effect on blood pressure; consider and exclude more common causes of hypotension; allergic reactions may cause cardiovascular collapse and necessitate vasopressors	Decreased blood pressure	Check for allergies to narcotics; maintain airway, and support respirations as indicated; administer IV fluids and epinephrine as ordered.
Nausea/ vomiting	Incidence 17%-35%. Rostral spread of drug, stimulating vomiting center in the medulla	Postoperatively, occurs 4-6 hours after administration; sometimes associated with coughing and turning	Check for patency of nasogastric tube; assess patient for abdominal distention. Treat with antiemetics: 2.5-10 mg droperidol IM or 10 mg metroclopramide IV; be alert to sedative effect of antiemetics. Carefully titrated naloxone (0.08-0.12 mg) may also be effective to

			decrease nausea and vomiting without interrupting analgesic effect.
Urinary retention	Incidence 22%-68%. Common side effect of narcotics. Increased incidence in males; appears to be dose-related. When local anesthetic administered, distended bladder does not cause discomfort or urge to void; with use of epidural narcotics, mechanism is more complex; may be related to relaxation of detrussor muscle in floor of bladder	Lack of urge to void, bladder distension; symptoms usually occur in first 24-48 hours and resolve spontaneously	Monitor intake/output carefully. If no indwelling catheter, assess for bladder distension. Catheterize prn. Titrate naloxone (0.08-0.12) every 2-3 minutes.
Pruritus	Incidence 28%-100%. Associated with epidural narcotics and dose-related; may continue for duration of analgesia; increased incidence in pregnancy; may be related to narcotic moving rostrally in CSF to trigeminal nerve; not related to drug preservatives; may increase with increased body temperature	Rash, wheals, or edema usually occurs over the face and neck area. Not an antigen-antibody reaction but may mimic allergic response	Relieve with antihistamine (eg, diphenhydramine HCl 25-50 mg IV) or titrate naloxone every 2-3 minutes. May worsen with coadministration of steroids and may necessitate limiting therapy. Nalbuphine HCl may be given as agonist. Usual dose 5-10 mg IV every 4-6 hours prn.

Abbreviations: ABG, arterial blood gas; *LOC*, level of consciousness; *PRN*, as needed; *PT*, prothrombin time; *PTT*, partial thromboplastin time.
(Courtesy of Naber L, Jones G, Halm M: *Crit Care Nurse* 14:69-72, 77-83, 1994.)

TABLE 2.—Drugs Used for Epidural Analgesia

Opioid	Dose	Onset of action	Duration	Infusion
Morphine	1-10 mg	30-60 minutes	6-24 hours	0.5-2.0 mg/hour
Fentanyl	50-200 μg	10-15 minutes	4-5 hours	50-100 μg/hour

(From Naber L, Jones G, Halm M: *Crit Care Nurse* 14:69-72, 77-83, 1994. Courtesy of Wild L, Coyn C: *Am J Nurse* 4:30, 1992.)

Pharmacology.—Narcotics commonly used are morphine and fentanyl citrate (Table 2). There are 5 routes of administration (Table 3).

Nursing and Research Issues.—Nursing education and technical skills must be updated as new pain management techniques are developed. Clinical research issues that need to be addressed include side effects, complications, patient awareness and involvement, cost-effectiveness, family anxiety, quality of life, and efficacy.

Conclusion.—Postoperative pain creates many harmful effects. Epidural analgesia can shorten hospital stay, decrease mortality rate, and improve the quality of life. Proper patient selection and good nursing management can control or prevent side effects. Critical care nurses need to update their knowledge and technical skills regarding pain control management.

▶ This is a description of another technology that is becoming increasingly used for pain management in several patient populations; postoperative, trauma, oncology, and chronic pain. The author does an excellent job of describing the technique, clarifying the complications that can arise and exploring how to recognize and treat them. This study is another example of the increased attention being given by critical care nurses to pain and its management.—A.K. Jacox, R.N., Ph.D.

TABLE 3.—Epidural Administration

Route	Technique	Advantages	Disadvantages
Intermittent dosing	Injection of narcotic bolus at timed interval	Based on patient need	Requires personnel to dose catheter; inconsistent analgesia and adverse effects related to fluctuating blood level
Continuous infusion	Delivery of narcotics at a constant rate by use of an infusion pump	More consistent analgesia and effects due to constant opioid blood level	Malfunctioning of equipment
Patient-controlled analgesia	Delivery of fixed rate of narcotics by infusion pump	Patients may administer extra bolus doses as needed	Method remains investigational for epidural narcotics
Implanted port	Port implanted just under skin, with catheter tunneling from epidural space	May be accessed for bolus or continuous infusion; useful for long-term pain control	Surgical procedure; potential for infection
Implanted infusion pump	Device implanted into subcutaneous pocket of abdomen to provide continuous infusion of analgesia via epidural catheter	Useful for long-term pain control	Requires major surgery and careful patient selection; potential for infection

(Courtesy of Naber L, Jones G, Halm M: *Crit Care Nurse* 14:69–72, 77–83, 1994.

COMPLICATIONS AND SIDE EFFECTS

Respiratory Depression Associated With Patient-Controlled Analgesia: A Review of Eight Cases

Etches RC (Univ of Alberta, Edmonton, Canada)

Can J Anaesth 41:125–132, 1994 131-95-7–24

Introduction.—Intravenous patient-controlled analgesia (PCA) often is viewed as an effective alternative to conventional IM opioid analgesia and as being free of respiratory depression. There is little actual evidence, however, that severe respiratory depression occurs less frequently than when epidural opioids are used.

Series.—Severe respiratory depression developed in 8 patients receiving PCA, and 3 other patients were brought to the author's attention. All patients had received morphine and at least 1 dose of naloxone. Three patients were not considered further because respiratory problems had begun shortly after surgery, before any opioid had been delivered by PCA. The incidence of severe respiratory depression associated with PCA in this population was 0.5%. Most of the patients who were cared for by the acute pain management service were adults undergoing major general or orthopedic operations.

Risk Factors.—Two of the patients were elderly women. Three had received other infusions concurrently. One patient's respiratory function was compromised, and 1 received sedative hypnotic therapy at the same time as PCA. Use of a background infusion with PCA increases the risk for development of severe respiratory depression. It often proves difficult to use PCA safely in the elderly and in patients with sleep apnea.

Conclusion.—Intravenous PCA provided in the context of a comprehensive pain management service compares favorably with IM and spinal opioids with respect to incidence of severe respiratory depression.

► The incidence of respiratory-related critical events associated with IV PCA in this study was 5 times as high as that reported in Abstract 131-95-7-27. Some of the same risk factors (concurrent use of a background infusion and concomitant administration of sedatives or hypnotic medications with the opioid) were identified in both studies. There is need for more of these kinds of studies conducted in various patient populations to document the incidence of side effects and complications and to identify preventive measures whenever possible.—A.K. Jacox, R.N., Ph.D.

Treatment of High-Dose Intrathecal Morphine Overdose: Case Report

Sauter K, Kaufman HH, Bloomfield SM, Cline S, Banks D (West Virginia Univ, Morgantown)

J Neurosurg 81:143–146, 1994 131-95-7-25

Purpose.—Patients given intrathecal morphine infusion for pain who have received accidental overdoses have been reported. The successful treatment of an accidental intrathecal injection of a 450-mg bolus of morphine was documented.

Case Report.—Woman, 45, with failed-back syndrome, had a 2-port subcutaneous infusion device implanted to deliver morphine at the T-8 vertebral level for pain relief. The drug reservoir port refilled the pump reservoir every 10 weeks for delivery of morphine sulfate, 6 mg/day. A nurse accidentally injected 450 mg of morphine sulfate into the side port, which accessed the intrathecal space. The patient became drowsy and hypertensive, and tonic-clonic seizures, intracerebral hemorrhage, and respiratory failure developed. The patient was given IV naloxone, nitroprusside, diazepam, and succinylcholine. She also received mechanical ventilation for 4 days. A lumbar catheter was installed to drain CSF. After 13 days, the patient had improved sufficiently to be discharged. At 6 months she has shown no neurologic deficits.

Conclusion.—Complications of morphine overdose were managed symptomatically, with good outcome. Non-neurosurgical caregivers should be taught how implantable infusion devices function and how life-threatening consequences can result from improper filling of devices.

▶ Sophisticated health care technology is rapidly moving into settings other than hospitals. This case report describing a home health care nurse's confusion in not knowing the difference between a drug reservoir port and the port accessing the intrathecal space is important. It emphasizes the need for attention to the educational needs of home health care nurses as they use such technology to care for patients outside the acute care setting.—A.K. Jacox, R.N., Ph.D.

Constipation as a Side Effect of Opioids

Canty SL (Elmhurst Mem Hosp, Ill)

Oncol Nurs Forum 21:739–745, 1994 131-95-7–26

Background.—Opioid analgesics are the most widely used and effective agents for control of cancer pain. However, morphine and opioid antagonists have important effects on the CNS and bowel. The bowel effects, including decreased biliary and pancreatic secretions, decreased gastrointestinal (GI) motility, and increased water and electrolyte absorption, contribute to the common problem of constipation. A clear understanding of the mechanisms of opioid binding in the GI tract and its effects on the bowel can help in selecting measures to control or prevent constipation. These mechanisms, as well as the assessment and management of opioid-related constipation, were reviewed.

Opioid Effects on the GI Tract.—Opioid-related constipation is a dose-dependent effect; tolerance to constipation is rare. The intestinal effects of opioids may occur through altered propulsion of the bowel contents, increased water absorption, or decreased secretions. Opioid effects on propulsion occur through inhibition of synaptic transmission in the CNS and enteric nervous system. Binding of opioid receptors in these systems results in a decrease in the stimulus that creates the propulsive contraction, decreasing gastric motility and causing constipation. Delayed transit time increases the duration of exposure of the intestinal contents to the mucosal lining, increasing water and sodium absorption and resulting in drier stool. Exposure to the mucosal lining is also lengthened because of decreased biliary, pancreatic, and intestinal secretions. Constipation may cause complications such as abdominal discomfort, nausea, fullness, or even diarrhea; rectal tears and fissures caused by passing hard, dry stool; and hemorrhoids related to straining.

Assessment and Treatment.—For patients receiving opioid treatment, assessment includes the patient's bowel habits, fluid intake, diet, exercise, and medications. The assessment findings are used to create an individualized treatment plan. Nonpharmacologic measures instituted at the beginning of opioid treatment can help to prevent constipation. These include increasing fluid and dietary fiber intake to soften stool; regular exercise, if possible, to stimulate GI motility; and establishing a regular toileting routine. Effective pain control may enhance the patient's ability to be active. Laxatives work through 3 general mechanisms: Osmotic laxatives cause fluid retention in the colon, increasing stool bulk and softness; those acting directly on the mucosa decrease net water absorption; and those that enhance intestinal motility decrease transit time, thus decreasing salt and water absorption. Laxative options include saline and osmotic laxatives, bulk-forming laxatives, surfactant laxatives, stimulants, phenolphthalein, athraquone, castor oil, and lubricants. Other available pharmacologic therapies include glycerin and bisacodyl suppositories and various types of enemas.

Conclusion.—Management of opioid-related constipation is focused on prevention and control. Understanding the mechanisms of this problem can aid in helping the patient to maintain an acceptable pattern of elimination, thus maintaining or improving quality of life. Nursing implications for dealing with opioid-related constipation are presented, including a decision tree that displays possible pharmacologic treatments.

▶ Constipation is a common side effect of long-term opioid use. This clearly written discussion should be useful to nurses working with patients with cancer and others who may be receiving long-term opioid therapy. Description of various types of laxatives and a decision tree for administering them add to the value of this article.—A.K. Jacox, R.N., Ph.D.

Respiratory-Related Critical Events With Intravenous Patient-Controlled Analgesia

Ashburn MA, Love G, Pace NL (Univ of Utah, Salt Lake City)

Clin J Pain 10:52–56, 1994 131-95-7-27

Purpose.—Although patient-controlled analgesia (PCA) is widely used, it has potentially lethal complications. Respiratory-related critical events in patients receiving IV PCA therapy on an acute-pain service were studied.

Methods.—The records of 3,785 patients who received IV PCA therapy for 11,521 patient-care days over 2½-years were studied. Additional information was obtained in instances of respiratory critical events, which led to or could have led to adverse outcomes.

Results.—Fourteen critical events occurred, or about 1 per 1,000 patient-care days. Eight critical events were caused by programming errors due to the design of the PCA device, and the device was subsequently removed from service. Two critical events occurred when family members activated the device, 2 were caused by clinical errors, and one each occurred when the patient or a family member tampered with the device. Four events, which included respiratory arrest in 2 patients, pulmonary aspiration in 1, and sedation hypoxemia hypercarbia in 1, required additional treatment with naloxone, ventilation or mask oxygen, and intensive care. All 14 patients had an uneventful recovery.

Conclusion.—Intravenous PCA requires constant and active monitoring by physicians and nurses and an active quality assurance program. The routine use of a continuous infusion might increase the risk for a respiratory-related adverse event. Its use should be limited to patients for whom the risk is warranted. Patients and families must realize that only the patient should activate the device. If anyone else is seen activating it, it should be immediately removed.

▶ The 0.1% incidence of serious respiratory-related critical events in patients receiving IV PCA illustrates the possibility of complications occurring even when pain is managed by a pain service. This study shows the contributions of a thoughtfully designed quality assurance program in detecting problems in care delivery and changing policy. This description of actions taken to minimize the possibility of adverse incidents occurring is an excellent example of institutional responsibility for safe and effective pain management.—A.K. Jacox, R.N., Ph.D.

Specific Drugs

Giving Fentanyl for Pain Outside the OR

Willens JS (Villanova Univ, Pa)
Am J Nurs 94:24–28, 1994 131-95-7–28

Introduction.—Although some nurses have expressed concern about the potency of fentanyl and its appropriateness for clinical use, it is no more difficult or dangerous to administer than other potent drugs that nurses administer regularly. It is similar to morphine and is effective in management of severe pain.

Routes of Administration.—Because fentanyl has a short duration of action and is associated with less respiratory depression and histamine release, it can be used either for continuous IV infusion or patient-controlled analgesia (PCA). A bolus of 50–100 μg is recommended to initiate a continuous IV infusion of 15–50 μg/hr. After an initiating bolus of

50–100 μg, the PCA dose is usually 20–100 μg, with a lockout time of 3–10 minutes. Fentanyl can also be given as a continuous epidural infusion or epidural PCA for postoperative pain management. A fentanyl transdermal patch, available in 4 doses (25, 50, 75, and 100 μg/hr), is used to control chronic, severe pain, such as in patients with cancer.

Mode of Action.—Fentanyl differs from morphine in that it is lipophilic, whereas morphine is hydrophilic. Therefore, fentanyl has a much faster time of onset and peak effect than morphine does, as well as a shorter duration of action.

Adverse Effects.—Like morphine, fentanyl can produce delayed-onset respiratory depression, especially in elderly patients or patients who have also received intraoperative intrathecal morphine, midazolam, other anti-anxiety agents, or CNS depressants. Therefore, respiration should be assessed hourly for 12 hours after fentanyl administration and then every 4 hours. Respiratory depression can be reversed with IV naloxone. Other adverse effects include hypotension, pruritus (to a lesser extent, however, than with morphine), urinary retention, nausea and vomiting (especially with the transdermal patch), and constipation.

Conclusion.—Frequent pain assessments are required to arrive at the optimal dose. The adverse effects of fentanyl are similar to those with morphine and are generally treated in the same ways. Fentanyl, although potent, is safe when given in small doses.

▶ This concise, well-written article does an excellent job of describing the use of fentanyl. It contains good descriptions of the mechanisms by which fentanyl operates and provides many practical suggestions for administering it and monitoring the patient after its use.—A.K. Jacox, R.N., Ph.D.

Evaluation of Intravenous Ketorolac Administered by Bolus or Infusion for Treatment of Postoperative Pain: A Double-Blind, Placebo-Controlled, Multicenter Study

Ready LB, Brown CR, Stahlgren LH, Egan KJ, Ross B, Wild L, Moodie JE, Jones SF, Tommeraasen M, Trierwieler M (Univ of Washington, Seattle; Waikato Analgesic Research, Hamilton, New Zealand; St Joseph Hosp, Denver)

Anesthesiology 80:1277–1286, 1994 131-95-7–29

Purpose.—Previous studies have shown a reduction in morphine requirements in patients given IM ketorolac for postoperative analgesia after major surgery. Intravenous ketorolac is not yet marketed in the United States, but its safety has been documented. The analgesic efficacy and safety of IV ketorolac for postoperative analgesia were evaluated in a double-blind, randomized, multicenter trial.

Methods.—The study population consisted of 201 adult patients undergoing major surgery. Sixty-five were randomized to receive a ketorolac infusion; 68, an IV ketorolac bolus; and 68, placebo during the first

24 postoperative hours. All patients had access to supplemental IV morphine with a patient-controlled analgesia (PCA) pump. Pain intensity was assessed at study entry and at 2, 4, 6, and 24 hours, with categorical pain intensity scores and visual analogue scale (VAS) scores. The amount of morphine used during the 24-hour study was also measured.

Results.—Sixty-five (32%) patients did not complete the study. Categorical pain intensity scores and VAS pain scores in both ketorolac groups were significantly lower at various time points during the study than were those in the placebo group. The average amount of PCA morphine used in the ketorolac infusion group was significantly lower than that used in the placebo group, but the difference in morphine use between the bolus group and the placebo group did not reach statistical significance. There were no significant differences in sedation scores among the 3 groups at any time, but vomiting was significantly less frequent in both ketorolac groups. Study observers reported less nursing difficulty in the ketorolac infusion group. Overall patient and observer ratings were statistically greater for both ketorolac groups.

Conclusion.—Patients receiving PCA morphine after major surgery will use less morphine if they are also given an IV ketorolac infusion. Intravenous ketorolac infusion and IV ketorolac bolus doses both improve the response to PCA morphine compared with placebo.

▶ This well-conducted study showed that a nonsteroidal analgesic combined with an opioid and administered IV resulted in less opioid use. An interesting finding was the high number of adverse events identified in the 3 study groups, with ketorolac resulting in significantly less vomiting and fewer patients with elevated temperature.—A.K. Jacox, R.N., Ph.D.

Nondrug Interventions

Cognitive-Behavioral Interventions for Children's Distress During Bone Marrow Aspirations and Lumbar Punctures: A Critical Review

Ellis JA, Spanos NP (Univ of Ottawa, Ont, Canada; Carleton Univ, Ottawa, Ont, Canada)

J Pain Symptom Manage 9:96–108, 1994 131-95-7–30

Purpose.—Children with cancer must undergo essential but painful procedures such as bone marrow aspiration and lumbar puncture. Age, sex, coping skills, and general fear of medical procedures and the extent of parental anxiety affect how much pain the child feels. Furthermore, it is difficult to distinguish between the associated anxiety and the pain itself. The distress does not decrease over time but sometimes increases. Procedural pain in children is not being effectively or consistently managed at many hospitals and oncology centers. What is the role of pharmacologic and behavioral interventions in easing procedural pain?

Pharmacologic Methods.—Minimal pharmacologic intervention consists of local anesthetic at the site of lumbar puncture or bone marrow aspiration. This entails a distressing needlestick. Use of an anesthetic cream comprising a eutectic mixture of local anesthetics alleviates the pain of the needlestick.

A survey found that the most common drugs used to control pain were IM meperidine, promethazine, and chlorpromazine. This combination is unacceptable for use in many children, because it can be overly sedating. Some children feel a heightened loss of control when their anxiety is accompanied by drowsiness.

Conscious sedation and general anesthesia have been used in Europe and are now more widely used in North America. Specifically, IV midazolam alone or in combination with fentanyl is safe and effective for controlling pain and distress. Conscious sedation has the advantage that children do not remember the procedure, which thereby averts a cycle of increasing anxiety with each procedure. However, hypoventilation and consequent hypoxemia pose a risk. Patients must be carefully monitored, and access to supplemental oxygen, resuscitation equipment, and experienced personnel are essential. It might be impractical for smaller facilities to have an anesthesiologist present at every procedure. Conscious sedation adds time, technology, and inconvenience to what are otherwise simple procedures.

Behavioral Methods.—Cognitive-behavioral therapy includes attention diversion, reinforcement, imagery, behavioral rehearsal, and filmed modeling. This therapy significantly lowered the pain of bone marrow aspiration when the anticipatory phase, the procedural phase (the aspiration), and the recovery phase were considered together. However, when the procedural phase was considered separately, cognitive-behavioral therapy was no different from oral diazepam in lowering pain. Diazepam lowered anticipatory distress but not procedural distress. Therefore, different types of interventions might be useful at particular times before, during, or after the procedure. Combining oral diazepam with cognitive-behavioral therapy led to less stress reduction than with cognitive-behavioral therapy alone. Perhaps diazepam interfered with learning and focusing on behavioral tasks during bone marrow aspiration. Finally, children did not subsequently use the coping strategies they learned from cognitive-behavioral therapy unless they were told to do so.

Hypnosis has been shown to reduce the pain experienced by children undergoing bone marrow aspiration or lumbar puncture. However, hypnosis does not appear to add more value than other procedures such as distraction or guided imagery. In addition, hypnosis has not been clearly defined and has been unambiguously implemented in clinical studies, which precludes a firm conclusion about its value.

Conclusion.—Ideally, conscious sedation and cognitive-behavioral strategies would both be available. The best method to help children during painful procedures probably is a combination of pharmacologic and behavioral support. Either alone probably will not meet the needs of all children.

By the time they are 7 years old, children can better explain their fears and needs. At that age, they might choose among distraction, imagery, or conscious sedation. Younger children might routinely be given conscious sedation for all procedures. Future research could examine which specific intervention works before, during, and after painful procedures. But the particular strategy might not be so important as the ability of children to understand what works best for them and what kind of support they can expect. Children who apparently cope well on their own could also be studied in the future. These children could be compared with others who report high levels of pain and distress even when aided by interventions intended to relieve pain.

► This well-written review of interventions to relieve pain and distress during bone marrow aspiration and lumbar puncture focuses on the need to combine pharmacologic and nonpharmacologic interventions. The authors thoughtfully analyzed the literature to identify which interventions affect pain and distress before, during, and after the procedure. This kind of analysis of what interventions work best during the course of an illness or treatment is greatly needed.—A.K. Jacox, R.N., Ph.D.

Ice Freezes Pain? A Review of the Clinical Effectiveness of Analgesic Cold Therapy

Ernst E, Fialka V (Univ of Exeter, England)

J Pain Symptom Manage 9:56–59, 1994 131-95-7–31

Background.—Cooling of the body surface is often used to treat musculoskeletal pain. The evidence for the clinical efficacy of ice and its possible mechanisms were reviewed.

Effects of Cold Therapy and Possible Modes of Action.—To date, data on the short-term analgesic effect of ice provide some indication of the efficacy of this form of therapy. However, there are surprisingly few hard data. Previous studies have lacked methodologic rigor, leading to the conclusion that this method is not scientifically proved. Nevertheless, clinical experience suggests that ice can provide short-term control of some types of pain, especially pain originating from the musculoskeletal system. Studies of the effects of serial applications are methodologically flawed and difficult to interpret. None of the studies have included a control group. Thus, the existence of analgesic effects from serial cold treatment remains to be established. Possible mechanisms by which cryotherapy may increase the pain threshold include an antinociceptive effect on the gate control system, reduction in nerve conduction, decrease in muscle spasm, and prevention of edema after injury.

Conclusion.—Although cooling is an attractive approach to the treatment of musculoskeletal pain, there is little scientific evidence to show its efficacy. All clinical studies assessing this modality have serious flaws.

Further studies are needed to provide scientific proof of the efficacy of this treatment and to test which types of pain respond best.

▶ This is an excellent review of the sparse and somewhat dismal literature studying the effects of ice on the reduction of pain. There is much written regarding the presumed effectiveness of ice in reducing pain, particularly acute pain related to the musculoskeletal system, and there are many theories regarding how the cold may operate to reduce pain. The authors, however, could not find a single well-designed study that tested this. This area is in great need of well-designed research studies to improve our understanding of whether—and under what circumstances—the application of ice is effective in reducing pain.—A.K. Jacox, R.N., Ph.D.

Spinal Cord Stimulation for Relief of Ischemic Pain in End-Stage Arterial Occlusive Disease

Rickman S, Wuebbels BH, Holloway GA Jr (Maricopa Med Ctr, Phoenix, Ariz)
J Vasc Nurs 12:14–20, 1994 131-95-7–32

Purpose.—In patients with advanced peripheral arterial occlusive disease, pain is the most common symptom and most often causes the patient to seek medical attention. If surgical revascularization is not an option for these patients, amputation of the affected limb may be the only alternative for pain relief. Spinal cord stimulation is under investigation as a means of not only relieving the pain associated with peripheral arterial occlusive disease but also of actually improving microcirculatory blood flow. Pain relief may occur through blocking of pain signals, as described in the gate-control theory of pain; other theories have also been advanced. The pain relief and vascular results of spinal cord stimulation in peripheral arterial occlusive disease were assessed in a nonrandomized, prospective study.

Methods.—The study included 25 patients who underwent implantation of a spinal cord stimulator at 6 North American hospitals. One component of the intervention was patient education about the test procedure, the surgery, and how to use the stimulator. All patients had end-stage arterial occlusive disease that was not amenable to surgical treatment either because of poor surgical risk, poor vessel runoff, or inadequate vessels with which to perform bypass. Common causes included arteriosclerosis with or without diabetes, thromboangiitis obliterans, Raynaud's disease, and embolic occlusive disease. The scale of the Ad Hoc Committee on Reporting Standards of the Society for Vascular Surgery and the Society for Cardiovascular Surgery was used to classify the patient's pain as grade I, II, or III. The patients were followed up for at least 6 months after stimulator implantation. Treatment failure was defined as foot amputation or heroic bypass surgery.

Results.—Treatment with spinal cord stimulation was successful in 67% of patients with grade II pain (pain at rest but no ulcers). For grade

III pain (pain at rest and foot lesions), the success rate was only 38%. At a mean follow-up of 1 year, average pain relief was 80% in both groups. The treatment successfully relieved pain even in patients with severe foot ischemia and yielded dramatic improvements in quality of life when successful. Risk factors for failure of spinal cord stimulation were the lack of significant pain relief during a trial stimulation period, the presence of foot ulcers greater than 2 cm in diameter, and the presence of areas of dry gangrene greater than 2 cm in diameter or any areas of wet gangrene.

Conclusion.—Spinal cord stimulation can effectively relieve pain and avert amputation for many patients with end-stage peripheral arterial occlusive disease. Dramatic improvements in quality of life are possible, including less interrupted sleep and increased ability to walk, perform self-care, and enjoy social interactions. In two thirds of patients with grade II pain, a stimulator implantation produces a successful result, so these patients can probably undergo the procedure without a trial period. Those with grade III pain should undergo a 5- to 7-day trial screening period. Clinical management requires close cooperation between the pain and vascular surgery services.

▶ There are too few studies that test combinations of modalities for their affectiveness in managing pain. A positive aspect of this study is that it reports on the combination of a surgical procedure and patient education regarding that procedure. Unfortunately, because of the lack of a control or even a comparison group, it is not possible to evaluate the effectiveness of the intervention or the significance of the reported successes in treatment.—A.K. Jacox, R.N., Ph.D.

Pain in Special Populations or Settings

Younger and Older Populations

Outcomes in Treatment of Pain in Geriatric and Younger Age Groups

Cutler RB, Fishbain DA, Rosomoff RS, Rosomoff HL (Univ of Miami, Fla; South Shore Hosp, Miami Beach, Fla)

Arch Phys Med Rehabil 75:457–464, 1994 131-95-7–33

Purpose.—Because of continuing uncertainty as to whether patients older than 65 years with chronic pain benefit as much as younger patients from management at a pain center, a large number of patients were asked to rate their pain when admitted to a pain center and again when discharged.

Methods.—The 153 patients, who were older than 65 years of age, were compared with 126 middle-aged patients (45–64 years of age) and with 191 younger patients (age 21–44 years). No fewer than 43 rating scales were used to evaluate the pain and the patient's functional status, behavioral variables, and management goals. Change scores were compared using analysis of covariance and pairwise post hoc tests.

Results.—The geriatric patients improved on all but 1 of the 43 self-rating scales, and the degree of improvement on 37 scales was significant, most often at a level of 0.001. The elderly patients differed significantly from the other age groups on most baseline variables, and their scores when admitted were better than those for the younger patients. Geriatric patients exhibited significantly better change on 2 scales and significantly worse change on 4.

Conclusion.—Geriatric patients with chronic pain clearly benefit from multidisciplinary treatment at a chronic pain center. At the same time, they appear to be a distinct group in many respects and for this reason should be considered separately in outcome studies.

▶ Demonstrating how patients of various ages respond differently to treatment in a pain center is an important outcome of this study. Finding that older patients present differently from younger and middle-aged patients on admission to a pain treatment center and demonstrating the lack of a linear relationship between age and pain severity scores add to the value of the study.—A.K. Jacox, R.N., Ph.D.

Cognitive Status and Postoperative Pain: Older Adults

Duggleby W, Lander J (Garden Grove Village, Edmonton, Alta, Canada)

J Pain Symptom Manage 9:19–27, 1994 131-95-7–34

Purpose.—Pain is inadequately managed in older persons. Although health practitioners believe that pain management in older persons should differ from that in younger persons, no compelling evidence suggests that older persons experience pain any differently. The relations among age, postoperative pain, analgesic intake, and mental status were studied in older adults.

Methods.—Sixty adults (24 men) with an average age of 65 years (range, 50–80 years) were studied. They had undergone total hip replacement, which entails moderate to severe postoperative pain. They had no other serious illnesses that interfered with anesthesia or surgery. The visual analogue scale (VAS) for pain assessment and the Mini-Mental Status Questionnaire, an instrument widely used in North America to screen for acute confusion and dementia, were administered various times on the day of surgery and during the next 4 days. Analgesic intake was noted.

Results.—Age was unrelated to pain, analgesic intake, or mental status. Pain significantly decreased over time, particularly between the day of surgery and the day after surgery. One third of patients continued to have moderate to severe pain on the fourth day after surgery. More than one third of patients had diminished mental status, usually observed on the first 2 days after surgery. Pain, not analgesic intake, was the major predictor of decreased mental status.

Conclusion.—Pain was poorly managed in this group of older adults. Pain, not analgesic intake, might lead to decline in mental status. Improvements in care and additional research are needed.

▶ This carefully conducted descriptive study provides empirical data to challenge several assumptions regarding pain in the elderly. The finding that the major predictor of mental status decline (acute confusion) was pain, not analgesic intake, provides further evidence of the negative physiologic consequences of unrelieved pain. The researchers' successful use of the VAS in this population and their thoughtful discussion of the potential relationships among pain, fatigue, lack of sleep, and mental status contributed to the value of this research report.—A.K. Jacox, R.N., Ph.D.

Surgical Patients

Dimensions of Procedural Pain and Its Analgesic Management in Critically Ill Surgical Patients

Puntillo KA (Univ of Calif, San Francisco)

Am J Crit Care 3:116–122, 1994 131-95-7–35

Purpose.—Endotracheal suctioning and chest tube removal both are among the most common procedures performed in critically ill patients, but pain from these procedures and the resultant psychological effects have not been thoroughly studied. When asked, cardiothoracic patients report that, after burning, pain is the most common sensation related to chest tube removal. Accordingly, a study was planned to document the degree of pain from endotracheal suctioning and chest tube removal in surgical ICU patients and to examine the relation between procedural pain and analgesic administration.

Methods.—Thirty-five patients undergoing cardiac surgery at a large teaching hospital in whom an endotracheal or chest tube had been placed within 3 days of admission to the ICU participated in assessment of pain with chest tube removal. Forty-five patients undergoing cardiac and abdominal vascular surgery participated in assessment of pain with endotracheal tube suctioning. Intensity of pain was rated on a 10-cm horizontal numerical scale, and the extent of pain was measured with use of a body outline diagram. The McGill Pain Questionnaire-Short Form word list served to assess pain sensation and affect.

Results.—Scores for the extent of pain were low for both endotracheal tube suctioning and chest tube removal. Scores of pain sensation and affect were relatively low. Pain intensity was less with endotracheal tube suctioning. Comparable language was used to describe the 2 procedures, except that more patients described their response to chest tube removal as "fearful." The patients generally received little analgesia before the procedures, and the amount of medication given did not closely correlate with the magnitude of pain.

Conclusion.—Despite the limitations of this study, including an overrepresentation by males, the author demonstrates that there is a prominent emotional component of procedure-related pain. Nurses who suction endotracheal tubes and help in removing chest tubes, in addition to providing pharmacologic support, are in a position to offer psychological support that will augment the effect of analgesia. It will be helpful to communicate to patients the types of sensation they may experience. If distress from pain exceeds pain intensity, it might be appropriate to use relaxation techniques in conjunction with medication before starting a painful procedure.

▶ Reporting on pain associated with endotracheal tube suctioning and chest tube removal is a good example of the kind of descriptive studies needed to provide a basis for the formulation and testing of intervention to deal with the pain.—A.K. Jacox, R.N., Ph.D.

Patterns of Prescribing and Administering Drugs for Agitation and Pain in Patients in a Surgical Intensive Care Unit

Dasta JF, Fuhrman TM, McCandles C (Ohio State Univ, Columbus)

Crit Care Med 22:974–980, 1994 131-95-7-36

Purpose.—Critically ill patients who receive mechanical ventilation frequently feel pain, anxiety, or agitation. There is considerable variation in the drugs prescribed to treat these emotional problems and possibly some prescribing errors. This study was conducted to assess the drug-prescription patterns for anxiety, agitation, muscle relaxation, and pain, the clarity of written orders, and the accuracy of transcribing those orders in a surgical ICU.

Methods.—A group of 221 patients (average age, 57 years) was admitted for abdominal surgery, cancer treatment, vascular surgery, transplant, surgery, trauma, or other causes. Approximately 52% required mechanical ventilation. For 91% of patients, drugs were prescribed, most commonly morphine sulfate, but also benzodiazepine and vecuronium.

Results.—A total of 2,103 doses of various drugs were administered. On 403 of 448 orders, drugs were prescribed to be given as needed, with no specific indications on 42% of these orders. More than 80% of the diazepam orders and almost 50% of the hydromorphone, lorazepam, and morphine orders were written in this way. Doses for most drugs were written as a range. On 17% of orders, the way nurses transcribed drug orders onto administration forms was different from the original order; that is, they added or left out words. In almost 3% of dosing administrations, a check mark rather than the actual dose was recorded. On average, only 27% of the maximum daily dose was administered.

Conclusion.—Drugs are frequently prescribed to be given "as needed," and inadequate indications for use are provided. Most patients receive less than the maximum doses of medication. Transcription errors are made when drugs are prescribed "as needed." Drugs are sometimes administered without noting the exact dose. Physicians need to be educated about order writing, and more research needs to be conducted on the prescribing habits of physicians.

▶ Like many other areas of clinical practice, pain management is interdisciplinary in nature, and the resolution of problems related to pain management necessitates interdisciplinary exploration. This interesting study by a pharmacist, a physician, and a nurse represents an excellent way to identify the basis for problems of inadequate treatment of patients.—A.K. Jacox, R.N., Ph.D.

Pain and Its Control in Patients With Fractures of the Femoral Neck While Awaiting Surgery

Roberts HC, Eastwood H (Southampton Gen Hosp, England)

Injury 25:237–239, 1994 131-95-7-37

Purpose.—For patients with fracture of the femoral neck, surgical treatment within 24 hours is recommended. Analgesia and immobilization of the affected leg are used to manage pain while the patient is awaiting surgery. Most of these fractures occur in elderly persons, who have decreased sensitivity to cutaneous and visceral pain. Painless fracture of the femoral neck has even been reported in the elderly. No studies have examined the effect of age on pain appreciation in patients with this type of fracture, however. Preoperative pain and its control in patients with fracture of the femoral neck were analyzed, including the effect of age.

Methods.—One hundred consecutive patients (80 women, 20 men; mean age, 80 years) with acute fractures of the femoral neck were interviewed before they underwent surgery. Two standard methods were used to assess the patients' subjective level of pain: a verbal rating scale and a Grimace Chart, which shows faces of persons experiencing pain. The medical and nursing staff perception of patient pain also was assessed in terms of the preoperative analgesia given. The patients' mental state was assessed, as well.

Results.—Only 2 patients reported no pain. Most of the others felt a great deal of pain: 89 patients reported a pain rating of 7 or greater on a scale of 0–10. Perception of pain was unaffected by the intracapsular vs. extracapsular nature of the fracture and by patient age. With one of the subjective assessments, elderly patients with preserved mental function felt greater pain; with the other method, patients taking the usual prefracture analgesia reported less pain.

Conclusion.—Elderly patients with fractures of the femoral neck experience considerable pain while awaiting surgery. They also appear to receive inadequate analgesia for their reported levels of pain. Regular nursing assessment of the degree of pain these patients feel before surgery, along with medical review of the prescribed analgesia is suggested. At a time when the benefits of traction for fracture of the femoral neck are being questioned, the optimal pain relief regimen for this common condition may warrant reconsideration.

▶ The authors cited research indicating decreased sensitivity to cutaneous and visceral pain in elderly people, but they noted that no studies had been done on the effect of age on perception of pain in patients with fractures of the femoral neck. Once again, the findings illustrate the tremendous gap between what clinicians think about pain and what is known through research. The study showed that 98 of 100 patients with femoral neck fractures had pain, with 89 reporting pain levels of 7 or more of a possible 10. The statement that the preoperative analgesia given to patients appears to have been inadequate was supported by the observation that one third of the 98 patients reporting pain received no analgesia despite the fact that movement during the process of admission to the hospital is a major cause of pain. In spite of the greatly increased knowledge of pain and its management in the past few decades, descriptions of this kind of serious undertreatment of pain are all too common.—A.K. Jacox, R.N., Ph.D.

Pain: Its Mediators and Associated Morbidity in Critically Ill Cardiovascular Surgical Patients

Puntillo K, Weiss SJ (Univ of California, San Francisco)
Nurs Res 43:31–36, 1994 131-95-7–38

Purpose.—Pain that is not managed adequately can result in significant physiologic and psychological stress and can negatively affect patient recovery. The factors that influence postoperative pain in critically ill patients undergoing surgery and the relationship of pain magnitude to patient morbidity were investigated.

Methods.—Seventy-four patients were assessed in the first few days after cardiac and abdominal vascular surgery. The effects of patient age, sex, and personality adjustment as well as analgesic administration on the degree of pain were determined.

Findings.—Pain intensity was moderate and did not decline during the period studied. Minimal distress resulted from physical sensations and emotional tension associated with pain. Although small amounts of analgesics were given, the amount of analgesic administered was the main consistent mediator of pain magnitude after surgery. Neither age nor personality adjustment affected the degree of any pain dimension. Women and patients undergoing abdominal vascular surgery reported more disturbing physical sensations related to pain. Patients with greater pain intensity had a significantly higher incidence of postoperative atelectasis.

Conclusion.—Although the small amounts of analgesic given may have stabilized the pain experience, they were apparently insufficient to minimize the intensity of the pain. By contrast, the relatively low magnitudes of pain sensation and pain affect reported by the patients indicate that the sensory disturbances and emotional distress associated with the pain may have been minimal.

▶ The authors of this well-conducted study did a nice job of documenting the effects of age, personality characteristics, and analgesic administration on pain in critically ill cardiovascular surgical patients. They documented, once again, the undertreatment of pain, this time in critically ill patients. Their finding that patients with greater pain intensity had a higher incidence of atelectasis is a very specific indication of the negative consequences of unrelieved pain.—A.K. Jacox, R.N., Ph.D.

Chest Pain

Differentiating Chest Pain: Advanced Assessment Techniques

Kernicki JG (Texas Woman's Univ, Houston)

Dimens Crit Care Nurs 12:66–76, 1993 131-95-7-39

Introduction.—Although the most common forms of chest pain are caused by anxiety-tension syndrome, coronary artery disease, and pleuropericardial disease, patients with other forms of chest pain are often seen for emergency treatment. Some of these less common forms of chest pain may be caused by cocaine use, the harvesting of the internal mammary artery for coronary artery bypass, mitral valve prolapse, 5-fluorouracil therapy, tachyarrhythmias, or gastric irritation. These forms may be recognized by characteristic cues (Table 1).

Pathogenesis.—Inflammation, obstruction or restriction, or distention or dilation may cause pain. The experience of pain is neurologically mediated by A delta fibers, which conduct impulses quickly, creating sharp, localized pain, and C fibers, which conduct impulses slowly, creating dull, diffuse, persistent pain.

Characteristic Cues.—Cocaine use, because it stimulates thromboxane production and platelet aggregation, may cause coronary artery vasospasm, sympathomimetic activation, or thrombosis; myocarditis also may develop. In 70% of patients who undergo coronary artery bypass procedures with internal mammary artery grafting, chest pain may occur as long as 22 months after the procedure. Both the descriptions of pain and the postulated causes for this form of chest pain vary. About half of patients with mitral valve prolapse experience chest pain of varying types, often associated with fatigue, weakness, dizziness, or dyspnea. Patients given 5-fluorouracil may experience coronary artery vasospasm, and this may lead to intimal hyperplasia. The pain may occur during or

TABLE 1.—Differential Cues for Assessment of Chest Discomfort

Cue	Possible Condition
• Area is usually size of palm of hand; related to effort	Ischemic heart disease
• Pain increases with inspiration or position change	Musculoskeletal origin of pain- Pericarditis
• Experience of pain with light touch of sternum over manubrium	Internal mammary artery used for coronary artery bypass procedure
• Pain is finger-point localized	Costochondritis
• Burning sensation of face and chest; Feeling of heaviness on chest	Gastrointestinal Irritation
• Pain sudden in onset	Pulmonary embolism
• Systolic click associated with chest discomfort	Mitral valve prolapse

(Courtesy of Kernicki JG: *Dimens Crit Care Nurs* 12:66–76, 1993.)

several hours after the infusion. Chest pain associated with tachyarrhythmias occurs as a tight sensation over the precordium. Monosodium glutamate can cause burning chest pain, similar to that of angina pectoris.

Conclusion.—Newer causes of chest pain are occurring as new surgical procedures, new trends in drug use, and new therapies are developed. Critical care nurses must be adept at eliciting information about pain (Table 2), interpreting the multicultural verbal and nonverbal expressions of pain, and recognizing the characteristic cues of distinct forms of pain (Table 3).

▶ This article, which describes types of chest pain not previously seen with any high degree of frequency, is similar to Abstract 131-95-7-41 in its description of symptoms emerging as a consequence of treatments. The types of chest pain described include those resulting from recreational use of cocaine and those caused by new cardiac surgical procedures and other therapies. The author suggests ways to differentiate various sources of chest pain, giving the physiologic basis for the type of pain experienced. As new pain-related clinical conditions emerge and new treatments are developed with increasing rapidity, this kind of description is important.—A.K. Jacox, R.N., Ph.D.

TABLE 2.—Chest Pain Questions Based on PQRST Mnemonic

P = Precipitating factors
Have you had this type of pain before?
What were you doing before you experienced the discomfort?

Q = Quality
Can you describe the pain to me?
What does it feel like?

R = Region, Radiation
Show me where is the pain?
How large an area is involved?

S = Associated Symptoms
In addition to the pain, what else did you experience?

T = Temporal Relations
Were you awakened by the pain?
Does it feel as if it is always present?
Have you found anything that might ease the pain?

(Courtesy of Kernicki JG: *Dimens Crit Care Nurs* 12:66–76, 1993.)

TABLE 3.—Comparison of Pain Characteristics

Precipitating Factors	Quality	Region	Associated Symptoms	Time and Response
ISCHEMIC HEART DISEASE PAIN CHARACTERISTICS				
Effort related activity	Tightness	Retrosternal	Profuse sweating	Gradual onset builds up to maximum
Excitement	Burning	Size of palm of hand	Weakness	Ceases with activity abatement
Large meals	Deep	Radiates to left shoulder, left hand, especially 4th - 5th finger, epigastrium, trachea, larynx	Shortness of breath	Nitroglycerine
Emotional stress	Constrictive	Never involves region above level of eye	Nausea, vomiting	Rest
COCAINE INDUCED CHEST PAIN				
Use of cocaine	Heaviness Pressure	Substernal Radiates to both arms	Palpitations Diaphoresis, nausea, dizziness, syncope, dyspnea	1 to 6 hours after use Relief with nitroglycerine
INTERNAL MAMMARY ARTERY HARVESTING INDUCED CHEST PAIN				
Internal mammary artery harvesting	Mild-severe	Anterior chest	Tenderness on palpation of sternum	Persistent
	Burning	Radiates over whole chest wall, always at site of graft	Hyperesthesia along incisional line	Shooting pain lasting for several seconds and occurring several times a day
	Prickling	Radiates to neck or axilla	Numbness	Variable response to Transcutaneous electric nerve stimulation (TENS)
	Dull		Delayed healing of sternum Allodyhia	
MITRAL VALVE PROLAPSE CHEST PAIN				
Prolapsed mitral valve	Localized tenderness	Center or left chest wall	Fatigue	Fleeting or lasts for days

	Dull - aching quality	Non-retrosternal	Weakness	Relief in recumbent position
			Midsystolic click (apical)	Nonresponsive to sublingual nitroglycerine
			Systolic murmur Unexplained dyspnea Palpitations	
5-FLUOROURACIL THERAPY AND CHEST PAIN				
Infusion of 5-fluorouracil (5-FU)	Mild to severe	Central	Nausea, vomiting	Several hours after I.V. bolus or as continuous infusion
		Radiates to left shoulder, left arm	Tachycardia	Good response to cardioactive drug
			Hypertension	No chest pain between treatment. Relieved by nitroglycerine
TACHYARRHYTHMIAS AND CHEST PAIN				
Anxiety, digitalis toxicity, exercise, organic heart disease	Sharp, stabbing, aching	Precordial	Weakness	Paroxysmal in onset
	"Skipped beat"		Fatiguability, lethargy, palpitations	Brief to hours Terminated by Antiarrhythmics. Direct current shock Vagal maneuvers
			Vertigo, weakness	
MONOSODIUM GLUTAMATE INDUCED CHEST PAIN				
Food ingestion high in monosodium glutamate	Burning	Retrosternal	Nausea, vomiting	Shortly after meal
		Face	Facial pain	Several hours post meal

(Courtesy of Kernicki JG: *Dimens Crit Care Nurs* 12:66–76, 1993.)

Cancer and HIV

Pain as an Early Symptom in Cancer

Vuorinen E (Kymenlaakso Central Hosp, Kotka, Finland)

Clin J Pain 9:272–278,1993 131-95-7–40

Purpose.—Between 40% and 87% of patients with cancer have pain, and more than 70% of these patients can be relieved of pain if appropriate analgesics and other techniques are used. Prevalence of pain, causes of pain, and the relevance of other symptoms in the early stages of cancer were investigated.

Methods.—A group of 378 patients with newly diagnosed cancer (0–6 months after diagnosis) was asked to respond to a multiple-choice questionnaire on pain and other symptoms. Patients were presented with a list of the most common symptoms associated with cancer: pain, weight loss, nausea, vomiting, insomnia, confusion, anorexia, fatigue, dyspnea, constipation, and hiccup.

Results—Two hundred forty (64%) patients responded to the questionnaire. Of these, 66 (28%) patients reported pain and were examined in the pain clinic. Thirty had pain caused by direct tumor growth, and 44 had pain secondary to cancer or its treatment. The pain was unrelated to cancer in 12 of 66 patients; 15 patients had 2 or more different types of pain simultaneously. Some 31% of the tumors in the study were located in the genitourinary organs, and 26% in the breast (table). The prevalence of pain among patients with various cancers differed substantially, from 50% among patients with lung cancer to 18% among patients with breast cancer. In answering the question concerning the first symptoms of their cancer, 39 (21.9%) patients had not noticed any symptoms, 27% had poor general condition, 23% had weight loss, and 24% reported pain.

Primary Tumor Sites

	Basic sample		Those who answered questionnaire		Those who had died	
Cancer site	No.	%	No.	%	No.	%
Genitourinary	100	26	73	31	15	18
Gastrointestinal	82	22	38	16	36	42
Breast	78	21	63	26	1	1
Hematological	41	11	26	11	7	8
Lung	34	9	14	6	18	21
Skin*	15	4	13	5	1	1
Other	28	7	13	5	8	9
Total	378	100	240	100	86	100

* Basal cell carcinomas excluded.
(Courtesy of Vuorinen E: *Clin J Pain* 9:272–278, 1993.)

Conclusion.—Awareness of pain and its management at early stages of cancer are essential. In earlier studies 19% to 48% of patients had pain as a symptom preceding diagnosis, which shows that pain is not only a problem in terminal cancer but at all stages of the disease.

► This is another study describing the prevalence of pain in patients with cancer, this time in Finland. The author did a competent job of describing pain in the sample but commented that "so far no validated or generally accepted methods have been published to measure symptoms in cancer other than pain." This statement ignores the reports on ways to measure symptoms other than pain (1), and it illustrates the need for a careful literature review so that subsequent research takes full advantage of the research that precedes it.—A.K. Jacox, R.N. Ph.D.

Reference

1. Bergner M, Bobbitt RA, Carter WB, et al: The Symptom Impact Profile: Development and final revisions of the health status measure. *Med Care* 19:787–805, 1981.

Patterns of Mucositis and Pain in Patients Receiving Preparative Chemotherapy and Bone Marrow Transplantation

McGuire DB, Altomonte V, Peterson DE, Wingard JR, Jones RJ, Grochow LB (Johns Hopkins Oncology Ctr, Baltimore; Univ of Connecticut, Farmington; Johns Hopkins Univ, Baltimore)

Oncol Nurs Forum 20:1493–1502, 1993 131-95-7–41

Purpose.—Oral mucositis, a well-known side effect of preparative regimens for bone marrow transplantation (BMT), is a common cause of pain associated with treatment. Patterns of oral mucositis and pain were explored in a selected group of patients undergoing BMT.

Methods.—Forty-seven patients undergoing allogeneic and autologous BMT and receiving high-dose chemotherapy without total-body irradiation were studied. Nine anatomical regions of the patients' mouths were assessed daily for extent and severity of mucositis from 9 days before BMT to 21 days after BMT. The McGill Pain Questionnaire-Short Form was used to measure oral pain.

Findings.—Mucositis developed in 89% of patients. On average, it began 3 days after transplantation, lasted 9.5 days, and resolved by 12.6 days after transplantation. Eighty-six percent of the patients reported pain that began a mean 4.5 days after transplantation, lasted 6.5 days, and resolved by 11 days after transplantation.

Conclusion.—In the initial weeks after BMT, oral cavity regions at high risk for mucositis should be systematically assessed to enable early detection and intervention. Assessment and management of mucositis-related oral pain should also be done.

▶ This well-conducted study describing patterns of mucositis in patients undergoing BMT and receiving high-dose chemotherapy illustrates an interesting and increasingly common clinical phenomenon. As new treatments for disease and illnesses are developed, the treatments themselves often produce serious side effects that must be managed. Early research on interventions generally focuses on their efficacy to deal with the target problem and may not fully describe other consequences of the intervention. The symptoms that arise from interventions very often are managed by nurses and represent a fertile area for nursing research.—A.K. Jacox, R.N., Ph.D.

▶ This article is significant in 2 respects. First, the publication relates the importance of evaluating treatment-related toxicities. In this study, mucositis developed in almost 90% of patients, and 86% had symptoms. It is important to note that treatment-related toxicities can result in secondary morbidity-like infection, especially when the mucosal surface is compromised in these immunodeficient patients. Symptoms may result from either the initial treatment-related toxicity or secondary morbidity. The second significant aspect of the article is to indicate that these toxicities should be anticipated and treated prophylactically. In the same manner that chemotherapy-associated emesis is treated prophylactically, painful treatment-related toxicities, like mucositis, also should be expected and prevented. Because of this, an infusion of analgesics is administered and a patient-controlled analgesia pump is frequently inserted during BMT to relieve the symptoms of mucositis. Tolerance can be improved and morbidity reduced with aggressive management of expected treatment-related toxicities. These are especially important considerations in patients with cancer, who are often debilitated and immunocompromised as a result of their disease or therapy.—N.A. Janjan, M.D.

Evaluation of Recalcitrant Pain in HIV-Infected Hospitalized Patients

Anand A, Carmosino L, Glatt AE (Nassau County Med Ctr, East Meadow, New York; State Univ of New York, Stony Brook; Catholic Med Ctr of Brooklyn and Queens, Jamaica, New York)

J Acquir Immune Defic Syndr 7:52–56, 1994 131-95-7–42

Purpose.—There is little information about the chronic, severe pain commonly experienced by patients with HIV. The epidemiology, clinical features, and treatment of severe chronic pain in patients with HIV were assessed.

Methods.—Of 24 patients, 23 were adults (average age, 32.6 years) and one was an 18-month-old infant.

Results.—Fourteen patients were IV drug users. Fourteen patients had pain at multiple sites, most frequently in the legs, followed by the abdomen, mouth, and chest. Twelve patients had pain for longer than 6 months, and all had a severity grade of ≥7 according to the pain control service examination. The 21 surviving patients had relief of severe pain within 2 weeks of beginning around-the-clock opiate analgesia. There were no major adverse reactions. Side effects such as constipation and nausea were treated easily.

Conclusion.—Severe pain is an undertreated problem for patients infected with HIV. Pain specialists are useful in helping patients deal with this problem. With careful monitoring, opioid analgesics administered around the clock can be safe and effective therapy.

▶ This study of HIV-infected patients with severe chronic pain identifies many of the problems inherent in dealing with pain in this relatively new disease. Before referral to the pain control service, fewer than half the patients had their pain assessed by their physicians, all were receiving analgesics ordered "as needed," and all had pain ≥ 7 on a 0–10 scale. After aggressive treatment with oral opioids and fentanyl patches, there was a significant reduction in pain, there was no difference between the amount of analgesic required for pain relief by substance-abusing and non–substance-abusing patients, and several patients who had been depressed had improvement in mood. The study demonstrates that severe pain in this population can be managed successfully through rather simple means.—A.K. Jacox, R.N., Ph.D.

Spinal Cord Injury

Understanding Chronic Pain After Spinal Cord Injury

Segatore M (Mem Univ of Newfoundland, Canada)

J Neurosci Nurs 26:230–236, 1994 131-95-7–43

Introduction.—After spinal cord injury, patients have a range of sensory experiences, including acute pain, nonpainful phantom sensations, and chronic pain that persists indefinitely. Chronic pain can be disabling and lead to chemical dependency, severe depression, and even suicide. Pain from injury to peripheral and central neural structures has unique characteristics that distinguish it from persistent acute pain and phantom sensations. The structural and functional foundations of pain, including background for discussion of the pathogenesis of acute and chronic pain after spinal cord injury, were reviewed.

Neural Injury Pain.—Chronic pain arising from injury to or pathologic changes that affect a variety of peripheral and central nervous structures (Table 1), is far more common than chronic nociceptive or somatic pain. Neural injury pain is a variant of chronic pain that occurs after injury to the spinal cord (central structure), and the spinal roots and cauda equina (peripheral structures). Characteristic features of this sensation

TABLE 1.—Neurologic Conditions Associated With Neural Injury Pain

Peripheral neuropathies
Neuralgia of the head and face (eg. trigeminal and glossopharyngeal neuralgia)
Post-herpetic neuralgia
Guillain-Barré
Spinal cord injury
Cerebrovascular accident
Epilepsy
Parkinson's disease
Transverse myelitis

(Courtesy of Segatore M: *J Neurosci Nurs* 26:230-236, 1994.)

include absence of ongoing tissue injury and burning electrical sensations (Table 2).

Incidence and Natural History.—Neural injury pain is believed to be the most common type of chronic pain after a spinal cord injury. In 1 study, 53% of patients had neural injury pain and 30% of patients reported severe pain. Neural injury pain usually appears within the first year after injury, but it can appear immediately or much later. It affects patients with every level of injury but may be most prevalent in those with incomplete lesions of the conus medullaris and cauda equina. The pattern and intensity of pain vary.

Summary.—Neuropathic and central pain is poorly understood and poorly treated; consequently, survivors of spinal cord injuries often seek health care. Current efforts in neurophysiology, neurochemistry, pharmacology, and clinical sciences add daily to the understanding of the human nervous system. Affected individuals should remain optimistic about

TABLE 2.—Clinical Features of Neural Injury Pain

Absence of on-going tissue injury
Burning electrical sensations
Delayed onset
Present in deafferented areas
Lancinating or paroxysmal bursts
Allodynia or hyperpathia

(Courtesy of Segatore M: *J Neurosci Nurs* 26:230-236, 1994.)

the emergence of increasingly more effective treatment that will target the sensory, cognitive, and emotional aspects of their pain.

► This article, which describes what is known about chronic pain after spinal cord injury, should be useful in sensitizing clinicians who work with such patients to the likelihood of their experiencing this kind of pain. Unfortunately, there is little discussion of the implications for pain management.—A.K. Jacox, R.N., Ph.D.

Organizational and Policy Issues

Effect of Insurance Status on Pain Medication Prescriptions in a Hematology/Oncology Practice

Holcombe RF, Griffin J (Louisiana State Univ, Shreveport)

South Med J 86:151–156, 1993 131-95-7-44

Purpose.—Insurance status may affect the pattern of pain medication prescription. This possibility was studied in private practices in northern Louisiana that were composed mainly of indigent patients with hematologic disorders or cancer.

Methods.—The case-control study with retrospective chart review included 710 active patients with all types of insurance status. The amount and type of pain medication prescribed and the diagnosis were noted.

Results.—The proportion of Medicaid patients who received pain medications was significantly greater than that of Medicare patients, privately insured patients, uninsured patients covered by the state hospital system, and the overall patient population. Medicaid patients, especially those with solid tumors, were prescribed the most expensive class of pain medications at a significantly greater rate than were other patients (table).

Conclusion.—In this practice, the amount and type of pain medications given to Medicaid patients, who have prescription drug coverage, differed significantly from those given patients without prescription drug coverage. Alternative methods of financing prescription medications for indigent patients who are ineligible for Medicaid should be considered.

► This study and the other two studies in this section are different from other studies in this chapter in that they report on organizational and policy issues rather than on the effects of a specific clinical approach or assessment instrument in a clinical population. This study, which shows how the payment source affects the amount and type of pain medication prescribed, is a good example of why we need more studies describing the influence of health policy on treatment and outcomes. Unfortunately, outcomes of the treatments in terms of pain relief were not reported in this study. Most studies compare the effectiveness of different treatments; this study compared the costs of different treatments. Ideally, we will see more studies that compare both costs and effectiveness.—A.K. Jacox, R.N., Ph.D.

Pain Medication Class and Cost

Class	*Trade Name*	*Generic Name*	*Cost/100*	*No./Month*	*Cost/Month*
1	MS contin	Sustained-release MSO_4, (30 mg)	$69.60	120	$83.50
2	Percocet*	Oxycodone 5 mg/acetaminophen	21.20	180	38.16
3	Darvocet*	Propoxyphene 100 mg/acetaminophen	18.70	180	33.66
4	Tylenol No. 3*	Codeine 30 mg/acetaminophen	15.00	180	27.00
5	Motrin 600	Ibuprofen 600 mg	16.40	120	19.68
6	MS Elixir*	Liquid MSO_4 10 mg/5 mL	9.70/100 mL	300 mL	29.10
7	Meperidine*	Meperidine 50 mg	23.00	120	27.60

Abbreviations: Cost/100, cost to patient of 100 tablets (or 100 mL); *No./month*, average number of pills (or mL) used over the course of 1 month; *Cost/month*, average monthly cost to patient; *Mso₄*, morphine sulfate.

*Generic.

(Courtesy of Holcombe RF, Griffin J: *South Med J* 86:151–156, 1993.)

The Oncology Nursing Society: Commitment and Activities Promoting Cancer Pain Relief

Spross JA, Moore P (Oncology Nursing Society, Pittsburgh, Pa)

J Pain Symptom Manage 8:376–380, 1993 131-95-7–45

Introduction.—The Oncology Nursing Society (ONS) has more than 23,000 members, and its mission is to promote excellence in oncology nursing by studying, researching, and exchanging information, experiences, and ideas that lead to improved oncology nursing. In caring for patients in pain, oncology nurses strive to ensure that the patient communicates changes in comfort level; identifies measures to modify psychosocial, environmental, and physical factors that increase comfort; describes the source of discomfort, treatment, and expected outcome; and describes appropriate interventions.

Position Paper.—In 1990, the ONS board of directors approved the position paper that details 11 position statements, including the statement that patients, including children, with cancer pain have a right to obtain optimal pain relief. Nurses caring for patients with cancer pain must exercise leadership in identifying and assessing cancer pain and in planning, implementing, coordinating, and evaluating the interdisciplinary management of cancer pain. Basic nursing education programs should include theoretical and clinical curriculum content on cancer pain and its management. Patient education is an essential element of cancer pain management and a primary responsibility of nurses. Cancer pain and pain management are research priorities for oncology nurses and the ONS. The ONS is committed to initiating legislative and health policy activities that will overcome obstacles in cancer pain management.

Pain Management Technology.—Pain management is central to oncology nursing as a profession. Pain, a symptom that affects as many as 90% of patients with cancer, interferes with all dimensions of quality of life. Most cancer pain can be relieved with oral analgesic agents. Technology is not inherently good or bad; it can benefit and advance pain relief. The ONS will form liaisons with other professional groups and policy organizations to define the use of technology in pain management.

Conclusion.—The ONS structure enables it to support the goal of cancer pain relief, from the broadest national policy-making activities to the provision of care by a nurse to a patient and family.

▶ The description of the numerous activities undertaken by the ONS in its efforts to promote relief of cancer pain is impressive. This report indicates the kind of effort that is necessary in changing attitudes and behaviors of nurses and other clinicians in ways that improve pain management for patients. The ONS has been aggressive in its efforts to improve pain management. It is an effort that could well be emulated by organizations of clinicians dealing with other clinical conditions.—A.K. Jacox, R.N., Ph.D.

▶ The ONS position paper represents a significant statement of support for the treatment of cancer-related pain. From a policy perspective, this publication is also important for nursing practice, because *Guidelines* and position papers influence standards of care. Documents like this, which recognize standards of practice, serve to increase knowledge, affect attitudes, influence therapy, and guide quality assurance efforts related to the management of cancer pain. This written commitment from the ONS substantially adds to the support given by other organizations in recognizing the need for and promoting the relief of cancer-related pain.—N.A. Janjan, M.D.

The Pain Resource Nurse Training Program: A Unique Approach to Pain Management

Ferrell BR, Grant M, Ritchey KJ, Ropchan R, Rivera LM (City of Hope Natl Med Ctr, Duarte, Calif)

J Pain Symptom Manage 8:549–556, 1993 131-95-7–46

Problem: Inadequate Pain Management.—Nurses play a central role in assessing and managing pain. However, nursing education has traditionally devoted minimal time to pain management. Nurses also often lack basic knowledge in this area, such as types of analgesics and the risk for opioid addiction. However, nurses are interested in learning more.

Action: The Pain Resource Nurse (PRN) Training Program.—A unique, 40-hour training program was developed, implemented, and evaluated at the City of Hope National Medical Center. The program sought to prepare 1 staff nurse on each shift and on each unit to be a resource for pain management. The comprehensive curriculum included definitions and assessment of pain; pharmacologic and surgical approaches to pain management; nondrug comfort measures such as acupuncture, application of heat and cold, and massage; clinical practice; and discussion of ethical and cultural issues. Nursing and hospital administration supported the program and encouraged the participants in their new role. Twenty-six nurses with average of 9 years of nursing experience participated.

Results: Increased Skill in Pain Management.—Comparison of test results before and after the program showed that participants learned much about pain management. At a 3-month evaluation, almost all of the participants reported improved attitudes toward patients with pain. They spent more time teaching patients and co-workers about pain management. However, participants continued to have difficulties with co-workers and physicians in implementing their PRN role. This created barriers to implementing standards of pain management.

Next Step: Expanding the Program.—The PRN program continues to be evaluated and can be expanded to other clinical settings.

▶ These authors describe an interesting way to approach improvement of pain management at an institutional level. The inclusion of details of the curriculum for the training program should be useful to those who wish to initiate this or a similar program in their own institutions.—A.K. Jacox, R.N., Ph.D.

Subject Index*

A

* *All entries refer to the year and page number(s) for data appearing in this and previous editions of the* Year Book.

B

D

E

G

I

J

K

L

N

P

Q

R

S

T

U

V

W

X

Z

Author Index

A

B

C

T

U

V

W

Y

Z